The Metabolic Syndrome and Obesity

The Metabolic Syndrome and Obesity

by

George A. Bray, MD

Pennington Biomedical Research Center
Louisiana State University System
Baton Rouge, LA

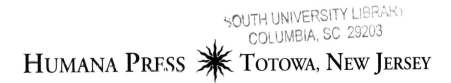
HUMANA PRESS ✳ TOTOWA, NEW JERSEY

Due diligence has been taken by the publishers, editors, and author of this book to assure the accuracy of the information published and to describe generally accepted practices. The author has carefully checked to ensure that the drug selections and dosages set forth in this text are accurate and in accord with the standards accepted at the time of publication. Notwithstanding, as new research, changes in government regulations, and knowledge from clinical experience relating to drug therapy and drug reactions constantly occurs, the reader is advised to check the product information provided by the manufacturer of each drug for any change in dosages or for additional warnings and contraindications. This is of utmost importance when the recommended drug herein is a new or infrequently used drug. It is the responsibility of the treating physician to determine dosages and treatment strategies for individual patients. Further it is the responsibility of the health care provider to ascertain the Food and Drug Administration status of each drug or device used in their clinical practice. The publisher, editors, and author are not responsible for errors or omissions or for any consequences from the application of the information presented in this book and make no warranty, express or implied, with respect to the contents in this publication.

This publication is printed on acid-free paper. ∞
ANSI Z39.48-1984 (American Standards Institute) Permanence of Paper for Printed Library Materials.

Cover design by Karen Schulz

Production Editor: Amy Thau

For additional copies, pricing for bulk purchases, and/or information about other Humana titles, contact Humana at the above address or at any of the following numbers: Tel.: 973-256-1699; Fax: 973-256-8314; E-mail: orders@humanapr.com, or visit our Website: http://humanapress.com

Photocopy Authorization Policy:
Authorization to photocopy items for internal or personal use, or the internal or personal use of specific clients, is granted by Humana Press Inc., provided that the base fee of US $30.00 per copy is paid directly to the Copyright Clearance Center at 222 Rosewood Drive, Danvers, MA 01923. For those organizations that have been granted a photocopy license from the CCC, a separate system of payment has been arranged and is acceptable to Humana Press Inc. The fee code for users of the Transactional Reporting Service is: [978-1-58829-802-7/07 $30.00].

Printed in the United States of America. 10 9 8 7 6 5 4 3 2 1

eISBN: 978-1-59745-431-5

Library of Congress Cataloging in Publication Data
Bray, George A.
 The metabolic syndrome and obesity/ by George A. Bray.
   p. ; cm.
 Includes bibliographical references and index.
 ISBN 1-58829-802-7 (alk. paper)
 1. Obesity. 2. Metabolic syndrome. I. Title.
 [DNLM: 1. Obesity. 2. Metabolic Syndrome X. WD 210 B827o 2007]
 RA645.O23B73 2007
 616.3'98--dc22
                                        2006024452

Introduction

Thirty years ago, I published my first monograph on obesity (Bray, 1976). Many things have changed in these 30 years, but many have remained the same. Preparation of *The Metabolic Syndrome and Obesity* has given me a chance to survey the changes to the field and to present an update of the scientific information. In retrospect, I conclude that a major component of the current "epidemic" of overweight is not medical, not genetic, not psychological, and will not be effectively treated by "lifestyle" changes that require individual choices.

We are all influenced by the prices of the goods we buy. With the reduction in food prices and distortion of commercially profitable products resulting from federal subsidies of corn, sugar, and rice, the food industry has been able to produce cheap, good-tasting, energy-dense foods and can sell them cheaply in large portion sizes. In contrast, foods like fruits and vegetables receive little in the way of subsidies, and are thus more expensive; thus we buy less. Providing more "healthy" food alternatives, as some advocate, will put items with "higher costs" on the shelves and is, in my view, unlikely to alter consumer choices as long as good-tasting, energy-dense foods remain cheap.

HISTORICAL CONTEXT FOR OBESITY

Obesity was already a problem before my first monograph was published. Between the writing of that monograph and *The Metabolic Syndrome and Obesity*, I was fortunate enough to find a short book in French, written by an American from Cincinnati named Worthington. The book summarized the history of obesity up to 1875 (Worthington, 1875). Obesity as a clinical problem has been described in medical writings from the Egyptian, Babylonian, Chinese, Indian, Meso-American, and Greco-Roman medical traditions (Bray, 2004). Causes for obesity were proposed and many treatments suggested. However, the problem is still with us, meaning that we neither understand it nor have effective therapy for its treatment. This statement also applies to the interval between my first monograph and this book. We have greatly increased our knowledge, as I outline here, as well as our treatments, yet at this writing the problem continues to get worse.

Numerous books dealing with obesity have been published. The first books dedicated solely to the subject of obesity in the English language were published in 1727 (Short, 1727) and 1760 (Flemyng, 1760). These volumes were followed by books in French, German, and many other languages during the next two centuries, until the first American monograph dealing with obesity was published by Rony (1940).

By the time Rony wrote his book, the basic concept of energy conservation and metabolism had been well established. Just prior to the French Revolution, Lavoisier (1789) had clearly confirmed that metabolism was similar to a slow oxidation and that more energy was consumed by human beings during exercise and after a meal. Some 50 years later, the Law of Conservation of Energy (First Law of Thermodynamics) was clearly stated independently by two Germans, Hermann von Helmholtz and Robert Mayer. Their work and the calorimeter developed earlier by Lavoisier stimulated the American Wilbur Atwater to develop the first effective human respiration calorimeter and to show that the Law of Conservation of Energy applied to human beings as it did to other animals.

While all of this basic science was developing, the first popular diet, a high-protein diet, was published in Great Britain in 1863 by William Banting in a small pamphlet titled "Letter on Corpulence, Addressed to the Public" (Banting, 1863). His publication excited the same fervor as some of the modern popular diet books that are reviewed in *The Metabolic Syndrome and Obesity*.

Another important contribution to the science of obesity from the era prior to World War II was the recognition that it could be caused by many distinct diseases. The first clear-cut examples were the presence of hypothalamic tumors that produced overweight, and are often associated with visual problems and endocrine dysfunction. Shortly afterward, Harvey Cushing (1912) showed that a pituitary tumor could also produce weight gain.

Finally, the life insurance industry has done its best to convince the public, based on its analysis of life insurance data, that being overweight was dangerous to health and tended to shorten life span. Beginning in the early 20th century, the life insurance industry published a number of studies making this point and showing that even modest increases in excess weight were associated with shortening of life span over many years.

LESSONS LEARNED ABOUT OBESITY
IN THE PAST 30 YEARS

The National Institutes of Health (NIH) is an evolving group of institutes designed to combat specific problems. In the late 1960s, the Fogarty International Center for Preventive Diseases was formed in honor of Congressman Fogarty, a Congressional Representative from the State of Rhode Island who had been a long-time and vocal supporter of expanded support for the NIH. One of the first activities of this new center was to organize a series of conferences on preventive medicine. The second of these conferences was on "obesity" because it was perceived to be a major public health issue, even in 1970. This conference was held at NIH in 1973, and the proceedings published in 1975.

The impetus to the field from the Fogarty Conference on Obesity led to the first in a series of international congresses on obesity. The first of these was held in London in 1974 and others were held at 3-year intervals until 1986 and then at 4-year intervals since. In addition to the development of these international meetings came the publication of the first volume of *International Journal of Obesity* in 1977.

The first edition of my monograph entitled *The Obese Patient* was published in 1976, and provided for me an opportunity to survey the field in which I had been working. At the same time, and without adequate recognition at the time, US agricultural policies were undergoing changes that made some food products cheaper. It was also the time when the "isomerase" process was developed that allowed the starch from corn to be converted to "fructose," thus producing high-fructose corn syrup, which is cheap to make and has displaced much of the sucrose used in foods and essentially all of the sucrose used to sweeten soft drinks and fruit drinks. As food prices fell, they represented a smaller fraction of household budget allowing more people to eat out and to enjoy the tasty, energy-dense foods provided by the increasing number of fast-food outlets.

The US government has been surveying the weight status of the American public in periodic surveys beginning in 1960. Between 1960 and the time of my first monograph in 1976, there had been a slow rise in the prevalence of obesity, which was comparable to the increase from other figures dating back to the Civil War in the 19th century. Between the survey completed between 1976 and 1980 and the next one dating from 1988 to 1994, the prevalence of obesity began to rise more rapidly. This increased rate at which people are becoming overweight has led some to label this as an "epidemic."

The major biological advance since 1976 has been the discovery of leptin. This peptide is produced in fat cells. Its absence produces massive obesity as found in the leptin-deficient, genetically obese ob/ob mice and in leptin-deficient human beings. Defects in the leptin receptor are responsible for three other varieties of animal obesity (fatty rat, Koletsky rat, and the diabetes mouse). Similar defects have been shown to produce obesity in human beings. In addition to the leptin-related genes, the other genes that produce obesity in animals have been shown to play a role in human obesity. One gene in particular, the one that encodes for the melanocortin-4 receptor, has been found to be defective in up to 5% of markedly overweight youngsters. This is one of the most frequent genetic causes of a chronic human disease yet reported.

Just prior to the Fogarty Center Conference in 1973, a report appeared showing that behavior-modification strategies could be used to treat overweight subjects. As this technique was explored in detail, it became one of the three pillars, along with diet and exercise for treatment of overweight people. Because of the response to behavioral strategies, obesity has been labeled a lifestyle disease. Efforts have been made to adapt these behavioral techniques for prevention of weight gain at the population level, but the effectiveness has been disappointing, to say the least. Behavior strategies are cognitive strategies, in that they require obese individuals to do something active—diet, exercise, and modify the way they live. As the literature clearly shows, these cognitive strategies do not translate well in preventive studies, and the weight that is initially lost using them is usually regained.

One of the most striking developments of the last 30 years has been the internet. This procedure for communication has now been applied to deliver behavioral management of obesity and offers promise of further important additions in the future.

The alternative to the cognitive approaches of lifestyle intervention is the use of noncognitive strategies—strategies that do not require continuing individual involvement. One example is fluoride used for dental caries. When fluoride was added to the water supply, dental caries were dramatically reduced without activity of the individual. One noncognitive strategy would be to use the fact that human beings are price-sensitive, and that using pricing strategies enhances the choice of appropriate foods.

At the time of my first monograph, the fat cell was viewed as a cell whose primary responsibility was the storage of fat. That view has now dramatically changed. With the discovery of leptin, it became clear that the fat cell had a much more significant function. Fat cells are part of the largest endocrine tissue in the body. They produce numerous peptides, which are released into the circulation and act on other cells. Among these are cytokines, peptides involved in regulating blood pressure, cell growth, regulation of triglyceride, metabolism, and blood clotting.

The past 30 years has also seen a plethora of new drugs introduced into the treatment of many diseases. One consequence of this new armamentarium is that some of these medications produce weight gain. One clear message for physicians who see overweight patients is to evaluate whether they are taking medications that produce weight gain.

Central adiposity as a risk factor for health was initially identified nearly 100 years ago, but it wasn't until 1982 that it became widely appreciated that people with central adiposity were at risk for diabetes and heart disease. Waist circumference has become the standard for assessing central adiposity. Increased waist circumference is also a criterion for the diagnosing the metabolic syndrome—a syndrome that is composed of a number of cardiovascular and diabetes risk factors, including high blood pressure, impaired fasting glucose, low levels of high-density lipoprotein cholesterol, and high levels of triglycerides.

Recently, the duration of sleep has been recognized as a factor related to obesity. Children and adults who sleep only short periods of time are more likely to be overweight. Metabolic studies provide a basis for understanding the changes produced by sleep.

Several prospective multicenter trials have shown that diets can influence disease risk. The Dietary Approaches to Stop Hypertension (DASH) diet trial compared the effect of three diets on blood pressure. One diet was the standard American diet, a second was a diet enriched with fruits and vegetables aimed at increasing magnesium and potassium levels to the 75th percentile of normal. The third diet—the DASH or Combination Diet—was enriched with fruits, vegetables, low-fat dairy products, but also had lowered total fat intake, more fiber, higher protein from vegetable sources, and reduced intake of calorically sweetened beverages and other sweets. Blood pressure was significantly reduced in people following the DASH diet. Another large clinical trial showed that a lifestyle-intervention program with reduced fat and exercise could significantly delay the onset of diabetes in people with impaired glucose tolerance (The Diabetes Prevention Program).

Obesity remains a stigmatized condition. Prejudice and dislike for the obese individual are commonplace. The efforts, particularly of women, to lose weight cost billions of dollars per year. This is captured in this poem from Ogden Nash:

The human body is composed
of head and limbs and torso
Kept slim by gents
At great expense
By ladies even more so.

As the prospective studies described here indicate, weight loss of modest degrees (5–10%) can produce a significant reduction in risk factors and thus a significant clinical benefit. In addition to this clinical benefit from weight loss, there is a self-image or cosmetic benefit. Weight loss improves quality of life. When the degree of weight loss is not sufficient to produce a cosmetic benefit from the patient's perspective, the patient may not be willing to pay the cost and continue the effort needed to maintain the clinical benefit that is evident to the physician.

Surgery for obesity has its roots in the 1960s, but the current popularity is the result of the lowered risk related to the use of laparoscopic techniques. Using laparoscopy for surgical treatment of the very overweight patient has reduced the risk and increased the number of treated patients. It is estimated that in 2005 more than 100,000 had this surgery. The mortality has been reduced and many of the complications associated with open surgical techniques have been reduced.

It is against this background of immense change over 30 years that I offer this new volume *The Metabolic Syndrome and Obesity* for your consideration.

George A. Bray, MD

REFERENCES

Banting, W. (1863). Letter on corpulence, addressed to the public. London: Harrison and Sons.
Bray, G. A. (1976). The Obese Patient: Major Problems in Internal Medicine. Philadelphia: WB Saunders.

Bray, G. A. (2004). Historical framework for the development of ideas about obesity. In G. Bray & C. Bouchard (Eds.), Handbook of Obesity: Etiology and Pathophysiology. New York, Marcel Dekker.

Cushing, H. W. (1912). The pituitary body and its disorders. Clinical states produced by the disorders of the hypophysis cerebri. Philadelphia: J. B. Lippincott.

Flemyng, M. (1760). A discourse on the nature, causes, and cure of corpulency. Illustrated by a remarkable case. Read before the Royal Society November 1757. London: L. Davis and C. Reymers.

Rony, H. R. (1940). Obesity and Leanness. Philadelphia: Lea & Febiger.

Short, T. (1727). A discourse concerning the causes and effects of corpulency together with the method for its prevention and cure. London: J. Roberts.

Worthington, L. S. (1875). De l'obesite. Etiologie, therapeutique et hygiene. Paris: E. Martinet.

Contents

I | THE PROBLEM

1 Definitions and Prevalence

KEY POINTS

- Overweight and central adiposity can be assessed clinically with the body mass index (BMI) and the waist circumference.
- Other measures of body fat and visceral fat are more precise but do not improve much on the clinical value of BMI and waist circumference.
- Overweight has been increasing slowly during most of the 20th century, but showed a 50% increase over the last 20 years.
- Children are also becoming overweight at an alarming rate.
- Women have a higher prevalence of overweight than men.
- Ethnic differences exist in the prevalence of overweight.
- Central adiposity measured by the waist circumference is a key element in the diagnosis of the metabolic syndrome.
- The relationship of central adiposity to health risks is more recent than that for increased body weight and risks to health.

INTRODUCTION

Overweight in the United States has been called an "epidemic" because it now affects nearly two-thirds of the adult population and a growing number of children (Hedley et al. 2004; Jolliffe, 2004). The World Health Organization (WHO) has also labeled overweight as an "epidemic" because worldwide it may affect more than 300 million

From: *The Metabolic Syndrome and Obesity*
By: G. A. Bray © Humana Press Inc., Totowa, NJ

people (WHO, 2000). The increased health risks and increased demands on the health care system for advice and treatment are a result of this epidemic. Thus a set of ground rules that define overweight and obesity and provide a risk–benefit approach to selecting treatments are needed. Thus, we need to treat obesity seriously.

As noted later, "obesity" is a "stigmatized" disease and a pejorative term. No one wants to be called "obese," and many people who are obese deny the problem rather than label themselves "obese." In a survey of patient preferences, Wadden et al. (2004) found that "overweight" was the preferred term. For this volume, I thus adopt the term *overweight* when describing the condition that I have previously called "obese." As noted later, the term *overweight* will be refined to provide quantitative grades of over-weight similar to those often used for obesity. In addition, I will use the term *clinically overweight* to refer to individuals who manifest one or more of the many disease states that can be associated with overweight.

The issue of overweight is ancient. It can be identified in all of the medical traditions in recorded history and in prehistoric artifacts (Bray, 2007). Both the Greek physician, Hippocrates, who is often called the Father of Medicine from his work 2500 years ago, and the Roman physician, Galen, described overweight patients and approaches to treating them. The literature has continued to expand. The first medical monographs in English dealing exclusively with overweight were published in 1727 (Thomas Short) and 1760 (Malcolm Flemyng). Despite this long history, the problems associated with overweight only continued to increase through the end of the 20th century and into the beginning of the 21st century.

In contrast to the long history dealing with overweight itself, the issues surrounding fat distribution are barely a century old. The recognition that the location of body fat contributed to the risk of disease was noted by the Life Insurance Companies in the early 20th century (America, 1901–1903). This theme was picked up nearly half a century later by Professor Vague, working in Marseille, France at the end of World War II (Vague, 1956). He noted that patients with "upper" body fat were at greater risk for diabetes and heart disease than patients with "lower" body fat. Using a technique that measured fat distribution from circumferences and skinfold thicknesses, he pro-vided a quantitative measure of central adiposity. However, it was still another 35 years before this concept received strong support. Using a simple measure of the waist circumference divided by the hip circumference, groups of investigators in the United States (Kissebah et al., 1982) and Sweden (Lapidus et al., 1984; Larsson et al., 1984) showed that those with upper body fat were at greater risk for heart disease, diabetes, and early death.

It soon became clear that a number of risk factors for heart disease were associated with central adiposity, which was in turn related to insulin resistance. In a seminal paper in 1988, Reaven established the concept that insulin resistance might underlie a number of risk factors for ill health, including the risk for diabetes and hypertension. He called this association of risk factors "Syndrome 'X'," but it has subsequently had a number of labels (Table 1) including the metabolic syndrome or dysmetabolic syndrome. Measuring insulin resistance is not easy and three definitions of the metabolic syndrome were developed to try and provide a functional definition. The common elements of the metabolic syndrome are an increased central adiposity measured by increased waist circumference, low levels of high-density cholesterol, elevated levels of triglycerides

Table 1
Synonyms for the Metabolic Syndrome

Metabolic syndrome	Dysmetabolic syndrome
Syndrome X	Insulin resistance syndrome
Plurimetabolic syndrome	Syndrome X plus
Android obesity	Deadly quartet
Glucose intolerance, Hypertension, Obesity (GHO) syndrome	Insulin resistance/hyperinsulinemia syndrome
Syndrome of affluence	Cardiovascular and metabolic syndrome
Reaven syndrome	Proatherogenic syndrome
Metabolic cardiovascular syndrome	MetSyn

Adapted from Leslie (2005).

(triacylglycerols) and high glucose. The definition of the metabolic syndrome is discussed in more detail later.

DEFINITIONS

With this introduction, let me define obesity, overweight, central adiposity, and the metabolic syndrome. Not all readers may be familiar with some of the current terminology and I have prepared an appendix of definitions in addition to what is provided in the text. Obesity refers to an increase in body fat, a measurement that is not easily done in clinical practice because interpretation of body fatness depends on such factors as gender, age, ethnic group, and level of physical activity. Overweight is an increase in body weight relative to some standard and has become a surrogate for "obesity" both clinically and epidemiologically. Central adiposity refers to conditions where fat is located more in the abdominal area than on the hips, thighs, or arms. The metabolic syndrome is a collection of measurements that reflect resistance to the action of insulin and that have central adiposity as a key component.

METHODS OF MEASURING BODY WEIGHT AND BODY FAT

Methods for determining body composition, including the fraction that is fat, and the standards to define degrees of overweight and central adiposity have improved over the past 25 years, greatly increasing the accuracy and ease of measuring body compartments and defining the degree of "overweight" in patients (N.A., 1996; Gordon and Chumlea, 1988; Heymsfield et al., 2004; Lohman, 1992; Seidell and Rissanen, 1997). For children, many of the same methods can be used, except those involving radiation (Veldhuis et al., 2005).

Weight and Height

Weight and height should be determined with calibrated scales and stadiometer. Electronic scales have largely replaced mechanical ones. Height and weight can be measured accurately and can be used to determine the body mass index (BMI). The BMI was introduced by Quetelet in 1835 based on his statistical evaluation of changes in people's weights (Quetelet, 1835). The BMI is defined as the body weight divided by the square of the height (wt/ht^2), and is usually expressed in metric terms (kg/m^2). It can also be calculated in metric units using pounds and inches if the following formula is used: BMI = 703 × {weight (lbs)/[height(inches)]^2}. Table 2 contains the

Table 2
Body Mass Index (BMI): Using Either Pounds and Inches or Kilograms and Centimeters

BMI (kg/m^2)

Inches	19	20	21	22	23	24	25	26	27	28	29	30	31	32	33	34	35	36	37	38	39	40	Cm
58	91	95	100	105	110	115	119	124	129	134	138	143	148	153	158	162	167	172	177	181	186	191	147
	41	**43**	**45**	**48**	**50**	**52**	**54**	**56**	**58**	**61**	**63**	**65**	**67**	**69**	**71**	**73**	**76**	**78**	**80**	**82**	**84**	**86**	
59	94	99	104	109	114	119	124	128	133	138	143	148	153	158	163	168	173	178	183	188	193	198	150
	43	**45**	**47**	**50**	**52**	**54**	**56**	**59**	**61**	**63**	**65**	**68**	**70**	**72**	**74**	**77**	**79**	**81**	**83**	**86**	**88**	**90**	
60	97	102	107	112	118	123	128	133	138	143	148	153	158	164	169	174	179	184	189	194	199	204	152
	44	**46**	**49**	**51**	**53**	**55**	**58**	**60**	**62**	**65**	**67**	**69**	**72**	**74**	**76**	**79**	**81**	**83**	**85**	**88**	**90**	**92**	
61	100	106	111	116	121	127	132	137	143	148	153	158	164	169	174	180	185	190	195	201	206	211	155
	46	**48**	**50**	**53**	**55**	**58**	**60**	**62**	**65**	**67**	**70**	**72**	**74**	**77**	**79**	**82**	**84**	**86**	**89**	**91**	**94**	**96**	
62	104	109	115	120	125	131	136	142	147	153	158	164	169	175	180	186	191	196	202	207	213	218	158
	47	**50**	**52**	**55**	**57**	**60**	**62**	**65**	**67**	**70**	**72**	**75**	**77**	**80**	**82**	**85**	**87**	**90**	**92**	**95**	**97**	**100**	
63	107	113	118	124	130	135	141	146	152	158	163	169	175	180	186	192	197	203	208	214	220	225	160
	49	**51**	**54**	**56**	**59**	**61**	**64**	**67**	**69**	**72**	**74**	**77**	**79**	**82**	**84**	**87**	**90**	**92**	**95**	**97**	**100**	**102**	
64	110	116	122	128	134	140	145	151	157	163	169	174	180	186	192	198	203	209	215	221	227	233	162
	50	**52**	**55**	**58**	**60**	**63**	**66**	**68**	**71**	**73**	**76**	**79**	**81**	**84**	**87**	**89**	**92**	**94**	**97**	**100**	**102**	**105**	
65	114	120	126	132	138	144	150	156	162	168	174	180	186	192	198	204	210	216	222	228	234	240	165
	52	**54**	**57**	**60**	**63**	**65**	**68**	**71**	**74**	**76**	**79**	**82**	**84**	**87**	**90**	**93**	**95**	**98**	**101**	**103**	**106**	**109**	
66	117	124	130	136	142	148	155	161	167	173	179	185	192	198	204	210	216	223	229	235	241	247	168
	54	**56**	**59**	**62**	**65**	**68**	**71**	**73**	**76**	**79**	**82**	**85**	**87**	**90**	**93**	**96**	**99**	**102**	**104**	**107**	**110**	**113**	
67	121	127	134	140	147	153	159	166	172	178	185	191	198	204	210	217	223	229	236	242	248	255	170
	55	**58**	**61**	**64**	**66**	**69**	**72**	**75**	**78**	**81**	**84**	**87**	**90**	**92**	**95**	**98**	**101**	**104**	**107**	**110**	**113**	**116**	
68	125	131	138	144	151	158	164	171	177	184	190	197	203	210	217	223	230	236	243	249	256	263	

BMI table — weights by height and BMI (italics = pounds and inches; bold = kilograms and centimeters)

Height	19	20	21	22	23	24	25	26	27	28	29	30	31	32	33	34	35	36	37	38	39	40
68 (lb)	*124*	*131*	*138*	*144*	*151*	*157*	*164*	*171*	*177*	*184*	*190*	*197*	*203*	*210*	*217*	*223*	*230*	*236*	*243*	*249*	*256*	*263*
173 (kg)	**57**	**60**	**63**	**66**	**69**	**72**	**75**	**78**	**81**	**84**	**87**	**90**	**93**	**96**	**99**	**102**	**105**	**108**	**111**	**114**	**117**	**120**
69 (lb)	*128*	*135*	*142*	*149*	*155*	*162*	*169*	*176*	*182*	*189*	*196*	*203*	*209*	*216*	*223*	*230*	*237*	*243*	*250*	*257*	*264*	*270*
175 (kg)	**58**	**61**	**64**	**67**	**70**	**74**	**77**	**80**	**83**	**86**	**89**	**92**	**95**	**98**	**101**	**104**	**107**	**110**	**113**	**116**	**119**	**123**
70 (lb)	*132*	*139*	*146*	*153*	*160*	*167*	*174*	*181*	*188*	*195*	*202*	*209*	*216*	*223*	*230*	*236*	*243*	*250*	*257*	*264*	*271*	*278*
178 (kg)	**60**	**63**	**67**	**70**	**73**	**76**	**79**	**82**	**86**	**89**	**92**	**95**	**98**	**101**	**105**	**108**	**111**	**114**	**117**	**120**	**124**	**127**
71 (lb)	*136*	*143*	*150*	*157*	*164*	*172*	*179*	*186*	*193*	*200*	*207*	*215*	*222*	*229*	*236*	*243*	*250*	*258*	*265*	*272*	*279*	*286*
180 (kg)	**62**	**65**	**68**	**71**	**75**	**78**	**81**	**84**	**87**	**91**	**94**	**97**	**100**	**104**	**107**	**110**	**113**	**117**	**120**	**123**	**126**	**130**
72 (lb)	*140*	*147*	*154*	*162*	*169*	*176*	*184*	*191*	*199*	*206*	*213*	*221*	*228*	*235*	*243*	*250*	*258*	*265*	*272*	*280*	*287*	*294*
183 (kg)	**64**	**67**	**70**	**74**	**77**	**80**	**84**	**87**	**90**	**94**	**97**	**100**	**104**	**107**	**111**	**114**	**117**	**121**	**124**	**127**	**131**	**134**
73 (lb)	*144*	*151*	*159*	*166*	*174*	*181*	*189*	*197*	*204*	*212*	*219*	*227*	*234*	*242*	*250*	*257*	*265*	*272*	*280*	*288*	*295*	*303*
185 (kg)	**65**	**68**	**72**	**75**	**79**	**82**	**86**	**89**	**92**	**96**	**99**	**103**	**106**	**110**	**113**	**116**	**120**	**123**	**127**	**130**	**133**	**137**
74 (lb)	*148*	*155*	*163*	*171*	*179*	*186*	*194*	*202*	*210*	*218*	*225*	*233*	*241*	*249*	*257*	*264*	*272*	*280*	*288*	*296*	*303*	*311*
188 (kg)	**67**	**71**	**74**	**78**	**81**	**85**	**88**	**92**	**95**	**99**	**102**	**106**	**110**	**113**	**117**	**120**	**124**	**127**	**131**	**134**	**138**	**141**
75 (lb)	*152*	*160*	*168*	*176*	*184*	*192*	*200*	*208*	*216*	*224*	*232*	*240*	*248*	*256*	*264*	*272*	*280*	*288*	*296*	*304*	*312*	*320*
190 (kg)	**69**	**72**	**76**	**79**	**83**	**87**	**90**	**94**	**97**	**101**	**105**	**108**	**112**	**116**	**119**	**123**	**126**	**130**	**134**	**137**	**141**	**144**
76 (lb)	*156*	*164*	*172*	*180*	*188*	*197*	*205*	*213*	*221*	*230*	*238*	*246*	*254*	*262*	*271*	*279*	*287*	*295*	*304*	*312*	*320*	*328*
193 (kg)	**71**	**74**	**78**	**82**	**86**	**89**	**93**	**97**	**101**	**104**	**108**	**112**	**115**	**119**	**123**	**127**	**130**	**134**	**138**	**142**	**145**	**149**
BMI	19	20	21	22	23	24	25	26	27	28	29	30	31	32	33	34	35	36	37	38	39	40

The BMI is shown as **italic underlined** numbers at the top and bottom of the table. To determine your BMI, select your height in either inches or cm and move across the row until you find your weight in pounds or bottom. Your BMI can be read at the top or bottom. The **bold** is for kilograms and centimeters. (Copyright 1999 George A. Bray.)

The italics are for pounds and inches.

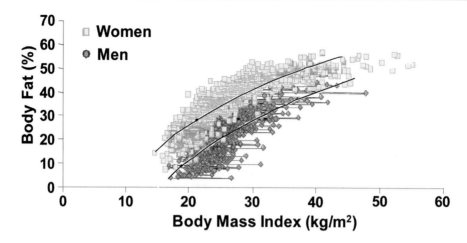

Fig. 1. Relationship of body mass index to body fat mass in men and women.

BMI values for various heights and weights in pounds and inches, as well as in kilograms and meters.

One concern with the use of the BMI is that it does not account for people with increased muscle mass, such as football players, weight lifters, and others who use weight lifting as part of their exercise program. This is indeed a fair concern, but in the field of "overweight," which is the subject of this book, this is not a problem. For most Americans, and indeed those around the world, the BMI is a reasonably good reflection of their degree of fatness *see* Fig. 1; Gallagher et al., 2000). It is fairly easy to exclude the others. When sedentary people are evaluated, a high BMI is almost certainly a sign of increased body fatness. The BMI has a positive association between height and adiposity among children and is better than other height–weight relationships for this group as well as adults (Freedman et al., 2004).

In order to give BMI some relation to everyday life, I have included the BMI data published in the *Wall Street Journal* on July 23, 2002 to show the BMI of several prominent Americans (*see* Table 3).

Waist Circumference and Central Adiposity

The circumference of the waist is the second essential anthropometric measurement. It can be determined by using a nonextensible tape measure (metal or plastic) that is placed around the waist. At least two definitions of "waist" are used. One method uses the level of the umbilicus. The problem with this one is that in very overweight people the "umbilicus" may be quite low. The other is half way between the last rib and the suprailiac crest, which is my preferred method because it uses stable landmarks.

INSTRUMENTAL METHODS USED TO MEASURE
BODY COMPOSITION

The number and precision of methods for measuring body composition (*see* Table 4) has improved greatly over the past 25 years (Heymsfield et al., 2004; Sjostrom et al., 1986), but some of these methods are expensive and used primarily in research settings.

Table 3
Body Mass Index (BMI) Values of Some Prominent Americans

Name	BMI	Name	BMI
Sylvester Stallone	34	Rebecca Lobo	22
Arnold Schwarzeneger	33	Venus Williams	22
Sammy Sosa	30	Demi Moore	22
Harrison Ford	29	Lisa Leslie	20
George Clooney	29	Julia Roberts	18
Bruce Willis	29	Hilary Swank	18
Mike Piazza	27	Nicole Kidman	17
Brad Pitt	27	Madonna	17
Michael Jordan	25	Gwynneth Paltrow	16

From the *Wall Street Journal* (July 23, 2002).

Table 4
Instrumental Methods of Body Composition

Method	Cost	Ease of use	Can measure regional fat	External radiation
Hydrodensitometry	$$	Easy	No	—
Air displacement plethysmography	$$$$	Easy	No	—
DXA	$$$	Easy	+	tr
Isotope dilution	$$	Moderate	No	—
Impedance (BIA)	$$	Easy	+	—
^{40}K counting	$$$$	Difficult	No	—
Conductivity (TOBEC)	$$$	Difficult	±	—
CT scan	$$$$	Difficult	++	++
MRI scan	$$$$	Difficult	++	—
Neutron activation	$$$$+	Difficult	No	+++
Ultrasound	$$	Moderate	+	—

BIA, bioelectric impedance analysis; TOBEC, total-body conductivity; +, special equipment; $, inexpensive; $$, some expense; $$$, expensive; $$$$, very expensive; tr, trace.

Others, particularly dual-energy X-ray absorptiometry and bioelectric impedance, have found wider clinical and epidemiological use.

Dual-Energy X-Ray Absorptiometry

DXA instruments were developed for determination of bone mineral content (BMC) as part of an evaluation of osteoporosis. The method requires the subject to lie supine on a table. Two very low-energy X-ray beams of different energy are passed through the body. The beams are attenuated to estimate lean body mass, body fat, and BMC (Heymsfieldet al., 2004). DXA has replaced underwater weighing in many laboratories as the gold standard for determining body fat and lean body mass (Bray et al., 2002). The advantages of DXA are that it can be safely applied to individuals weighing up to 150 kg (300 lb) and it is easy to use, and with appropriate standards, it is very accurate. On the other hand, it is expensive, with instruments that must be calibrated regularly costing between $40,000 and $100,000. The weight limits of the table prevent measurement for individuals weighing more than 150 kg. The reproducibility of DXA is 0.8% for bone, 1.3% for density, 1.7% for fat, and 2% for body weight. The radiation exposure with this procedure is barely higher than normal background radiation, and well below that of a chest X-ray (DeLany et al., 2002).

Density

Determining body density and partitioning it into fat and nonfat compartments, based on the fact that fat floats and the nonfat components sink, was the gold standard of body composition until the advent of DXA (Heymsfield et al., 1997). Its advantages are that it is highly reproducible, easy to perform, and requires only a good balance. Its disadvantage is that some individuals are unable or unwilling to completely submerge in water. Measurement of pulmonary residual volume at the time of the test is an important secondary method required to increase the accuracy of this procedure.

Whole Body Plethysmography (Bod Pod)

Air displacement using body plethysmography is similar in principle, but does not require submersion. This method allows calculation of the specific gravity from volume and weight of the body and thus for estimating fat and non-fat components of the body (Elia and Ward, 1999). In a comparison of air displacement (Bod Pod) versus water displacement (underwater weighing) Ginde et al. (2005) found that the underwater displacement (underwater weight) and air displacement were highly correlated (r = 0.94) with a standard error of the estimate of 0.0073. Bland-Altman analysis, asking how well the methods estimated fat, showed no significant bias between the two methods. Thus, air displacement appears to be an important new instrument for measurement of body fat in a two-compartment model.

Isotope Dilution

Estimating body water by injecting a tracer amount of isotopic water (D_2O, $H_2^{18}O$, ^3H_2O) or some other chemical that mixes completely in body water (thiocyanate), makes it possible to calculate body fat and thus partition body weight into body water and nonwater compartments. Body fat can then be calculated by assuming a value of the percent of water in lean tissue. For adults, this figure is 73%, but it is lower in children. This method, density, and DXA have comparable accuracy (Bray, 2002).

Bioelectric Impedance

Measurement of the resistance and impedance of the body between predetermined points on the leg and arm or between feet and arms has been widely used to determine water content (N.A., 1996). With proper training and careful placement of electrodes, highly reproducible measurements can be obtained. The instrument for this procedure costs between $2000 and $3000, and is portable. The advantages of this method are its relatively low cost and its ease of performance from the subject's point of view, as well as the ability to compare with other centers that use similar instrumentation. The disadvantages include that the impedance only adds a small amount of extra information to the other pieces of information, such as height and age, required for the equations. Second, the method is indirect because it only measures body water, which is used to estimate body fat. Several precautions are needed to obtain valid information from bioelectric impedence analysis (BIA). First, the instrumentation must be reliable. Second, the procedures must be standardized by using the same time of the day, the same ambient temperature, and standard placement of electrodes. Third, the subject should be similar to the populations from which the standard values are derived. Finally, the subject's water status should be stable because BIA measures water.

Infrared Reactance

This technique involves the application of an infrared signal over the biceps, where reflectance is read and acts as a signal for underlying fatness. No commercially acceptable unit yet embodies this technology, and it is not clinically recommended.

Total-Body Electrical Conductivity

Two instruments, one for adults and one for children, have been developed that use total-body conductivity (TOBEC). The principle is similar to the methods of evaluating fat content of meat through changes in electromagnetic fields that depend on the relation of fat and water. Like DXA, the TOBEC instrument is expensive, but it may be useful in a research setting, particularly for children (Heymsfield et al., 2004).

Multicompartment Methods

For laboratory purposes, a four-compartment model, including body weight, body water, body density, and BMC provides the best way to estimate fat (Bray, 2002; Heymsfield et al., 2004).

INSTRUMENTAL METHODS FOR MEASURING VISCERAL FAT

Patterns of body fat distribution between subcutaneous and internal or visceral compartments can be reliably determined by either computed tomography (CT) or magnetic resonance imaging (MRI) (Heymsfield et al., 2004; Seidell and Rissanen, 1997; Sjostrom et al., 1986). The most common procedure is to obtain a single cross-sectional slice at the interspace between the fourth and fifth (L 4–5) lumbar vertebrae. This slice can then be divided into the area above the abdominal muscles and the intra-abdominal fat and the amount of each quantitated. A second procedure involves taking several slices, often 8, with two below and five above the L 4–5 lumbar vertebrae and calculating the volume of visceral adipose tissue. This volumetric method reduces the error of measurement considerably because variations in gas patterns within the abdomen have less influence on the volume of fat than on a single slice (Heymsfield et al., 2004; Smith, 2005). Because of the expense, these techniques are not used for routine clinical determination of visceral fat. In a recent comparison of methods as predictors for the development of diabetes, it was found that the waist circumference was as good an index of fat distribution as the visceral or subcutaneous fat determined by CT (Heymsfield et al., 2004; Knowler, 2002).

Clinical Recommendations

Careful measurement of height, weight, and waist circumference are the essential measurements, indeed clinically vital signs, needed to begin evaluation of an overweight

Table 5
Classification of Overweight and Obesity as Recommended
by the National Heart Lung Blood Institute Guidelines

	BMI (kg/M²)	Obesity class	Disease risk[a] relative to normal weight and waist circumference	
			Men <102 cm Women < 88 cm	>102 cm >88 cm
Underweight	<18.5		–	–
Normal[b]	18.5–24.9		–	–
Overweight	25.0–29.9		Increased	High
Obesity	30.0–34.9	1	High	Very high
	35.0–39.9	2	Very high	Very high
Extreme obesity	≥40.0	3	Extremely high	Extremely high

[a]Disease risk for type 2 diabetes, hypertension, and cardiovascular disease.

[b]Increased waist can also be a marker for increased risk in normal weight individuals. (Source: National Institutes of Health, 1998.)

patient (*see* Chapter 5). This will provide the BMI, which is a measure of the risk associated with weight status and a measure of central adiposity that is needed to make the diagnosis of the metabolic syndrome. If the clinician is concerned about whether lean body mass is increased, DXA may be considered. Although impedance measurements are used in many clinical settings, they often underestimate fat. Most other techniques are for research use.

In this text, the term *overweight* will be used in place of "obesity" (*see* Table 5) To allow for the gradations achieved with grades I, II, and III obesity, I have chosen overweight to refer to the entire range above BMI of 25 kg/m² and overweight grades I–III to correspond to the BMI 30–34.9 kg/m², BMI 35–39.9 kg/m², and BMI > 40 kg/m², respectively. The term *clinically overweight* refers to individuals with a BMI > 25 kg/m² who have diabetes, hypertension, atherogenic dyslipidemia, or sleep apnea.

USE OF THESE METHODS TO DESCRIBE BODY COMPOSITION

The human body can be analyzed from many perspectives and one five-level model is shown in Fig. 2 (Wang et al., 1992). These five levels reflect improvements over the past five centuries in the methods of examining the human body. The initial studies of the human body during the Renaissance were done for artistic purposes, which required studies of the underlying anatomic structure.

Vesalius published the first modern anatomy of the human body in 1543. With the invention of the microscope in the 17th century, the tissue (level II) and cellular levels (level III) of the human body were gradually unveiled. This was followed in the 19th and 20th centuries by improvements in chemistry and physics that allowed for a molecular (level IV) and atomic (level V) understanding of body composition. A similar progression occurred in the study of human disease or pathology. It began with descriptions of illness in the "whole" patient and as techniques improved the diseases were gradually identified as affecting organs—thus organ pathology. Next came tissues and tissue pathology. Finally, cells and subcellular molecules gave rise to cellular and molecular pathology.

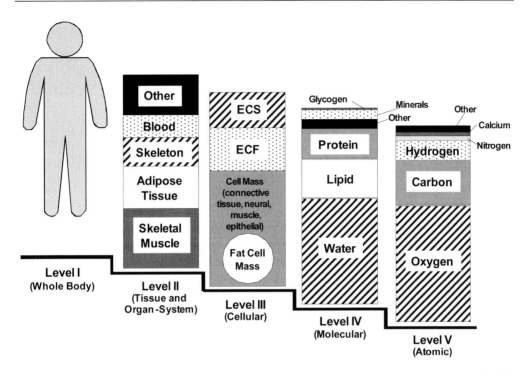

Fig. 2. A five–level model depicting the whole body as level I, the tissue and organ systems as level 2, the divisions of the body cell mass as level 3, the molecules that compose the body as level 4, and the atomic composition of those molecules as level 5. (Adapted from Wang et al., 1992.)

Whole Body (Level I)

The first level of analysis of body composition is the whole body (level I). Wang et al. (1992) identified at least 10 different measurable components, including stature (height), length of limbs, various circumferences including waist and hips, skinfold thickness at various sites (e.g., triceps, subscapular), body surface area (BSA), body volume, BMI, and body density.

Tissue and Organ Composition (Level II)

The division of the body into organs and tissues is the next obvious step. Five major tissues are shown in Fig. 2, including skeletal muscle, adipose tissue, skeleton, blood or hematopoietic tissues, and all others. The amount and location of adipose tissue are most important. As much as 80% of body fat is subcutaneous; however, fat also surrounds many organs and accumulates around the abdominal organs and this fat may have more pathological meaning for human disease. Fat in this latter category is most difficult to measure accurately except with expensive imaging techniques.

Cellular Composition (Level III)

A third level in the analysis of body composition is its cellular components. The body is composed of cells in all tissues and organs, which have intracellular fluid and are surrounded by extracellular fluids and solids. Figure 2 lists two major cellular categories. In group 1 are connective tissue cells, neural cells, muscle cells, epithelial cells, and in group 2, the fat cells that we are most concerned about in overweight individuals. One technique for measuring body cell mass uses the naturally occurring radioactive isotope of potassium (^{40}K). Because more than 95% of potassium is intracellular, the ability to measure an isotope of potassium provides an index of body cell mass. ^{40}K is a naturally occurring isotope of potassium, and its abundance can be determined with whole-body radiation counters. Total-body weight is the sum of all tissues, including muscle cells, connective tissue cells, epithelial cells, and neural cells. The metabolically active tissues, such as bone, adipose tissue, blood cells, and muscle, make up 75% of body weight (Sjostrom et al., 1986).

Molecular Composition (Level IV)

This part of the model is most widely used in clinical medicine. Water constitutes 60% or more of body weight in males, and 50% or more in females. Of this 60%, approximately 26% is extracellular and 34% intracellular. Lipids range from less than 10% of body weight in well-trained athletes to nearly 50% in very overweight patients. Of these lipids, 2–3% are essential structural lipids, and the remainder are nonessential stores of fat. Protein constitutes 15% of normal body composition, and minerals constitute 5.3%. Thus, water, lipid, protein, and minerals account for 99.4% of the molecular constituents of the body.

Several formulas can be used to describe body weight. The most widely used ones have two compartments: the sum of fat and the fat-free mass.

$$\text{Body weight} = \text{fat} + \text{fat-free mass (FFM)}$$

DXA partitions the body into three components:

$$\text{Body weight} = \text{fat} + \text{bone mineral mass} + \text{lean body mass}$$

More complex relations can be developed by subdividing FFM into other components. One four-compartment model is as follows:

$$\text{Body weight} = \text{fat} + \text{water} + \text{protein} + \text{bone mineral}$$

The amount of fat in the body varies more widely than any other single component. Table 6 shows the percent body fat for men and women at three levels of BMI and for three ethnic groups. Several things are obvious. First, at any level of BMI, women have more fat than men. At the designated overweight point (BMI = 25 kg/m²), women have 12% more fat than men. Ethnic and age differences are also evident. Asian men and women at the same BMI are generally fatter than blacks or whites. Body fat rises by 1 to 2% for each additional 20 years of age in each gender and in all three ethnic groups (Gallagher et al., 2000).

Data from dissection studies of the human body and from all indirect measures clearly show that women have a higher percentage of body fat than do men. Values of body fat below 10% have been reported in highly trained long-distance runners, but as the values get lower, the precision of the measurement worsens and the reliability of these numbers is sometimes questionable. At the other extreme, body fat can rise to more than 50% of total-body weight, but rarely above 60%. The very large majority of this fat is stored in droplets in the 40 to 90 billion adipocytes in the adult human body. A small quantity of lipid is associated with membrane structures and is considered essential.

Table 6
Variations in Percent Body Fat for Caucasians, African Americans, and Asians

	Females			*Males*		
	African American	*Asian*	*Caucasian*	*African American*	*Asian*	*Caucasian*
Age 20–39						
BMI						
18.5	20	25	21	8	13	8
25	32	35	33	20	23	21
30	38	40	39	26	28	26
Age 40–59						
BMI						
18.5	21	25	23	9	13	11
25	34	36	35	22	24	23
30	39	41	41	27	29	29

Adapted from Gallagher et al. (2000).

Proteins provide the structural and functional components of the body. Approximately 15% of the body is protein, but this varies with age and degree of physical training, and with a variety of clinical and hormonal states. Many minerals constitute the remainder of the body's molecular structure. Water, lipid, protein, and mineral account for more than 99% of the molecular constituents of the body.

Atomic Composition (Level V)

A final approach partitions the human body into its atomic components. If the standard or reference man is 70 kg, his weight would be 60% oxygen, 23% carbon, 10% hydrogen, 2.6% nitrogen, 1.4% calcium, and less than 1% assigned to all of the other atoms in the body, such as chloride, copper, fluoride, chromium, magnesium, potassium, phosphorus, sodium, sulfur, nickel, zinc, and others. Eleven elements thus account for more than 99.5% of body weight. Oxygen, carbon, hydrogen, nitrogen, and calcium account for more than 98% of total body mass. Less than 2% is attributable to the other atomic elements. The atomic components of clinical interest are nitrogen, calcium, magnesium, sodium, potassium, and chloride (Wang et al., 1992).

BODY COMPOSITION THROUGH THE LIFE SPAN

Whatever way is used to express the components that make up the body, the proportion will change during the life span. Several factors modify the level of body fat and body composition, including gender, age, level of physical activity, and hormonal status. Figure 3 shows data on body fat distribution by age for men and women (Kotani et al., 1994). Two important observations are evident from this figure. First, percentage of body fat steadily increases with age in both men and women. Women have a higher percentage of body fat than do men for a comparable height and weight at all ages after puberty. Second, visceral fat in women is lower during the reproductive years, but rises rapidly to nearly male levels in the postmenopausal years, when risk for cardiovascular

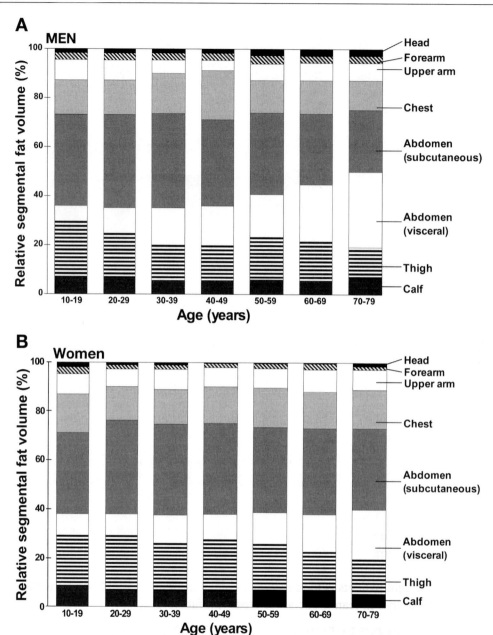

Fig. 3. (A) Changes in body fat over the lifetime of men using computed tomographic (CT) scans. The changes in abdominal fat and calf fat with age are particularly noteworthy. **(B)** Changes in body fat over the lifetime of women using CT. Note that abdominal visceral fat only begins to rise after the menopause. (Adapted from Kotani et al., 1994.)

disease (CVD) and other diseases increases sharply. Indeed, corrections for differences in body fat distribution correct for almost all of the differences in excess mortality of men over women, suggesting that the underlying factors leading to differences in fat distribution are significant in the risk of diabetes, heart disease, high blood pressure, and stroke in men.

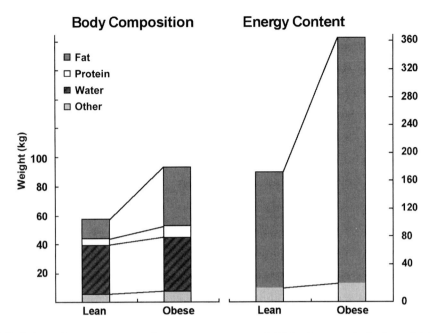

Fig. 4. Relation of energy stores to body compartments. A 30-kg increase in body weight occurs mainly as an increase in body fat with a small increase in protein and water (lean body mass). Because most body energy is stored in fat, the 30-kg (50%) increase in body weight produces a near doubling of body energy stores.

BODY FAT AND BODY ENERGY STORES

Using some of the methods described earlier, we can compare body composition and its energetic equivalent in men and women of two different weights. This is presented in Fig. 4, which shows the effect of a 30-kg increase in weight for the standard 70-kg man and the standard 56-kg woman. More than 66% of this increase in weight in men, and up to 90% in women, is accounted for by increased fat. The remainder is lean tissue that supports the extra fat. Because the extra stored triglyceride is energy-rich, the 30-kg increase in weight nearly doubles body energy stores. The therapeutic challenge for treating overweight patients is to reduce this excess energy stored in body fat without a disproportionate loss in lean tissue associated with fat storage.

CRITERIA FOR THE METABOLIC SYNDROME

When central adiposity was recognized as a key predictor of risk for diabetes and CVD, efforts began to identify the components that might lead to a diagnosis of the metabolic syndrome. Several definitions have now been proposed. Table 7 lists those from the National Cholesterol Education Program (NCEP), Adult Treatment Panel (ATP)-III, the International Diabetes Federation (IDF), and the WHO. Insulin resistance is an important part of this syndrome but it cannot be easily measured, so other criteria have been used to replace it. Atherogenic dyslipidemia is also important and can be defined by low levels of high-density lipoprotein (HDL) cholesterol and high triglycerides. The original WHO criteria were more complicated and more numerous than the other two. A modified version was presented by the US NCEP (Expert Panel, 2001) when the

Table 7
**Diagnostic Criteria for the Metabolic Syndrome According
to the WHO, ATP III, and the IDF**

	WHO	*ATP-III-revised*	*IDF*
Definition	Diabetes, or impaired fasting glucose, or impaired glucose tolerance, or insulin resistance (assessed by euglycemic clamp) plus two or more of the following:	Three or more of the following:	Central adiposity (criteria below are for Europid men and women; other waist criteria needed in other populations)
Adiposity level	Waist-to-hip ratio	Waist circumference	Waist circumference
Female	>0.85	>88 cm	>80 cm
Male	>0.90	>102 cm	>90 cm in europid female and male
	BMI >30 kg/m^2		
Fasting glucose		≥100 mg/dL^a	≥100 mg/dL or diagnosed diabetes
Microalbuminuria	≥20 ug/min or albumin/creatinine ratio 30 mg/g		
Triglycerides	≥150 mg/dL	≥150 mg/dL	≥150 mg/dL or treatment for this lipid abnormality
HDL-cholesterol			
Female	<39 mg/dL	<50 mg/dL	<50 mg/dL
Male	<35 mg/dL	<40 mg/dL	<40 mg/dL
Blood pressure	≥140/90 mmHg	≥135/85 mg/dL	≥135/85 mmHg or treatment for this abnormality

^{a}Revised ATP-III criteria lowered this from 110 mg/dL to 100 mg/dL
WHO, World Health Organization; ATP, Adult Treatment Panel; IDF, International Diabetes Federation.

organization published its ATP-III recommendations in 2001. The recommendations required that three of the five measures be abnormal to make the diagnosis. The IDF has simplified this even further by requiring an increased waist circumference and two of the other four criteria (*see* Chapter 10).

PREVALENCE OF OVERWEIGHT, CENTRAL ADIPOSITY, AND THE METABOLIC SYNDROME

Overweight is an increase in body weight relative to some standard. At least two techniques are available for evaluating the degree of overweight. The first to use is the life insurance table (Table 8). This approach was used through most of the 20th century. Relative weight derived from these tables is the weight of an individual compared to a table, usually the Metropolitan Life Insurance table (*see* Table 8). This method was the basis for comparing body weights in the initial years of the Framingham Heart Study, which started in 1948. BMI is the second method and is now the most widely used standard for determining overweight (*see* Table 2). It correlates more closely with body

Table 8
Metropolitan Life Insurance Tables Height and Weight Table
of 1983 for Women[a]

Height (ft & in)	Small frame	Large frame	Large frame
4′9"	99–108	106–118	115–128
4′10"	100–110	108–120	117–131
4′11"	101–112	110–123	119–134
5′0"	103–115	112–126	122–137
5′1"	105–118	115–129	125–140
5′2"	108–121	118–132	128–144
5′3"	111–124	121–135	131–148
5′4"	114–127	124–138	134–152
5′5"	117–130	127–141	137–156
5′6"	120–133	130–144	140–160
5′7"	123–136	133–147	143–164
5′8"	126–139	136–150	146–167
5′9"	129–142	139–153	149–170
5′10"	132–145	142–156	152–173
5′11"	135–148	145–159	155–176

[a]All measurements corrected for height without shoes and weight without clothes.

fat content than do other anthropometric relationships of height and weight, and thus is the preferred measure in epidemiological and population studies (*see* Fig. 1). Its advantages are ease of determination and the accuracy with which both height (stature) and weight can be measured. Its chief limitation is that, particularly in the normal BMI range (18.5–24.9 kg/m^2), the correlation with actual body fat content is sufficiently low that it is a poor guide to individual fat level. For BMI values above 25 kg/m^2 and especially those above 30 kg/m^2, BMI is a much better guide to the degrees of excess fat and risk to health.

The BMI is not a new concept. It originated more than a century ago. It was the brain child of Lambert-Adolphe-Jacques Quetelet (1835) who introduced the concept of the BMI as a tool to assess differences among human beings. His classic book titled *On the Development of Man and his Faculties*, was published when he was 39 years old. This work made him famous throughout Europe. A second edition of this volume was published in 1869. just 5 years before his death.

Table 5 lists BMI ranges and the relative risk associated with each as defined by the National Heart, Lung and Blood Institute. For this book, I substitute overweight for obesity. This concept of BMI and risk is explored in more detail in Chapters 3 and 5, which outline the clinical evaluation of overweight patients. A table for estimating BMI is shown in Table 2.

Population Changes

Using BMI, we can divide the population into groups and compare these groups across national boundaries, and examine time trends. The mean BMI for women is slightly lower than for men (26.6 kg/m^2 for men vs 25.5 kg/m^2 for women). The median BMI is 25.9 kg/m^2 for men and 25.1 kg/m^2 for women, resulting in greater skew, that

Table 9

Comparison of the Prevalence of Overweight Grade I (BMI > 30 kg/m²)
Using the Behavioral Risk Factor Surveillance System (BRFSS) Telephone
Survey vs the National Center for Health Statistics Surveys

Survey year	BRFSS telephone survey	National Center for Health Statistics direct measurement
1960–1962	N/A	14.6%
1971–1975	N/A	14.3%
1976–1980	N/A	14.5%
1988–1994 (1991)	12%	22.5%
1996	15.8%	N/A
1998	17.9%	N/A
1999–2000	19.8%	30.5%
1999–2002	21.3%	30.6%

BMI, body mass index; N/A, not available.

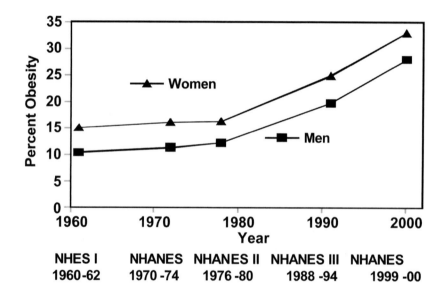

NHES I	NHANES	NHANES II	NHANES III	NHANES
1960-62	1970 -74	1976 -80	1988 -94	1999 -00

Fig. 5. Prevalence of a body mass index (BMI) above 30 kg/m² from 1960 to 2000. At all time intervals, women have a higher prevalence of overweight with a BMI above 30 kg/m², than men. (An update of this information is available in Ogden et al., 2006.)

is, the long upper tail is greater for women, giving them a higher percentage with a BMI above 30 kg/m² than for men.

The percentage of Americans with a BMI above 25 kg/m² or 30 kg/m² has been determined in several surveys by the US government, beginning in 1960 (Flegal et al., 2002). The data have been collected in two different ways. One is the use of telephone surveys conducted by state Departments of Health in collaboration with the Centers for Disease Control and Prevention (CDC) in Atlanta, Georgia. These surveys are now done annually and are called the Behavioral Risk Factor Surveillance System (BRFSS). The other approach is to directly measure height and weight in field

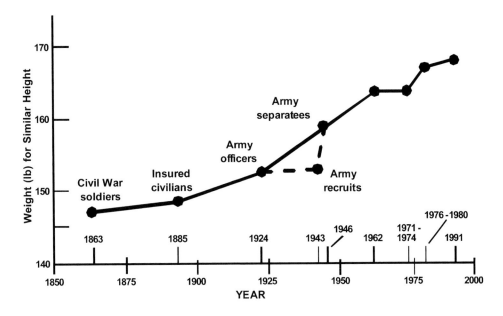

Fig. 6. Changes in the body weight of males since the Civil War (Bray, 1976).

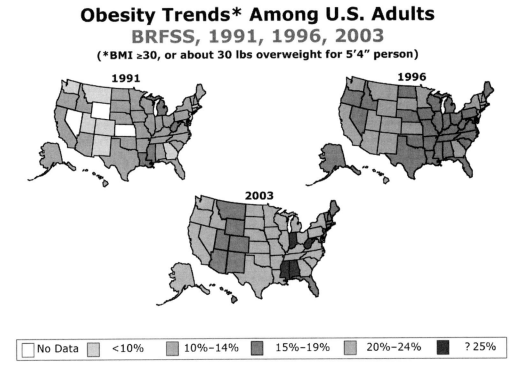

Fig. 7. Change in obesity trends among US adults using the telephone-based Behavioral Risk Factor Surveillance Survey (BRFSS). The BRFSS provides a graphic picture of the overall trends and regional disparities. (From U.S. Centers for Disease Control.)

surveys as is done by the National Health and Nutrition Examination surveys (NHANES) that began in 1960. A comparison of the results from these two surveys is shown in Table 9. It can be seen that the BRFSS data give a prevalence that is about two-thirds that of the NHANES surveys. This could be because people under-report their weight, overreport their height, or both during the telephone surveys. Data would suggest that they do a bit of both. When reading the literature on preva-lence of overweight in the United States, however, it is important to identify which method has been used.

The data on BMI above 30 kg/m^2 for men and women obtained from the surveys of the National Center for Health Statistics (NCHS) is plotted in Fig. 5. The percentage of men and women exceeding a BMI of 30 kg/m^2 steadily increased in each of the first three surveys. There was a striking rise between the third survey (1976–1980) and fourth survey (1988–1994).

The increase in percentage of men with a BMI above 30 kg/m^2 nearly doubled, and the percentage of women with a BMI above 30 kg/m^2 rose by more than 50%. The rise in body weight relative to height is not new (Bray, 1976). Figure 6 shows that body weight of American men for a given height has been rising since the Civil War. What is new in the NHANES data is the rate of this rise.

Using BRFSS, the prevalence of obesity among US adults increased from 12% in 1991 to 21.3% in 2002 (Fig. 7). Among class III overweight (i.e., people with a BMI >40 kg/m^2), the prevalence increased from 0.9% in 1991 to 2.3% in 2002, which is probably a significant underestimate, but shows the dramatic increase in trends.

The BRFSS collects a great deal of useful data relating to overweight in small slices of the American population. With this system, variations in the prevalence of overweight grade I (BMI >30 kg/m^2) ranged from 13.1% to 30.0% in different metropolitan statistical regions around the United States (Ford et al., 2005). For example, Memphis, Tennessee; Youngstown, Ohio; and San Antonio, Texas were at the top of the list and Honolulu, Hawaii; Nassau-Suffolk, New York; and Denver, Colorado were at the lowest end of the distribution of frequencies of overweight.

A 1998 survey showed that the percent of the population that was overweight in various states ranged from a low of 12.7% for Arizona to a high of 22.9% for West Virginia (Finkelstein et al., 2004). The striking thing was that in nearly 60% of the United States, the prevalence of overweight had increased by more than 50% since 1991. In 1991, the prevalence of a BMI above 30 kg/m^2 in a self-reported survey was less than 15% in 41 states. By 1998, the prevalence of overweight was more than 15% in nearly 80% of the United States.

The lifetime risk of developing overweight in the United States is significant. Using the data from the Framingham Heart Study, Vasan et al. (2005) calculated the 4-year risk and the long-term (10- to 30-year) risk of becoming overweight. They examined the effects for men and women at ages 30, 40, and 50 who had a normal BMI at each. The 4-year risk of becoming overweight, that is developing a BMI above 25 kg/m^2, was 14–19% in women and 26–30% in men. The 4-year risk for developing a BMI above 30 kg/m^2 if BMI was normal was 5–7% for women and 7–9% for men. Over the longer 30-year interval, the risks were similar in men and women, and varied somewhat with age, being lower if one was under 50 years of age. The 30-year risk was 50% of deve-loping overweight (BMI >25 kg/m^2), was 25% of developing a BMI above 30 kg/m^2, and 10% of developing a BMI above 35 kg/m^2.

Table 10
Prevalence of Overweight With a Body Mass Index of 30 kg/m² in Several Countries

		Prevalence of BMI >30 kg/m²	
Country	Years	Men	Women
Belgium (Ghent)	1989–1996	10	11
Germany (Augsburg)	1989–1996	21	22
Italy (Friuli)	1989–1996	17	19
United Kingdom (Glasgow)	1989–1996	23	23
Poland (Warsaw)	1989–1996	22	28
Russia (Moscow)	1989–1996	8	21
Argentina	1997	28	25
Mexico	1995	11	23
India	1988–1990	0.5	0.5
Malaysia	1990	8	6
Saudi Arabia	1996	16	24
Tunisia	1997	7	23
China	1992	1	2
Japan	1990–1994	2	3
Philippines	1993	3	2
South Africa (Cape Town)	1990	14	49
Western Cape (White)	1990	18	20
Durban (Indian)	1990	4	18

Adapted from Seidell and Rissanen (2002).

Class III overweight (i.e., those with a BMI >40 kg/m²), is a particular problem because it is one of the fastest growing groups of overweight individuals. These are also the individuals who are considered for bariatric surgery (*see* Chapter 11). In the most recent NCHS survey from 1999 to 2000, this group accounted for 4.9% of the adult population In men, 3.3% fell in this category compared with 6.4% of women over 20 years of age. The prevalence of a BMI above 40 kg/m² was highest in the non-Hispanic black population (9%) with much of this being non-Hispanic black women, in whom the prevalence was 13.5% (Hedley et al., 2004).

The epidemic of overweight is not confined to the United States, but can be identified in data from all over the world (Seidell and Rissanen, 1997). The data from several countries are shown in Table 10. The prevalence of overweight clearly is increasing worldwide in the Eastern and Western hemispheres, and above and below the equator. Despite the wide range, all data suggest that most populations have increased the percentage who are overweight over the past 20 years.

Metabolic Syndrome

Waist circumference as a measure of central adiposity has not been as frequently collected as height and weight, and there is less data. One thing is clear, however, and that is that the criteria, or cut-points, for waist circumference differ by gender and by ethnic group. Table 11 is a list of cut-points for waist circumferences for men and women in a few ethnic groups.

Table 11
Waist Circumference Cut Points by Gender and Ethnicity

Group	Waist circumference cut-points	
	Men	Women
United States	102 cm (40 in)	88 cm (35 in)
European (IDF)	94 cm (37 in)	80 cm (31 in)
Chinese and South Asian	90 cm (35 in)	80 cm (31 in)
Japanese	85 cm (33 in)	90 cm (35 in)

IDF, International Diabetes Federation.

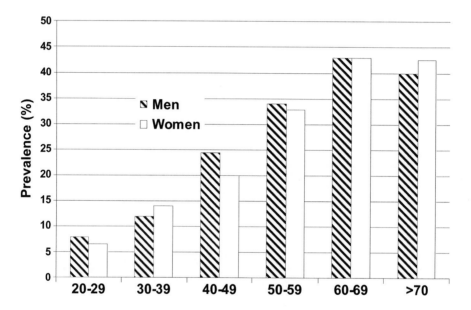

Fig. 8. Ethnic and gender differences in the prevalence of overweight. (Redrawn from Ford, 2002.)

The prevalence of the metabolic syndrome using the ATP-III criteria described in Table 7 has been estimated at 23.7% of the adult population or 47 million US adults (Ford et al., 2002). The prevalence increases with age, rising from 6.7% in those aged 20–29 years to 43.5% in those aged 60–69 and 42% in people older than 70 years (Fig. 8). There is an ethnic variation in this prevalence. The overall values are similar in men and women (24% vs 23.4%), but for African-American and Mexican-American women, the prevalence was 57 vs 31% for the men. The prevalence of the metabolic syndrome is increasing and is likely to lead to increases in the incidence of diabetes and CVD (Ford et al., 2004).

The metabolic syndrome is also a prevalent problem in other parts of the world. Table 12 summarizes the prevalence in several countries.

Central adiposity, as measured by the waist circumference, is the principal criterion now used to assess abdominal or visceral fatness. Although longitudinal data is limited, what there is suggests that it has increased, just as BMI has increased. Using data from

Table 12
Prevalence of the Metabolic Syndrome among
Men and Women From Countries Around the World

Country	Men	Women
Australia (>24 yr)	20%	17%
China (35–74 yr)	10%	13%
Finland (42–60 yr)	20%	23%
France (30–64 yr)	10%	8%
India (>20 yr)	8%	18%
Iran (>20 yr)	26%	42%
Ireland (50–69 yr)	22%	21%
Oman (>20 yr)	20%	23%
Scotland (45–64 yr)	28%	—
Turkey (>31 yr)	29%	40%
United States (>20 yr)	25%	29%

From Eckel et al. (2005), Ford et al. (2004), and Gu et al. (2006).

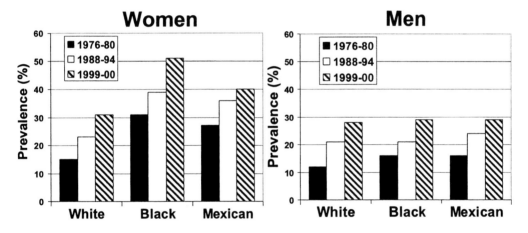

Fig. 9. Prevalence of the metabolic syndrome as defined by the National Cholesterol Education Program Adult Treatment Panel III (from Flegal et al., 2002).

the NHANES conducted between 1988 and 1994 and the more recent survey from 1999 to 2000, Ford et al. (2003) found that the age-adjusted waist circumference had increased in men from 96 cm to 98.9 cm and from 88.9 cm to 92.2 cm in women. These data suggested that the waist circumference distribution had shifted to the larger size. Using age-specific rates of high-risk waist sizes, the authors estimated that there are about 35 million men and 58 million women who have high-risk waist circumference measurements.

Using the measure of central adiposity and the other criteria provided by the NCEP, ATP-III, Ford et al. reported the prevalence of the metabolic syndrome. Overall, about 24% of adult Americans have the metabolic syndrome as diagnosed with the ATP-III criteria. There are both age-related and ethnic differences in its prevalence. Few young people have the metabolic syndrome, with the prevalence rising to more than 50% of those in their sixth decade. There are also ethnic differences. These are discussed next.

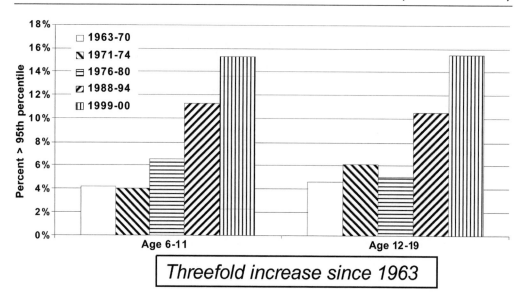

Fig. 10. Prevalence of overweight in children. (Redrawn from Ogden et al., 2006.)

Prevalence of Overweight in Women and Ethnic Groups

The distribution of increased weight is not equally divided among the population (Flegal et al., 2002). Figure 9 shows the percentages of whites, blacks, and Mexican Americans in the United States with a BMI above 30 kg/m². Both Mexican Americans, and black women in particular, have high percentages with a BMI above 30 kg/m². Using the National Health Interview Survey with self-reported height and weight, the prevalence of a BMI of 30 kg/m² or above was 16% among immigrants and 22% among US-born individuals. The prevalence was 8% among immigrants living in the United States for less than 1 year and 19% for those in the United States for at least 15 years. These differences were not accounted for by sociodemographic characteristics, illness burden, BMI, or access to health care among some subgroups of immigrants (Goel et al., 2004).

Prevalence of Overweight in Children

In children, overweight is defined as a weight above the 95th percentile for height and is comparable to an adult BMI of more than 30 kg/m². *At risk for overweight* is the term used in children for a weight between the 85th and 95th percentile and corresponds to an adult BMI range of 25–30 kg/m². The prevalence of overweight in children is also rising, according to surveys conducted since the 1960s (Fig. 10). In the surveys done between 1963 and 1970, 6- to 11-year-olds had a prevalence of overweight of 4.3% and in 12- to 17-year-olds the prevalence of overweight was only slightly higher at 4.6%. In the NHANES II survey conducted between 1976 and 1980 the prevalence of overweight was 7.5% for the 6- to 11-year-olds and 5% in the 12- to 17-year-olds. In the NHANES III survey from 1988 to 1991, the prevalence in the younger children rose to 13.5% and to 11.5% in the 12- to 17-year-olds (Troiano and Flegal, 1998). Using a different population of children, Strauss and Pollack (2001) showed that the yearly rate of increase in overweight children (BMI >95th percentile) in the National Longitudinal

Table 13
Prevalence of Overweight in the United States (%), 1999–2004

	1999–2000		2003–2004	
kg/m^2	>25	>30	>25	>30
All adults	64.5	30.5	66.3	32.2
Men	60.5	27.5	70.8	31.1
Women	61.9	33.4	62	33.2
Children	28.2	13.9	33.6	17.1

Adapted from Ogden (2006).

Survey of Youth (NLSY) was 3.23% in non-Hispanic white, 4.3% in Hispanics, and 5.85% in African-American youth. In the NHANES survey conducted between 1999 and 2002, the prevalence of overweight in 6- to 11-year-olds rose to 15.8% and in 12- to 19-year-olds it rose to 16.1% (Hedley et al., 2004). The burden of overweight is particularly prominent among some subpopulations in America. In the Indian Health Service, one report showed that 39.1% of boys and 38% of girls were overweight and 22% of boys and 18% of girls had BMI equivalent to 30 kg/m^2 or more (Zephier et al., 1999). In a study of 924 Indianapolis schoolchildren, Saha et al. (2005) found that the trajectory toward overweight differed by race with blacks at greater risk than whites. They suggest that race-specific guidelines may be needed to determine the highest risk children.

Weight status in childhood predicts weight later in life. In a review of 24 studies on the relationship of weight status in infancy and childhood to weight later on, Baird et al. (2005) and Kinra et al. (2005) found that in most studies, infants who were obese, or who were at the higher end of the distribution range were at higher risk, and that infants who grew more rapidly were also at increased risk of overweight. These relationships held for infants born between 1927 and 1994, indicating the consistency of the pattern. These earlier growth patterns in girls are associated with an earlier age of menarche (Pierce and Leon, 2005). An analysis of the development of overweight among children shows that not only have more children become overweight in the past three decades, but the overweight children have been getting even heavier (Jolliffe, 2004).

The most recent data show that the prevalence of overweight continues to rise in men and children, but may have stabilized in women. Table 13 compares the prevalence with a BMI between 25 and 29.9 kg/m^2 and for a BMI above 30 kg/m^2 (Ogden et al., 2006).

The metabolic syndrome is also a feature of overweight children. Because the set of measurements that are available differ from those in adults, different criteria are used in children. Caprio et al. identified the prevalence of the metabolic syndrome in children to be 38.7% in the moderately overweight and 49.7% in the very overweight using the following criteria: a BMI above the 97th percentile for age and gender, that is, a z-score greater than 2; a triglyceride above the 95th percentile for age, gender and ethnicity; an HDL-cholesterol above the 5th percentile for age, gender, and ethnicity; a systolic blood pressure and/or diastolic blood pressure above the 95th percentile for age and gender; and impaired glucose tolerance (Weiss et al., 2004).

In this chapter I have reviewed the methods for measuring body fat and for determining whether or not an individual is overweight. As should be clear, the prevalence of overweight has risen rapidly during the past 20 years. The reasons for this are not entirely clear, but will be explored to the extent possible in the next few chapters. The major thrust of the latter part of the book will be on the approaches that are available to help ameliorate the issue.

REFERENCES

America, A. S. o. (1901–1903). Transactions of the Actuarial Society of America 7:492–497.

Baird, J., et al. (2005). Being big or growing fast: systematic review of size and growth in infancy and later obesity. BMJ 331(7522): 929.

Bray, G. A. (1976). The Obese Patient: Major Problems in Internal Medicine. Philadelphia, PA: WB Saunders.

Bray, G. A. (2002). Predicting obesity in adults from childhood and adolescent weight. Am J Clin Nutr 76(3):497–498.

Bray, G. (2007). The Battle of the Bulge. Pittsburgh, PA: Dorrance.

Bray, G. A., et al. (2002). Prediction of body fat in 12-yr-old African American and white children: evaluation of methods. Am J Clin Nutr 76(5):980–990.

DeLany, J. P., et al. (2002). Energy expenditure in preadolescent African American and white boys and girls: the Baton Rouge Children's Study. Am J Clin Nutr 75(4):705–713.

Eckel, R. H., et al. (2005). The metabolic syndrome. Lancet 365(9468):1415–1428.

Elia, M. and Ward, L. C. (1999). New techniques in nutritional assessment: body composition methods. Proc Nutr Soc 58:33–38.

Expert Panel on Detection, Evaluation, and Treatment of High Blood Cholesterol In Adults. (2001). Executive Summary of The Third Report of The National Cholesterol Education Program (NCEP). JAMA 285(19):2486–2497.

Finkelstein, E. A., et al. (2004). State-level estimates of annual medical expenditures attributable to obesity. Obes Res 12(1):18–24.

Flegal, K. M., et al. (2002). Prevalence and trends in obesity among US adults, 1999–2000. JAMA 288(14):1723–1727.

Ford, E. S., et al. (2002). Prevalence of the metabolic syndrome among US adults: findings from the third National Health and Nutrition Examination Survey. JAMA 287(3):356–359.

Ford, E. S., et al. (2003). Trends in waist circumference among U.S. adults. Obes Res 11(10):1223–1231.

Ford, E. S., et al. (2004). Increasing prevalence of the metabolic syndrome among U.S. Adults. Diabetes Care 27(10):2444–2449.

Ford, E. S., et al. (2005). Geographic variation in the prevalence of obesity, diabetes, and obesity-related behaviors. Obes Res 13(1):118–122.

Freedman, D. S., et al. (2004). Inter-relationships among childhood BMI, childhood height, and adult obesity: the Bogalusa Heart Study. Int J Obes Relat Metab Disord 28(1):10–16.

Gallagher, D., et al. (2000). Healthy percentage body fat ranges: an approach for developing guidelines based on body mass index. Am J Clin Nutr 72(3):694–701.

Ginde, S. R., Geliebter, A., Rubiano, F., et al. (2005). Air displacement plethysmography: validation in overweight and obese subjects. Obes Res 13:1232–1237.

Goel, M. S., et al. (2004). Obesity among US immigrant subgroups by duration of residence. JAMA 292(23):2860–2867.

Gordon, C. C. and Chumlea, W. C. (1988). Stature, recumbent length, and weight. In Anthropometric Standardization Reference Manual (pp. 3–8). Champaign, IL: Human Kinetics Books.

Gu, D., et al. (2006). Body weight and mortality among men and women in China. JAMA 295(7):776–783.

Hedley, A. A., et al. (2004). Prevalence of overweight and obesity among US children, adolescents, and adults, 1999–2002. JAMA 291(23):2847–2850.

Heymsfield, S. B., et al. (1997). Evaluation of total and regional body composition. In G. Bray, C. Bouchard, and W. P. James (Eds.), Handbook of Obesity (pp. 41–77). New York: Marcel Dekker.

Heymsfield, S. B., et al. (2004). Evaluation of total and regional adiposity. In G. Bray, C. Bouchard, and W.P. James (Eds.), Handbook of Obesity (pp. 33–79). New York: Marcel Dekker.

Jolliffe, D. (2004). Extent of overweight among US children and adolescents from 1971 to 2000. Int J Obes Relat Metab Disord 28(1):4–9.

Kinra, S., et al. (2005). Early growth and childhood obesity: a historical cohort study. Arch Dis Child 90(11):1122–1127.

Kissebah, A. H., et al. (1982). Relation of body fat distribution to metabolic complications of obesity. J Clin Endocrinol Metab 54(2):254–260.

Knowler, W. C., et al. (2002). Reduction in the incidence of type 2 diabetes with lifestyle intervention or metformin. N Engl J Med 346(6):393–403.

Kotani, K., et al. (1994). Sexual dimorphism of age-related changes in whole-body fat distribution in the obese. Int J Obes Relat Metab Disord 18(4):207–202.

Lapidus, L., et al. (1984). Distribution of adipose tissue and risk of cardiovascular disease and death: a 12 year follow up of participants in the population study of women in Gothenburg, Sweden. Br Med J (Clin Res Ed) 289(6454):1257–1261.

Larsson, B., et al. (1984). Abdominal adipose tissue distribution, obesity, and risk of cardiovascular disease and death: 13 year follow up of participants in the study of men born in 1913. Br Med J (Clin Res Ed) 288(6428):1401–1404.

Lohman, T. G. (1992). Advances in Body Composition Assessment. Champaign, IL: Human Kinetics.

N.A. (1996). Bioelectrical impedance analysis in body composition measurement (Proceedings of a National Institutes of Health Technology Assessment Conference, Bethesda, MD, 1994). Am J Clin Nutr 64(3 Suppl):387S–532S.

National Institutes of Health. (1998). Clinical Guidelines on the identification, Evaluation, and Treatment of overweight and obesity in Adults—The Evidence Report. Obes Res 6(Suppl 2):51S–209S.

Ogden, C. L., Carroll, M. D., Curtin, L. R., McDowell, M. A., Tabak, C. J., Flegal, K. M. (2006). Prevalence of overweight and obesity in the United States, 1999–2004. JAMA 295(13):1549–1555.

Pierce, M. B. and Leon, D. A. (2005). Age at menarche and adult BMI in the Aberdeen children of the 1950s cohort study. Am J Clin Nutr 82(4):733–739.

Quetelet, L.-J.-A. (1835). Sur l'homme et le developpement de ses facultes, ou essai de physique sociale. Paris : Bachelier.

Quetelet, L.-J.-A. (1869). Physique sociale; ou, Essai sur le développement des facultés de l'homme. Brussels: C. Marquardt.

Reaven, G. M. (1988). Banting lecture 1988. Role of insulin resistance in human disease. Diabetes 37(12):1595–1607.

Saha, C., et al. (2005). Onset of overweight during childhood and adolescence in relation to race and sex. J Clin Endocrinol Metab 90(5):2648–2652.

Seidell, J. C. and Rissanen, A. M. (1997). Time trends in worldwide prevalence of obesity. In G. Bray, C. Bouchard, and W.P. James (Eds.), Handbook of Obesity (pp. 79–91). New York: Marcel Dekker.

Seidell, J. C. and Rissanen, A. M. (2002). Prevalence of obesity in adults: the global epidemic. In G. Bray, C. Bouchard, and W.P. James (Eds.), Handbook of Obesity New York: Marcel Dekker.

Sjostrom, L., et al. (1986). Determination of total adipose tissue and body fat in women by computed tomography, 40K, and tritium. Am J Physiol 250(6 Pt 1):E736–E745.

Smith, S. R., et al. (2005). Effect of pioglitazone on body composition and energy expenditure: a randomized controlled trial. Metabolism 54(1):24–32.

Troiano, R. P. and Flegal, K. M. (1998). Overweight children and adolescents: description, epidemiology, and demographics. Pediatrics 101(3 Pt 2):497–504.

Vague, J. (1956). The degree of masculine differentiation of obesities: a factor determining predisposition to diabetes, atherosclerosis, gout, and uric calculous disease. Am J Clin Nutr 4(1):20–34.

Vasan, R. S., et al. (2005). Estimated risks for developing obesity in the Framingham Heart Study. Ann Intern Med 143(7):473–480.

Veldhuis, J. D., et al. (2005). Endocrine control of body composition in infancy, childhood, and puberty. Endocr Rev 26(1):114–146.

Vesalius, A. (1543). De humani corporis fabrica. Basileae: ex off., Joannis Oporini.

Wadden, T. A., et al. (2004). Efficacy of lifestyle modification for long-term weight control. Obes Res 12 Suppl:151S–162S.

Wang, Z. M., et al. (1992). The five-level model: a new approach to organizing body-composition research. Am J Clin Nutr 56(1):19–28.

Weiss, R., et al. (2004). Obesity and the metabolic syndrome in children and adolescents. N Engl J Med 350(23):2362–2374.

World Health Organization. (2000). Obesity: preventing and managing the global epidemic. Report of a WHO consultation. World Health Organ Tech Rep Ser 894:i–xii, 1–253.

Zephier, E., et al. (1999). Prevalence of overweight and obesity in American Indian School children and adolescents in the Aberdeen area: a population study. Int J Obes Relat Metab Disord 23 Suppl 2:S28–S30.

2 How Do We Get Fat?

An Epidemiological and Metabolic Approach

KEY POINTS

- Positive energy balance is the essential ingredient required to store more body fat and become overweight.
- It is what the energy balance concept does not tell us that is important; for example, it doesn't explain genetic factors, gender differences in fatness, or effects of age or medications.
- An epidemiological model for developing overweight in response to the environment identified food, reductions in energy expenditure, viruses, toxins, and drugs as contributing mechanisms.
- The cost of food plays important role in food choices.
- A homeostatic model for control of food intake and energy expenditure helps isolate the specific places where mechanisms can be targeted for understanding and treating the problem.

INTRODUCTION

Research over the past two decades has provided an unprecedented expansion of our knowledge about the physiological and molecular mechanisms regulating body fat. Perhaps the greatest impact has resulted from the cloning of genes corresponding to the five mouse monogenic obesity syndromes and the subsequent characterization of the human counterparts to these syndromes. Extensive molecular and reverse genetic studies (mouse knockouts) have helped establish other critical pathways regulating body fat and food intake, as well as validated or refuted the importance of previously identified pathways.

From: *The Metabolic Syndrome and Obesity*
By: G. A. Bray © Humana Press Inc., Totowa, NJ

In this chapter, the rapidly expanding literature is reviewed from two perspectives. The first is an epidemiological approach, considering environmental agents that affect the human being. The second views body weight regulation from a "set-point" or homeostatic approach by considering the way in which one part of the metabolic system talks to another and how this system may be "overridden" by hedonic or pleasure centers. As part of the rapid growth in the biology of obesity, there have been many new terms introduced. Because all readers may not be equally familiar with this new lexicon, a glossary of terms is included in the Appendix to this chapter.

GENETIC FACTORS

The epidemic of overweight is occurring on a genetic background that does not change as fast as the epidemic has been exploding. It is nonetheless clear that genetic factors play an important role in its development (Perusse et al., 2005). One analogy for the role of genes in overweight is that "genes load the gun and a permissive or toxic environment pulls the trigger." Identification of genetic factors involved in the development of obesity increases yearly. From the time of the early twin and adoption studies more than 10 years ago, the focus has been on evaluating large groups of individuals for genetic defects related to the development of overweight. These genetic factors can be divided into two groups: the rare genes that produce excess body fat and a group of more common genes that underlie susceptibility to becoming overweight—the so-called "susceptibility" genes (Perusse et al., 2005).

Underlying the following discussion is the reality that genetic responses to the environment differ between individuals and affect the magnitude of the weight changes. Several genes have such potent effects that they produce overweight in almost any environment where food is available. Leptin deficiency is one of them. Most other genes that affect the way body weight and body fat vary under different environmental influences have only a small effect. That these small differences exist and differ between individuals accounts for much of the variability in the response to diet. A more detailed discussion of genetic factors affecting clinical expression in overweight individuals is presented in Chapter 4.

EPIGENETIC AND INTRAUTERINE IMPRINTING

Over the past decade, it has become clear that infants who are small for their age are at higher risk for metabolic diseases later in life. This idea was originally proposed by Dr. David Barker and is often called the Barker Hypothesis (Barker et al., 1993). Several examples illustrate its role in human obesity. The first was the Dutch winter famine of 1944, in which the calories available to Amsterdam were severely reduced by the Germans. During this famine, intrauterine exposure occurred during all parts of the pregnancy. Intrauterine exposure during the first trimester increased the subsequent risk of overweight in the offspring (Ravelli et al., 1999).

Two other examples that fall into the category of fetal imprinting are the increased risk of obesity in offspring of diabetic mothers (Dabelea et al., 1999) and in the offspring of mothers who smoked during the individual's intrauterine period (Power and Jefferis, 2002). In a study of infants born to Pima Indian women before and after the onset of diabetes, Dabelea et al. noted that the infants born after diabetes developed were heavier than those born to the same mother before diabetes developed (1999).

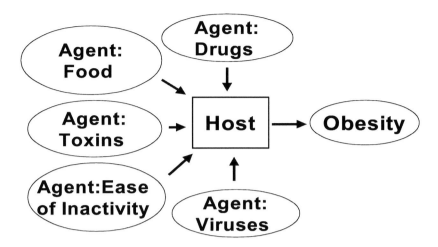

Fig. 1. Epidemiological model of obesity. In this model, the agent that produces obesity is food or food-related products. If food is in limited supply, obesity does not develop. The food that is ingested interacts with the host. In a susceptible host, the toxic effects of food produce obesity, the disease.

Smoking during pregnancy increases the risk of overweight at entry to school from just under 10% to more than 15% if smoking continued throughout pregnancy and to nearly 15% if it was discontinued after the first trimester, indicating that most of the effect takes place in the early part of pregnancy (Arenz et al., 2004; Toschke et al., 2003).

ENVIRONMENTAL AGENTS AND OVERWEIGHT: AN EPIDEMIOLOGICAL APPROACH

One view on the etiology of increased body fat is from the epidemiological or environmental perspective. The spectrum of defects is shown in Fig. 1. Here food, medications, viruses, toxins, and sedentary lifestyle are viewed as acting on the host to produce increased fat. However, we need to remember that there are genetic components for each of them.

Food as an Environmental Agent for Obesity

Energy is obtained from the foods we eat and the beverages we drink. Thus, without food there could be no life, let alone excess stores of fat. The cost of this food is important in determining food choices. In addition to cost and total quantity, food styles of eating and specific food components may be important in determining whether or not we become overweight.

COSTS OF FOOD

Economic factors may play an etiological role in explaining the basis for the intake of a small number of excess calories that leads to overweight over time. What we consume is influenced by the prices we have to pay for it. Over the recent past, particularly since the beginning of the 1970s, the price of foods that are high in energy density (fat and sugar rich) has fallen relative to other items. The consumer price index (CPI) has risen at the rate of 3.8% per year from 1980 to 2000 (Finkelstein et al., 2005) compared with the rise in food prices, which have risen only 3.4% per year. From 1960 to 1980, when there was only a small increase in the prevalence of overweight, food prices rose at a rate of 5.5% per year—slightly faster than the CPI, which grew at a rate of 5.3% per year. The relative prices of foods high in sugar and fat have decreased since the early 1980s compared with fruits and vegetables. For comparison, Finkelstein et al. note that between 1985 and 2000 the price of fresh fruits and vegetables rose 118%, fish 77%, and dairy 56%, compared with sugar and sweets, which rose only 46%, fats and oils 35%, and carbonated beverages only 20%. Is it any wonder that people with limited income eat more sugar- and fat-containing foods (Finkelstein et al., 2005)?

Human beings are price-sensitive when purchasing food or any other item. The lower the cost of an item, the more likely they are to buy it and the more of it they are likely to buy. Thus the cost of food is an important factor in the epidemic of overweight. From 1960 to 1980 the price of food rose less than the cost of other components in the CPI. Real wages also rose, providing additional money for consumption, some of which could buy a wider variety of healthy foods, such as fresh fruits and vegetables, fish, and dairy products. This was a time when the rise in the prevalence of overweight was slow. However, between 1985 and 2000, the relative cost of fruits and vegetables increased much faster than foods containing more fat and sugar, meaning that the food dollar could buy relatively more food energy if the foods contained more sugar and fat or more carbonated beverages. At the present time, it costs between $0.30 and $1.50 per 1000 kcal for fats/oils, sugars and grain; between $1 and $90 per 1000 kcal for meat, fish, and dairy products; and a similar amount for 1000 kcal of fruits or vegetables (Drewnowski and Darmon, 2005). Is it any wonder that inexpensive, good-tasting, energy-dense foods are widely consumed?

The food environment in which we live is determined more by food processors and supermarkets than by farmers or nutritionists. The largest supermarket in the United States is Wal-Mart. The groceries sold by Wal-Mart account for about one-fifth of the money spent on groceries at supermarkets. Wal-Mart's food prices are, on average, 14% lower than other chains where it markets, thus Wal-Mart is a major player in the lower prices people pay for food. Consumers can buy only what supermarkets offer to sell. In 2003, the 10 largest supermarkets had combined sales of $400 billion, with Wal-Mart having $130 billion of that. To the extent that they can provide lower energy-density (*see* p. 37) foods and smaller portion sizes at lower prices, there may be hope for moving the entire food industry toward a lower-weight America (Tillotson, 2005).

QUANTITY OF FOOD EATEN

Eating more food energy over time than we need for our daily energy requirements produces extra fat. In the current epidemic, the increase in body weight is, on average, 0.5 to 1 kg per year. The amount of net energy storage required by an adult to produce 1 kg of added body weight (75% of which is fat) can be calculated by using a few assumptions. One kilogram of adipose tissue contains about 7000 kcal (29.4 mJ) of energy. If the efficiency of energy storage is 50% with the other 50% being used by synthetic and storage processes, one would need to ingest 14,000 kcal (58.8 MJ) of food energy, which would equate to an extra 40 kcal per day (40 kcal/day × 365 days/year = 14,600 kcal; Hill and Peters, 1998). For simplicity, this can be rounded to 50 kcal per day or the equivalent of 10 teaspoons full of sugar.

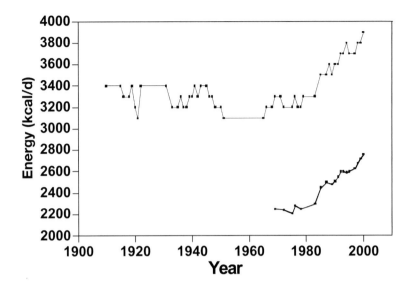

Fig. 2. Energy available for consumption over the 20th century with a correction for waste during the last quarter of the century (USDA food report, 1998).

Has the intake of energy increased? Figure 2 shows the energy intake available from the food supply and the estimated intake corrected for waste based on United States Department of Agriculture (USDA) calculations. The energy intake (kcal per day) was relatively stable during the first 80 years of the 20th century. During the last 20 years, however, there was a clear rise from about 2300 to about 2600 kcal per day, or an increase of 300 kcal per day. This is more than enough to account for the 50 kcal per day net (100 kcal gross) required to produce 1 kg weight gain each year.

The lifetime pattern of energy intake can be plotted from data obtained in the National Health and Examination Survey done by the US National Center for Health Statistics (Fig. 3). There is a rapid increase in food intake for both boys and girls during the first decade. As puberty begins, the energy intake increases more in males than females, reaching a peak during adolescence for both sexes. From age 20 onward there is a slow decrease in both sexes, but again males remain higher on average than females, in part, because males have a higher lean body mass than females (*see* Chapter 1).

Portion Size

Portion sizes have dramatically increased in the past 40 years (Nielsen and Popkin, 2003) and now need reduction. One consequence of the larger portion sizes is more food and more calories (Putnam and Allshouse, 1999). The USDA estimates that between 1984 and 1994 daily calorie intake increased by 340 kcal per day, or 14.7%. Refined grains provided 6.2% of this increase, fats and oils 3.4%, but fruits and vegetables only 1.4%, and meats and dairy products only 0.3%. Calorically sweetened beverages that contain 10% high-fructose corn syrup (HFCS) are made from these grain products. These beverages are available in containers with 12, 20, or 32 oz., which provide 150, 250, or 400 kcal if all is consumed. Many foods list the calories per serving, but the package often contains more than one serving. The increase in portion sizes is illustrated by comparing what is served in the fast food restaurants (Table 1). In 1954, the burger

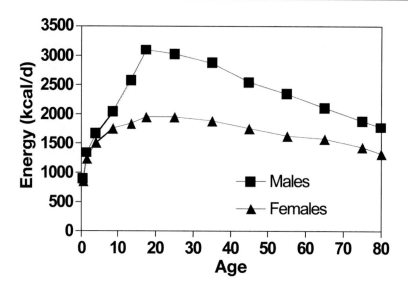

Fig. 3. Food intake over the 80-year lifespan of men and women. (Drawn from NHANES III data.)

Table 1
Change in Portion Sizes During the 20th Century

Item	Year	Ounces/kilocalories	Year	Ounces/kilocalories
Burger King® hamburger	1954	2.8/202	2004	4.3/310
McDonald's® fries	1955	2.4/210	2004	7/610
Coca Cola®	1916	6.5/79	2004	16/194
Movie popcorn	1950	3 cups/174	2004	21 cups/1700

Adapted from Newman, C. (2004).

served by Burger King weighed 2.8 oz. and had 202 kcal. In 2004, the size had grown to 4.3 oz. with 310 kcal. In 1955, McDonald's served French fries that weighed 2.4 oz. with 210 kcal. By 2004, this serving had increased to 7 oz. and 610 kcal. Popcorn served at movie theaters has grown from 3 cups containing 174 kcal in 1950 to 21 cups with 1700 kcal in 2004 (Newman, 2004). Nielsen and Popkin (2003) examined the portion sizes consumed by Americans and showed the increased energy intake associated with the larger portions of essentially all items examined. Guidance for intake of beverages suggests increased intake of water, tea, coffee, and low-fat dairy products with lesser consumption of beverages that contain primarily water and caloric sweeteners (Popkin et al., 2006). The importance of drinking water as an alternative to consuming calories is suggested in a recent study. There was an inverse relationship between water intake expressed per unit of food and beverage intake and total energy intake. When water intake was less than 20 g per gram of food and beverages, energy intake was 2485 kcal per day. At the highest quartile, when water intake was at or above 90 g per gram of food and beverage, energy intake fell to 1791 kcal per day. Thus, drinking water may be one strategy for lowering overall energy intake (Table 2) (Stookey et al., 2007).

Table 2
Effect of Drinking Water on Total Energy Intake

Quartile of drinking water	Water intake (g/g of food and beverage)	Energy intake (kcal)
1	<20	2485
2	20–50	2413
3	50–90	2235
4	≥90	1791

Adapted from Stookey, J. D., et al. (2007).

Portion size influences what we eat in both controlled and naturalistic settings. Using a laboratory setting, both normal and overweight men and women were given different amounts of a good-tasting pasta entrée. They ate 30% more when offered the largest size than when offered half the amount (1000 vs 500 g; Rolls et al., 2002). A similar finding was made when different-sized packages of potato chips were offered. Women ate 18% more and men 37% more when the package size was doubled (85 vs 170 g; Rolls et al., 2004).

Energy Density

Energy density interacts with portion size to affect how much is eaten. Energy density refers to the amount of energy in a given weight of food (kcal/g). The energy density of food is increased by dehydration, or by adding fat. Conversely, lower energy density is produced by adding water or removing fat. When energy density of meals was varied and all meals were provided for 2 days, the participants ate the same amount of food, but as a result got more energy when the foods were higher in energy density. In this experiment, they got about 30% less energy when the meals had low rather than high energy density (Bell et al., 1998; Stubbs et al., 1998). When energy density and portion size were varied, Rolls and her colleagues showed that both factors influence the amount that is eaten. The meals with low energy density and small portion sizes provided the fewest calories (398 vs 620 kcal; Kral et al., 2004).

The quantity of food consumed is also influenced by its proximity and container. In a variety of experiments, Wansink et al. showed that when food was located in close proximity subjects tended to eat more than when the food was further away. They also showed that people underestimate how much they eat and that individuals will pour out more of a beverage into a short, wide glass than into a tall, thin one. Moreover, they will drink more from the shorter glass (Wansink, 1996; Wansink et al., 2006).

Styles of Eating

Breast feeding is a case in which the style of eating can be associated with later weight gain. In infants, breast milk is their first food, and for many infants their sole source of nutrition for several months. There are now a number of studies showing that breast feeding for more than 3 months significantly reduces the risk of being overweight at entry into school and in adolescence when compared with infants who are breast fed less than 3 months (Rogers, 2003). This may be an example of "infant imprinting" (Gillman et al., 2006; Harder et al., 2005).

The composition of human breast milk may also play a role. The fats included in this nutritious food are obtained from the mother's fat stores. The composition of fat in

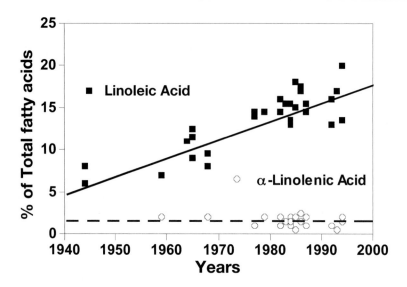

Fig. 4. Fatty acid composition of breast milk from World War II until the end of the 20th century. (Redrawn from Ailhaud and Guesnet, 2004.)

human breast milk has changed over the last 50 years of the 20th century. An analysis of samples taken over this time period showed that the quantity of linoleic acid has increased steadily. This fatty acid is common in fats from plants and probably reflects the increasing use of vegetable oils. In contrast, the quantity of the essential α-linolenic acid has remained constant (Ailhaud and Guesnet, 2004; Fig. 4). The way in which these fatty acids are metabolized differs with the linoleic acid, forming prostacyclin, which can act on receptors on the fat cell to modulate fat cell replication. It is conceivable that the changing fatty acid content of human breast milk may have modified the sensitivity to fats later in life.

RESTAURANTS AND FAST FOOD ESTABLISHMENTS

Eating outside the home has increased significantly over the past 30 years. There are now more fast food restaurants (277,208) than churches in the United States (Tillotson, 2004). The number of fast food restaurants has risen since 1980 from 1 per 2000 Americans to 1 per 1000 Americans. Of the 206 meals eaten out in 2002, fast food restaurants served 74% of them. Other important figures are that Americans spent $100 billion on fast food in 2001, compared with $6 billion in 1970. An average of three orders of French fries are ordered per person per week, and French fries have become the most widely consumed vegetable. More than 100,000 new food products were intro-duced between 1990 and 1998 (2002). Eating outside the home has become easier over the last four decades as the number of restaurants has increased, and the percent of meals eaten outside the home reflects this. In 1962, less than 10% of meals were eaten outside the home. By 1992, it had risen to nearly 35%, where it has remained (2002). However, in a telephone survey of body mass index (BMI) in relation to proximity to fast food restaurants in Minnesota, Jeffrey et al. found that eating at a fast food restaurant *was* associated with having children, a high-fat diet, and a high BMI, but not with the subjects' proximity to the restaurant (Jeffery et al., 2006).

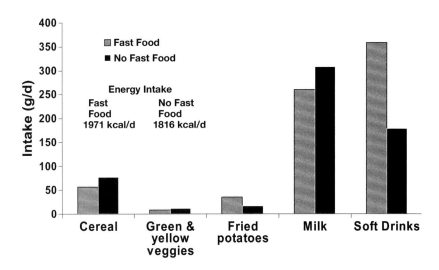

Fig. 5. Effect of consuming a fast food meal on one day with the food consumed on another non-fast food day. (Drawn from Paeratakul et al., 2003.)

Eating in a fast food restaurant also changes the foods consumed. Paeratakul et al. compared a day in which individuals ate at a fast food restaurant with a day when they did not. On the day when food was eaten in the fast food restaurant, individuals consumed less cereal, milk, and vegetables, but more soft drinks and French fries (Fig. 5; Paeratakul et al., 2003). Similar findings were reported by Bowman et al., who also reported that on any given day more than 30% of the total sample consumed fast food. In this national survey, several other features were also associated with eating at fast food restaurants, including being male, having a higher household income, and residing in the South (Bowman et al., 2004). Children who ate at fast food restaurants consumed more energy, more fat and added sugars, and more sweetened beverages than children who did not eat at fast food restaurants.

To test the effect of eating fast food in a controlled environment, Ebbeling et al. (2004) provided fast food in large amounts for a 1-hour lunch to normal and overweight adolescents. Overweight participants (weight higher than the 85th percentile for height) ate more (1860 kcal) than lean participants (1458 kcal) and the average intake was more than 60% of their estimated total daily energy requirements. During a second study, energy intake was significantly higher in the overweight subjects on the 2 days when the subjects ate fast food than on the 2 days when they did not (2703 vs 2295 kcal per day), a difference that was not observed in the lean adolescents. In a 15-year follow-up of the Coronary Artery Risk Development in Young Adults study, Pereira et al. (2005) found that the frequency of consuming fast food at baseline was directly associated with weight gain in blacks and whites. Increases in the frequency of consuming fast food during the 15 years of follow-up were also associated with increased risk of weight gain. It thus seems clear that eating at fast food restaurants increases the risk of ingesting more calories than are needed.

A decline in consumption of food at home is one consequence of the increase in eating out. To examine the relationship between frequency of family dinners and overweight status among 9- to 14-year-olds, Taveras et al. (2005) did a cross-sectional and longitudinal study of 14,431 boys ($n = 6647$) and girls ($n = 7784$). They found that the frequency of eating family dinner was inversely associated with the prevalence of overweight in the cross-sectional study, but did not predict the degree of weight gain in the longitudinal study.

NIGHT-EATING SYNDROME

The original description of the night-eating syndrome was published in a classic paper by Stunkard in 1955. Recent studies have refined this syndrome, which consists of individuals who eat more than 50% of their daily energy intake during the nighttime and is described in more detail in Chapter 4.

FREQUENCY OF FOOD INTAKE

For more than 40 years, there have been suggestions that eating fewer meals would be more likely to lead to obesity than eating many meals (Bray, 1976). One of the clear-cut effects of eating fewer meals is an increase in cholesterol (Bray, 1972). Crawley and Summerbell (1997) showed that among males, but not females, the number of meal-eating events per day was inversely related to BMI. Males with a BMI of 20 to 25 ate just over six times per day compared with less than six times for those with a BMI of more than 25 kg/m^2.

Eating breakfast would be associated with eating more frequently, and there are data showing that eating breakfast is associated with lower body weight. Eating breakfast cereal has been related to decreased BMI in adolescent girls. Using longitudinal data on adolescent girls, Barton et al. (2005) showed that as cereal intake per week increased from zero to three times per week, there was a small, but significant decrease in BMI.

FOOD COMPONENTS

There have been a number of significant changes in the quantities of different foods eaten during the time when the epidemic of overweight developed, and they have no doubt changed the intake of other nutrients as well. From 1970 to 2000, per capita intake of fats and oils increased from 56 to 77 lbs. per person, sugars from 139 to 172 lbs. per person, fruits from 241 to 280 lbs. per person, vegetables from 337 to 445 lbs. per person, grains from 136 to 200 lbs. per person, and proteins from 588 to 621 lbs. per person. Figure 6 plots some of the changes in various food groups using the USDA guide (USDA, 2006). It is clear that more food from all categories is being consumed, thus providing more energy to Americans with the resulting problem of overweight. Using data from the USDA, Frazao and Allshouse reported that whereas fruits and vegetable consumption increased 20% between 1970 and 2000, the consumption of calorie sweetened beverages rose 70% and the consumption of cheese rose 162% (2003).

CALORICALLY SWEETENED SOFT DRINKS

One of the consequences of the lower farm prices in the 1970s was a drop in the price of corn, which made the production of cornstarch (which is converted to HFCS) inexpensive. With the development of isomerase technology in the late 1960s that could convert starch into fructose, a very sweet molecule, the manufacture of soft drinks entered a new era. This is shown graphically in Fig. 7 (Bray et al., 2004). From the early 1970s through the mid-1990s, HFCS gradually replaced sugar in many manufactured products, and almost entirely replaced sugar in soft drinks manufactured in the United States. In addition to being cheap, HFCS is very sweet. We have argued that this

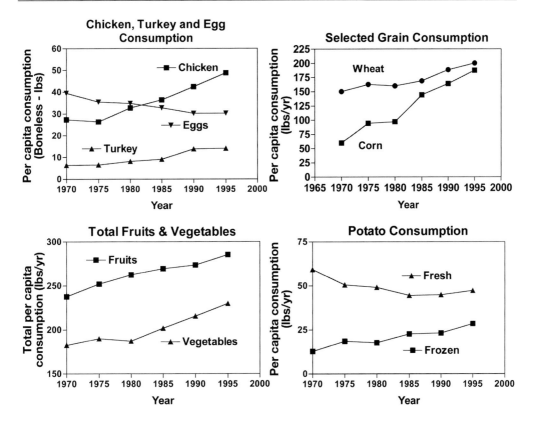

Fig. 6. Changes in consumption of selected food items from 1970 to 1995. (Drawn from USDA data.)

"sweetness" in liquid form is one factor driving the consumption of increased calories that are needed to fuel the current epidemic of obesity.

Fructose differs in several ways from glucose, the other half of the sucrose (sugar) molecule. Fructose is absorbed from the gastrointestinal (GI) track by a different mechanism than glucose. Glucose stimulates insulin release from the pancreas, but fructose does not. Fructose also enters muscle and other cells without depending on insulin, whereas most glucose enters cells in an insulin-dependent manner. Finally, once inside the cell, fructose can enter the pathways that provide the triglyceride backbone (glycerol) more efficiently than glucose. Thus, high consumption of fructose as occurs with the rising consumption of soft drinks and the use of high-fructose corn sweeteners may be a "fat equivalent" (Havel, 2002).

The relationship of soft drink consumption to calorie intake, body weight, and the intake of other dietary components has been examined in both cross-sectional and longitudinal studies (Vartanian et al., 2006). Of the 11 cross-sectional studies examining the relationship between caloric intake and soft drink consumption, 9 found a moderately positive association. Among the four longitudinal studies, the strength of the association was slightly stronger. The authors conclude that there is little caloric compensation when human beings drink soft drinks; that is, soft drinks are "added" calories and do not lower the intake of energy in other forms. The strengths of these relationships were stronger in women and in adults. Not surprisingly, the authors found that studies funded

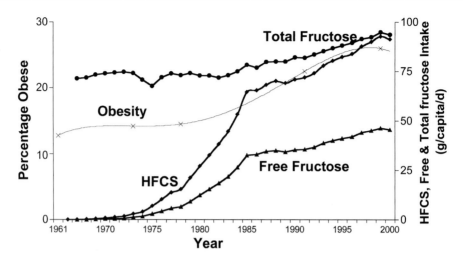

Fig. 7. Intake of high-fructose corn syrup and total fructose since 1970. (From Bray et al., 2004.)

by the food industry had weaker associations than those funded by independent sources. A critique of the relationship between soft drink consumption and the development of obesity in children has been published by Dietz (2006) (Table 3). There are five studies in children that have shown a positive relationship between soft drink consumption and weight gain (Berkey et al., 2004; Ludwig et al., 2001a; Striegel-Moore et al., 2006; Welsh et al., 2005). These are summarized in the following pargraphs. They make the case for reducing the consumption of calorie-sweetened beverages by children and adolescents overwhelmingly strong.

Several studies on the consumption of calorically sweetened beverages in relation to the epidemic of overweight have gotten significant attention (Bray et al., 2004). Ludwig et al. (2001a) reported that the intake of soft drinks was a predictor of initial BMI in children in the Planet Health Study. They went on to show that higher soft drink consumption also predicted an increase in BMI during nearly 2 years of follow-up. Those with the highest soft drink consumption at baseline had the highest increase in BMI. In one of the few randomized, well-controlled intervention studies, Danish investigators (Raben et al., 2003) showed that individuals consuming calorically sweetened beverages during 10 weeks gained weight, whereas subjects drinking the same amount of artificially sweetened beverages lost weight. Equally important, drinking sugar-sweetened beverages was associated with a small but significant increase in blood pressure. Women in the Nurses Health Study (Schulze et al., 2004) also showed that changes in the consumption of soft drinks predicted changes in body weight over several years of follow-up. In children, a study focusing on reducing intake of "fizzy" drinks and replacing them with water showed slower weight gain than those not advised to reduce the intake of fizzy drinks (James et al., 2004).

As soft drink consumption in the population has increased, the consumption of milk, a major source of calcium, has decreased (Fig. 8). Milk, particularly low-fat milk, is a valuable source of calcium for bone growth during the time of maximal bone accretion. Calcium is also a dietary nutrient that may be related to the development of overweight (Zemel et al., 2000). The level of calcium intake in population studies is inversely related

Table 3
Relation of Soft Drink Consumption to Risk of Increasing Body Weight

Author	Number of SS	Age range	Duration	Association
Phillips	132	9–10		Positive
Welsh et al., 2005	10,904	2–3	1 year	Positive
Berkey et al., 2004	12,192	9–14	Two 1-year periods	Positive
Ludwig et al., 2001a	548	11–12	Baseline and 2 years	Positive
Striegel-Moore et al., 2006	2371	9–10	9–10 years	Positive

SS, Subjects.

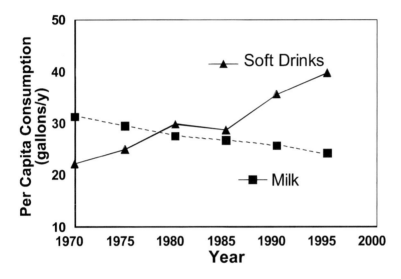

Fig. 8. The consumption of soft drinks and the relation of high-fructose corn syrup consumption to the epidemic of obesity. The declining consumption of milk in the United States between 1970 and 1997 and the rising consumption of soft drinks occurred this same period. (Drawn from USDA data.)

with being overweight (Davies et al., 2000; Pereira et al., 2002). In other epidemiological studies and in feeding trials, higher dietary calcium levels were also associated with a reduced BMI or reduced incidence of the insulin resistance syndrome (Pereira et al., 2005). Although intriguing, some investigators remain unconvinced that calcium or dairy products are beneficial for preventing weight gain or producing weight loss (*see* Chapter 9).

Fructose consumption, either in beverages or food, may have an additional detrimental effect. Fructose, unlike other sugars, increases serum uric acid levels. Nakagawa et al. propose that this increase occurs when fructose is taken into the liver where adenosine triphosphate is used to phosphorylate fructose to fructose-6-phosphate. The adenosine-5'-diphosphate can be further broken down into adenosine-5'-monophosphate and uric acid. Thus, the production of uric acid is a byproduct of the metabolism of fructose in the liver. The high levels of uric acid could set the stage for advancing cardiovascular disease, the authors propose, by reducing the availability of nitric oxide, which is crucial for maintaining normal blood pressure and normal function of the vessel walls (endothelium). If this hypothesis is borne out, it will provide another reason that nature

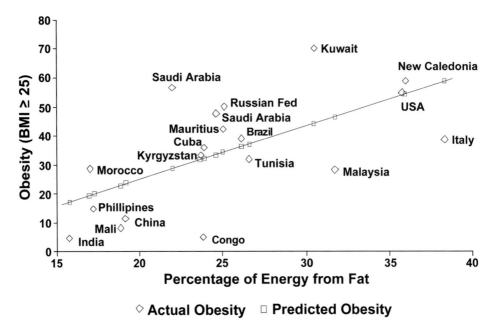

Fig. 9. Dietary fat intake in various countries and the prevalence of overweight. (From Bray and Popkin, 1998.)

preferred glucose over fructose as a substrate for metabolism during the evolutionary process (Nakagawa et al., 2006).

DIETARY FAT

Fat is another component of diet that may be important in the current epidemic (Astrup et al., 2000; Bray and Popkin, 1998). In epidemiological studies, dietary fat intake is related to the fraction of the population that is overweight (Fig. 9; Bray and Popkin, 1998). In experimental animals, high-fat diets generally produce fat storage. In humans, the relationship between dietary fat and the development of overweight is controversial. It is certainly clear that ingesting too many calories is essential for an increase in body fat. Because the storage capacity for carbohydrate is very limited, it must be oxidized first. Thus, when people overeat, they oxidize carbohydrate and store fat. When fat is a large component of a diet, foods tend to be energy-dense and thus over-consumption is easy to achieve.

Foods combining fat and sugar may be a particular problem because they are often very palatable and usually inexpensive (Drewnowski and Specter, 2004). The Leeds Fat Study shows that high-fat consumers have an increased incidence of overweight (Blundell and MacDiarmid, 1997). High fat content of foods increases their "energy density," meaning that they have more available energy for each unit of food. The reason is obvious from the energy contained in fats and carbohydrates. Each gram of fat has 9 kcal, whereas carbohydrates yield only 4 kcal/g. Thus, lowering the fat content or raising the quantity of water in foods are ways of reducing the energy density. Providing an increased number of palatable foods with low energy density would be valuable in helping fight the epidemic of overweight. Alcohol is particularly prob-

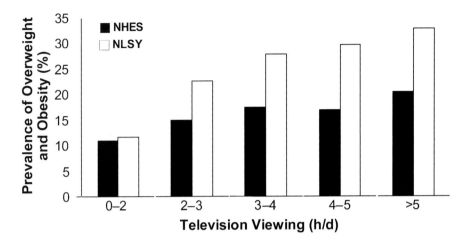

Fig. 10. Relationship of television viewing in children to prevalence of overweight (Redrawn from Dietz et al., 1985).

lematic in this regard. When a high-fat snack with alcohol is given before lunch, subjects consumed just under 200 kcal (812 kJ) more at lunchtime than when they were given an alcohol-free pre-lunch snack that was high in carbohydrates (Tremblay and St-Pierre, 1996).

Low Levels of Physical Activity

Epidemiological data show that low levels of physical activity and watching more television predict higher body weight (Hancox et al., 2004). Recent studies suggest that individuals in American cities who have to walk more than people in other cities tended to weigh less (Saelens et al., 2003). Low levels of physical activity also increase the risk of early mortality (Blair and Brodney, 1999). Using normal weight, physically active women as the comparison group, Hu et al. found that the relative risk of mortality increased from 1.00 to 1.55 (55%) in inactive lean women compared with active lean ones, to 1.92 in active overweight women, and to 2.42 in women who are overweight and physically inactive (2004). It is thus better to be thin than fat and to be physically active rather than inactive.

Television has been one culprit blamed for the reduced levels of physical activity, particularly in children. The first suggestion that TV viewing was associated with overweight was published by Gortmaker and Dietz. Using data from the National Health Examination Survey (Dietz and Gortmaker, 1985) and the National Longitudinal Study of Youth (Gortmaker et al., 1996), they found a linear gradient from 11 to 12% overweight in children watching 0 to 2 hours per day to more than 20 to 30% when watching more than 5 hours per day (Fig. 10). Since that time a number of studies have shown that children and adults who watch more television are more overweight. By one estimate, about 100 kcal of extra food energy is ingested for each hour of television viewing. In studies focusing on reducing sedentary activity, which largely means decreasing television viewing, there was a significant decrease in energy intake with increased activity (Epstein et al., 2005).

Although television receives a good deal of blame, there is some evidence that the major increase in viewing time occurred prior to the onset of the epidemic of overweight. In evidence reviewed by Cutler (2003), television viewing increased from 158 to 191 minutes, or 21%, between 1965 and 1975, when color television became available at low prices. In contrast, between 1975 and 1995, when the epidemic of overweight was in full swing, the increase was only 11% (from 191 to 212 minutes). Although the use of television grew more slowly, other electronic devices, particularly computers and more recently the Internet, have grown even faster. Television and other "screen" systems differ in that you can eat and watch television, but it is harder to do that when you need to respond to what is on the screen. The exposure to 10 or more commercials per hour, most of which are for fast foods, soft drinks, and other energy dense products, may be an additional component associated with television in the epidemic of overweight (Finkelstein et al., 2005).

Effect of Sleep Time and Environmental Light

Nine epidemiological studies have been published that relate shortness of sleep time with overweight. Six of these studies are cross-sectional in design, and three are longitudinal. The earliest of these studies was only published in 1992, but most were published after 2002. They include both children and adults. In a small, case–control study involving 327 short-sleepers compared with 704 controls, Locard et al. (1992) found that short-sleepers were heavier than the controls.

In two large cross-sectional studies in children, Sekine et al. (2002) and von Kries et al. (2002) found that there was a dose–response relationship between the amount of sleep and the weight of children when they entered school. von Kries et al. studied 6862 children aged 5 to 6 years whose sleeping time was reported in 1999 to 2000 by the parent, with follow-up in 2001 to 2002. Overweight in this study was defined as a weight for height greater than the 97th percentile. Children with reported sleeping time of less than 10 hours had a prevalence of overweight of 5.4% (95% confidence interval [CI] 4.1 to 7.0), those who slept 10.5 to 11.0 hours per night had a prevalence of 2.8% (95% CI 2.3 to 3.3), and those who slept more than 11.5 hours had a prevalence of overweight of 2.1% (95% CI 1.5 to 2.9) (Fig. 11). Among the 8274 children from the Toyama Birth Cohort in Japan (Sekine et al., 2002) there was a graded increase in the risk of overweight, defined as a BMI above 25 kg/m^2, as sleep time decreased. If the children who were reported to sleep more than 10 hours at age three had an odds ratio of 1.0, those who slept 9 to 10 hours had an odds ratio of 1.49, those with 8 to 9 hours an odds ratio of 1.89, and those children who reported to sleep less than 8 hours had an odds ratio for overweight of 2.87.

In a cross-sectional study of 383 11- to 16-year-old adolescents, Gupta et al. (2002) used 24-hour wrist actigraphy to assess sleeping. He found that for every 1 hour of sleep loss, the risk of overweight was increased by 8%. In the final study in children, Reilly et al. (2005) found that the reported duration of sleep at age three in 7758 children was related to their measured weight at age six.

A dose–response relationship between duration of sleep and body weight has also been reported by Vioque et al. (2000). As the amount of sleep increased from 6 to 9 hours per night, there was a small increase in overweight. The largest study of overweight and sleep is based on self reports from more than 1 million people aged 30 to 102 years

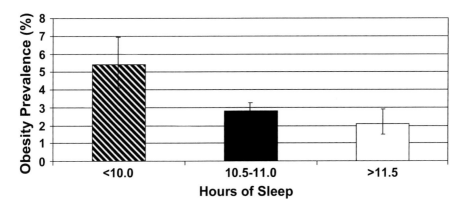

Fig. 11. Dose–response between the amount of sleep and the weight changes. (Drawn from von Kries et al., 2002.)

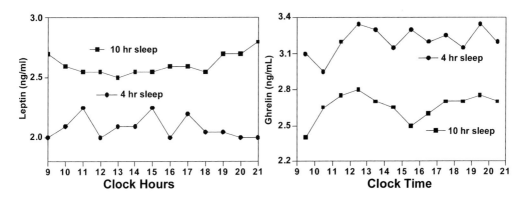

Fig. 12. Effect of short or long sleep duration on the ghrelin and leptin level in healthy volunteers who slept in a metabolic unit. (Readapted from Spiegel et al., 2004.)

and is consistent with the other studies (Kripke et al., 2002). Gangwisch et al. (2005), using the National Health and Nutrition Examination Survey study data, also found a relationship between sleep duration and overweight.

These epidemiological studies are buttressed by experimental studies (Spiegel et al., 2004). Manipulating sleep time in the laboratory has several endocrine consequences. First, it reduces glucose tolerance and increases insulin resistance. Second, it lowers leptin levels and raises ghrelin levels. This is shown in Fig. 12.

Another setting in which lighting plays a role in the development of weight gain is seasonal affective depressive syndrome. For some people, the shortening of the daylight hours with the onset of winter is associated with depression and weight gain. When the days begin to lengthen in the spring this symptom complex is reversed. Current evidence suggests that it is related to changing activity of the serotonin system and can be treated with exposure to light or by manipulating brain levels of serotonin pharmacologically.

Medications That Produce Weight Gain

Several drugs can cause weight gain, including a variety of hormones and psychoactive agents (Allison et al., 1999; *see* Chapter 4). The degree of weight gain is generally less than 10 kg and not sufficient to cause substantial overweight. Some of these drugs can also increase the risk of future type 2 diabetes mellitus.

Toxins

SMOKING

The rise of smoking from 1900 to 1970 and its decline during the last 30 years of the 20th century has been tracked by the Centers for Disease Control and Prevention (N. A., 1999). Weight gain after stopping smoking is gender-dependent, with men gaining an average of 3.8 kg and women 2.8 kg (Williamson et al., 1991). In a more recent analysis, men were found to gain 4.4 kg and women 5.0 kg (Flegal et al., 1995) and it was calculated that this gain could account for about one-fourth to one-sixth of the increased prevalence of overweight. Economists have calculated that a 10% increase in the price of cigarettes could increase BMI by 0.0251 kg/m^2 because of the decrease in smoking (Cutler et al., 2003). Snacks are the major component of food intake that rises when people stop smoking.

ORGANOCHLORINES

In human beings, we know that body fat stores many "toxic" chemicals and that they are mobilized with weight loss. Backman first showed in 1970s that organochlorines in the body decreased after bariatric surgery. The metabolic rate can be reduced by organochlorine molecules (Tremblay et al., 2004), and conceivably, prolonged exposure to many chlorinated chemicals in our environment has affected metabolic pathways and energy metabolism. Thyroid hormone synthesis is decreased, plasma T3 and T4 are decreased, thyroid hormone clearance is increased, and skeletal muscle and mitochondrial oxidation are reduced.

MONOSODIUM GLUTAMATE

Food additives are another class of chemicals that are widely distributed and may be involved in the current epidemic of overweight. In experimental animals, exposure to monosodium glutamate, a common flavoring ingredient in food, in the neonatal period will produce fatness (Olney, 1969).

Viruses as Environmental Agents

Several viruses produce weight gain in animals and the possibility that they do this in human beings needs more study. It has been known for many years that the injection of several viruses into the central nervous system could produce fatness in mice. The list of viruses now includes canine distemper virus, RAV-7 virus, Borna disease virus, scrapie virus, SMAM-1 virus, and three adenoviruses (types 5, 24, and 36). These observations were generally assumed to be pathological in nature and not relevant to overweight humans. However, the recent finding that antibodies to one of the adenoviruses (AM-36) are found in larger amounts in some overweight humans than in controls challenges this view. This viral syndrome resulting from AM-36 can be replicated in the ferret, a non-human primate. The features of the syndrome are modest increase in weight and a low cholesterol concentration in the circulation. Further studies are needed to establish that a syndrome of weight loss associated with low concentrations of cholesterol clearly exists in human beings. If so, this would enhance the value of the epidemiological model.

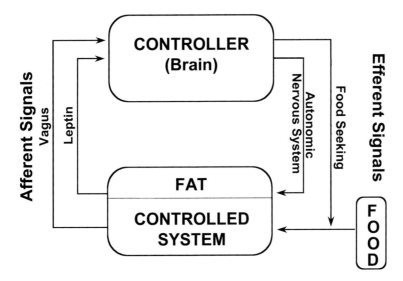

Fig. 13. A feedback model for obesity. The bottom of the figure represents the gastrointestinal (GI) track and the entry of food through the mouth. Vagal fibers carry information about taste and the size and activity of the gut to the brain. In addition, there are a variety of GI peptides that also act as signals about the size and content of the GI track. Other metabolic signals are provided by nutrients. The adipose organ produces leptin, which is a major signal for modulating food intake. The brain represented at the top consists of a receiver for external signals, a transducer, a comparator, and efferent signal generators that affect food intake and metabolism. (©1999 George A. Bray.)

REGULATION OF BODY FAT AS A PROBLEM OF HOMEOSTATIC ENERGY REGULATION WITH A HEDONIC OVERRIDE

A defect in the way the body responds to feedback signals is another way to view the problem of overweight. Such a system has four parts. The control center in the brain is analogous to the thermostat in a heating system. It receives information about the state of the animal or human, transduces this information into neurochemical signals, and activates pathways that lead to or inhibit feeding and the search for food. The signals that the brain receives come from the environment through sense organs and from the body through neural, nutrient, or hormonal signals. The response the brain makes includes both the activation and inhibition of motor systems and the modulation of the autonomic nervous system or hormonal control system. Outside of the brain is the so-called controlled system, which, for the purpose of this discussion, includes the digestive tract, which ingests, digests, and absorbs food; the metabolic systems in the liver, muscles, and kidneys that transform nutrients; and adipose tissue, which both stores and releases fatty acids and acts as a secretory endocrine organ. A feedback model is illustrated in Fig. 13 (Bray, 2003).

Digestion, Metabolism, and Fat Storage

The controlled system consists of the GI tract, liver, muscles, fat tissues, cardiovascular–pulmonary–renal system, and the supporting bone tissue. The ingestion, digestion, and absorption of food provides nutrients to the body and also provides signals from these nutrients to the vagus nerve, which provides the major neural control of GI function,

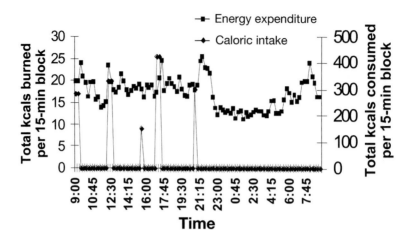

Fig. 14. Energy balance in one subject. This man spent 23 hours in a respiration calorimeter. His food intake is shown by the spikes and his energy expenditure by the connected lines. The goal was to come as close to energy balance as possible. Over 4 consecutive days, we were never closer than 25 kcal to energy balance and on three of the four measurements it was further away. Energy balance is probably a theoretical concept, not a practical consideration. (De Jonge, Bray, unpublished observations.)

and from hormones released by the GI tract. The nutrients that are absorbed can be metabolized to provide energy or stored as glycogen in liver, protein in muscle, or fat in adipose tissue.

The largest part of the energy we expend each day is for "resting" metabolism, which includes the metabolism of food; transport of sodium, potassium, and other ions across cell membranes; repair of DNA; synthesis of protein; beating of the heart; and functioning of the brain, liver, and kidneys. Energy expenditure is most strongly associated with fat-free body mass.

Increased body fat results from a positive energy balance, which results from a defect in the internal regulatory system. One assumption of this concept is that we are in energy balance. To examine this idea, we have attempted to produce a "zero" energy balance; that is, to get subjects as close as possible over a 24-hour time interval to balancing energy intake and expenditure so that there was no difference. Figure 14 shows the energy intake and expenditure of a normal male volunteer during 24 hours in our respiration calorimeters (De Jonge et al., unpublished observations). This system has a prediction algorithm that allows us to predict the 24-hour energy balance each 20 minutes using minute-to-minute measurements. We can thus adjust either food intake or exercise to achieve balance. In looking at this figure, the spikes reflect the intake of energy in 20-minute intervals. Energy expenditure is in 15-minute intervals and continues between meals, but drops during sleep to about 80% of daytime average. This individual spent 4 days in a row in the chamber. The closest we came to energy balance was ±100 kcal (±420 kJ). Based on this and a number of other studies, we conclude that day-to-day energy balance is either positive or negative. We do not achieve meal-to-meal or day-to-day energy balance. Rather, if we are to avoid weight gain, we must achieve this over a longer time interval.

There is some evidence that there is regulation over a period of several days. The first study to support this idea was by Edholm et al. (1955). They measured food intake

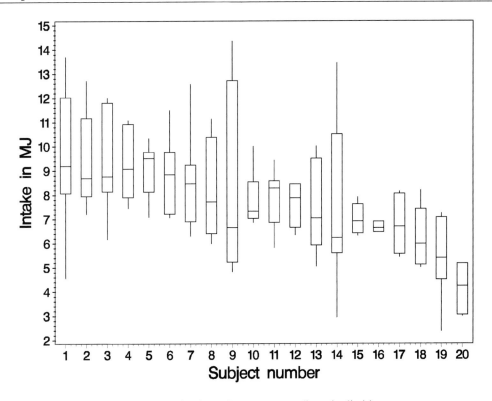

Fig. 15. Energy intake and energy expenditure in dietitians.

and energy expenditure in military recruits. There was no correlation of energy intake and energy expenditure from day to day, but over a period of several days there was a correlation between the two. We have conducted a similar study in dietitians. They were enrolled in a study to see whether they could accurately record food intake over a 7-day interval when energy expenditure was being measured by doubly labeled water (Champagne et al., 2002). Their energy intake was not significantly lower than their energy expenditure during this period of time. However, there were striking day-to-day variations in energy intake (Fig. 15). This box and whisker plot shows the 25th and 75th percentile for intake with the median intake. Some individuals varied by more than 1000 kcal per day (4180 kJ per day), whereas others had much smaller variations. When the day-to-day variations were examined, it became clear that there was a maximal relationship between intake and expenditure evident at days 3 and 4, but not at days 1, 2, or 5 (Bray et al., unpublished observations). This implies that there are signal systems operating over extended periods of time that are important in whether we can maintain energy balance long-term or whether the system is easily thrown off balance.

If we are to maintain a stable body weight, the metabolic mix of carbohydrate, fat, and protein that are oxidized by the body must equal the amounts of these nutrients taken in as food. That is, to maintain energy balance requires that the mix of foods we eat be completely metabolized or oxidized. The capacity for storage of carbohydrate as glycogen is very limited and the capacity to store protein is also restricted. Only the fat stores can readily expand to accommodate increasing levels of energy intake above those required for daily energy needs. Several studies now show that a high rate of carbohydrate oxidation, as measured by a high RQ (*see* Appendix), predicts future weight gain (Zurlo et al., 1990). One explanation is that when carbohydrate oxidation is higher than the intake of carbohydrate, carbohydrate stores are depleted. To replace these carbohydrates, an individual must eat more carbohydrates or reduce the oxidation of carbohydrates by the body, because the body cannot convert fatty acids to carbohydrates and the conversion of amino acids to carbohydrates mobilizes important body proteins (Flatt, 1995). Obese individuals who have lost weight are less effective in increasing fat oxidation in the presence of a high-fat diet than normal weight individuals, and this may be one reason why they are so susceptible to regaining weight that has been lost.

The final common pathway for retaining the energy from foods is in the mitochondrial chain of enzymes involved in oxidative phosphorylation. A growing number of studies have shown that the genes controlling these enzymes are not expressed at normal levels in people with diabetes, individuals with a family history of diabetes, or following ingestion of a high-fat diet (Patti and Kahn, 2004; Ukropcova et al., 2005). This defect in expression of genes for oxidative phosphorylation may underlie the susceptibility of some individuals to becoming overweight when eating a high-fat diet that is so prevalent in Western societies.

Physical activity gradually declines with age. To avoid becoming overweight as we age, we must gradually reduce our food intake or maintain a regular exercise program. A moderate level of exercise is beneficial in two ways. First, it reduces the risk of cardio-vascular disease and type 2 diabetes. Second, it facilitates the oxidation of fat in the diet (Smith et al., 2000). However, maintaining an exercise program is difficult for many people, particularly as they get older.

The concept of "energy wasting" through uncoupling proteins (UCPs) is one of the expanding basic science aspects of obesity. The original UCP-1 found in brown fat has a well-established role in helping newborn infants maintain body temperature (Appendix). Increased expression and/or activation of this protein uncouples oxidative phosphorylation, resulting in the conversion of energy to heat (thermogenesis). This molecule is important in human infants, but its importance in adults has been questioned because of the very low levels of brown fat (and hence UCP-1 expression) in adult humans. Recently, the identification of two additional UPCs (UCP-2 and UCP-3) that are highly expressed in adult human tissues has attracted considerable interest. These two UPCs, however, do not have the same effects as UCP-1. That is they do not seem to allow for heat dissipation by enhancing a mitochondrial proton leak. Rather, they appear to be involved in transport of fatty acids into cells.

THE FAT CELL

The fat cells in adipose tissue serve two major functions. First, they are the cells that store and release fatty acids ingested in the food we eat or synthesized in the liver or fat cell. Second, fat cells are a major endocrine cell, secreting many important metabolic and hormonal molecules (Fig. 16).

Before fat cells can undertake these functions, however, they must be converted from precursor mesenchymal cells to mature fat cells. In vitro studies have shown a two-stage process: proliferation followed by differentiation. The proliferative phase is initiated by hormonal stimulation with insulin and glucocorticoids. After the cells begin to grow, they enter a state of differentiation during which they acquire the genetic state of mature

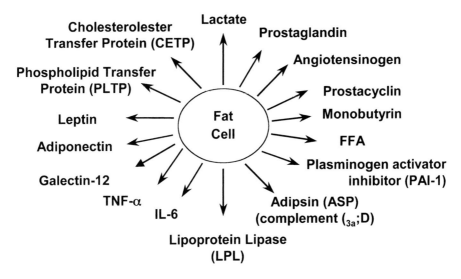

Fig. 16. The fat cell and its endocrine products.

fat cells that can store fatty acids, break down triglycerides, and make and release the many hormones that characterize the mature fat cell. Most of the fatty acids that are stored in human fat cells are derived from the diet, although these cells maintain the capacity for *de novo* synthesis of fatty acids (Hellerstein et al., 1993).

The discovery of leptin catapulted the fat cell into the arena of endocrine cells (Zhang et al., 1994; Fig. 16). The finding of a peptide released from adipose tissue that acts at a distance has refocused interest in the fat cell from a cell that primarily stores fatty acids to a cell with endocrine and paracrine functions (Appendix). In addition to leptin, this fat cell secretes a variety of peptides, including lipoprotein lipase, adipsin (complement D), complement C, adiponectin, tumor necrosis factor-α, interleukin-6, plasminogen activator inhibitor-1, angiotensinogen, bradykinin, and resistin, in addition to other metabolites, such as lactate, fatty acids, glycerol, and prostacyclin formed from arachidonic acid. This important endocrine tissue has thus greatly expanded its role. Adiponectin and resistin are recent addition to the growing list. Two adipocytokines, visfatin and vaspin, have been suggested to arise primarily in visceral adipose tissue, although this is not a settled issue (Fukuhara et al., 2005; Hida et al., 2005).

Messages to the Brain From the Environment and the Body

The brain receives a continuing stream of information from both the external and internal environment that play a role in the control of feeding. The external information provided by sight, sound, and smell are all distance signals for identifying food.

Taste and texture of foods are proximate signals generated when food enters the mouth. The classic tastes are sweet, sour, bitter, and salty, with "umami" as a fifth taste. In nature, most sweet foods also have vitamins and minerals because they come from fruits. Sour and particularly bitter foods often contain unwanted chemical compounds. The extreme example of this is "bait-shyness" or taste aversion, the property that some items have that produces a permanent rejection of future food with the same taste. This is a hard-wired response in the brain that overrides the usual feedback signals.

A taste for fats, specifically unsaturated fatty acids, may be a sixth taste. Receptors on the tongue can identify certain fatty acids. The discovery of taste receptors for poly-unsaturated fatty acids on the taste bud that involves a potassium rectifier channel offers an opening into modifying taste inputs into the food intake system (Gilbertson et al., 2005). An important advance was showing that the CD-36 receptor, which binds fatty acids, is the receptor for these fatty acids. These receptors are located on the lingual papillae of the tongue. Mice that do not have the CD-36 receptor do not prefer solutions enriched with long-chain fatty acids or a high-fat diet. These receptors are in close proximity to Ebner's glands, a source of lingual lipase, which will cleave triglycerides into fatty acids that can activate the CD-36 receptor. When this receptor is activated, there is a rise in flow of pancreatic secretions and an increase in their content (Laugerette et al., 2005).

Several GI peptides have been studied as potential regulators of food intake. Most of these peptides, including cholecystokinin, gastrin-releasing peptide, oxyntomodulin, neuromedin B, and polypeptide YY3-36, reduce food intake. Cholecystokinin was the first peptide shown to reduce food intake in animals and humans alike (Bray and Greenway, 2007). Investigation of the growth hormone secretogue receptor has led to the identification of a new GI hormone involved with the control of feeding. This peptide, called ghrelin, is produced in the stomach. It stimulates food intake in animals and human beings when given systemically or into the brain. The level is low in people who are overweight, suggesting that it may play a role in controlling appetite and weight gain.

Pancreatic peptides, including amylin, glucagon-like peptide (GLP)-1, and enterostatin, also modulate feeding. Amylin is produced in the β-cell of the pancreas along with insulin and they are co-secreted. In experimental studies, amylin has been shown to reduce food intake by acting on the amylin (calcitonin-like gene product) receptor. The major locations for this receptor are in the hindbrain and hypothalamus (Barth et al., 2004). Pramlintide is a commercial analog of amylin that is currently used to treat diabetes (*see* Chapter 9). Both glucagon and its 6-29 amino acid derivative, GLP-1, reduce food intake in animals and humans. GLP-1 works in the brain (Seeley et al., 1996) and after peripheral administration (*see* Chapter 9). Exenatide is a GLP-1-like peptide isolated from the salivary glands of the Gila monster. It has been approved for the treatment of diabetes (*see* Chapter 9).

Enterostatin, the pentapeptide signal portion of pancreatic co-lipase, is of interest because it selectively reduces fat intake in experimental animals. The beta-chain of the adenosine triphosphatase is the receptor for this small peptide. This peptide increases satiety in human beings and reduces food intake in baboons.

Nutrients may also be afferent signals to reduce food intake. A dip in the circulating level of glucose precedes the onset of eating in more than 50% of the meals in animals and human beings (Campfield and Smith, 2003). When this dip is blocked, food intake is delayed. The pattern recognized by this dip is independent of the level from which the drop in glucose begins. The small drop in glucose continues even when food is not available. The dip follows a small rise in insulin, suggesting a relationship of these two signals (Bray, 2003; Bray and Greenway, 2007).

The Brain and Food Intake

The brain plays the central role as receiver, transducer and transmitter of information from the peripheral organs (Berthoud, 2002). This control is accomplished through

Table 4
Neurotransmitters That Regulate Food Intake in the Brain

Increase	Decrease
Agouti-related peptide	α-Melanocyte stimulating hormone
Dynorphin	Corticotropin-releasing hormone
Endocannabinoids	Cholecsytokinin
Ghrelin	Cocaine amphetamine-regulated transcript
Melnin-concentrating hormone	Leptin
Neuropeptide Y	Amylin
Norepinephrine	Serotonin
Orexin A	Polypeptide YY3-3/Oxyntomodulin

sensory organs and internal signals that are integrated through central neurotransmitters that in turn activate neural, hormonal, and motor efferent pathways. These neurotransmitter systems include monoamines, amino acids, and neuropeptides (Table 4). Underlying the response to these modulators of feeding is a system that responds to fatty acid synthesis. A potent synthetic inhibitor of fatty acid synthase (C75) causes anorexia and a profound weight loss (Tu et al., 2005). This drug not only blocks formation of fatty acids by blocking fatty acid synthase, it enhances fatty acid oxidation by stimulating carnitine palmitoyltransferase-1. Associated with the changes in food intake were the induction of genes for anorexigenic control of metabolism and inhibition of genes involved in the stimulation of feeding.

Monoamines, such as norepinephrine, serotonin, dopamine, and histamine, as well as certain amino acids and neuropeptides, are involved in the regulation of food intake. The serotonin system has been one of the most extensively studied of the monoamine pathways (Bray, 2003; Bray and Greenway, 2007). Its receptors modulate both the quantity of food eaten and macronutrient selection. Stimulation of the serotonin receptors in the paraventricular nucleus reduces fat intake with little or no effect on the intake of protein or carbohydrate. This reduction in fat intake is probably mediated through 5-HT$_{2C}$ receptors, because its effect is attenuated in mice that cannot express the 5-HT$_{2C}$ receptor.

Stimulation of α$_1$ noradrenergic receptors also reduces food intake (Bray, 2003; Bray and Greenway, 2007). Phenylpropanolamine is an agonist acting on this receptor that has a modest inhibition of food intake. Some of the antagonists to the α$_1$ receptors that are used to treat hypertension produce weight gain, indicating that this receptor is also clinically important.

Stimulation of α$_2$ receptors increases food intake in experimental animals, and a polymorphism in the α$_{2a}$ adrenoceptor has been associated with reduced metabolic rate in humans. On the other hand, the activation of β$_2$ receptors in the brain reduces food intake. These receptors can be activated by agonist drugs (β-blockers), by releasing norepinephrine in the vicinity of these receptors, or by blocking the reuptake of norepinephrine.

Histamine receptors can also modulate feeding. Stimulation of the H$_1$ receptor in the central nervous system reduces feeding, which has been utilized experimentally by modulating the H$_3$ autoreceptor, which controls histamine release. When the autoreceptor is stimulated, histamine secretion is reduced and food intake increases. Blockade of this H_3 autoreceptor, on the other hand, decreases food intake. The histamine system is important in control of feeding because drugs that produce weight gain (*see* Chapter 4) are modulators of histamine receptors.

In animals, seasonally variable dopamine transmission in the suprachiasmatic nucleus appears to drive the storage of food at the appropriate time of year in anticipation of hibernation or migration. Loss-of-function mutations in the D2 receptor gene are associated with overweight in human beings, and dopamine-antagonists can induce obesity in humans. One suggestion is that this is through modulation of nutrient partitioning, with obesity in man or fat storage in migratory and hibernating species as the results (Pijl, 2003).

The opioid receptors were the first group of peptide receptors shown to modulate feeding. They also modulate fat intake. Both the μ and κ opioid receptors can stimulate feeding. Stimulation of the μ-opioid receptors increases the intake of dietary fat in experimental animals. Corticotrophin-releasing hormone and the closely related urocortin reduce food intake and body weight in experimental animals.

The endocannabinoid system is a most recent addition to the central controllers of feeding. Tetrahydrocannbinol, isolated from the marijuana plant, stimulates food intake. Isolation of the cannabinoid receptor was followed by identification of two fatty acids, anandamide and 2-arachadonylglycerol, that are endogenous ligands in the brain for this receptor. Infusion of anadamide or 2-arachadonylglycerol into the brain stimulates food intake. The cannabinoid-1 receptor is a pre-ganglionic receptor, meaning that its activation inhibits synaptic transmission. Antagonists to this receptor have been shown to reduce food intake and lead to weight loss (*see* Chapter 9). There is also a peripheral ligand, oleylethanolamide, which inhibits food intake.

The discovery of leptin in 1994 opened a new window on the control of food intake and body weight (Bray, 2003; Bray and Greenway, 2007; Zhang et al., 1994). This peptide is produced primarily in adipose tissue, but can also be produced in the placenta and stomach. As a placental hormone, it can be used as an indicator of trophoblastic activity in patients with trophoblastic tumors (hydatidiform moles or choriocarcinoma). Leptin is secreted into the circulation and acts on a number of tissues, with the brain being one of its most important targets. The response of leptin-deficient children to leptin indicates the critical role that this peptide plays in the control of energy balance.

To act on leptin receptors in the brain, leptin must enter brain tissue, probably by transport across the blood–brain barrier (Cowley et al., 1999). Leptin acts on receptors in the arcuate nucleus near the base of the brain to regulate, in a reciprocal fashion, the production and release of at least four peptides (Fig. 17). Leptin inhibits the production of neuropeptide Y (NPY) and agouti-related peptide (AGRP) while enhancing the production of pro-opiomelanocortin (POMC), the source of α-melanocyte-stimulating hormone (α-MSH) and cocaine–amphetamine-regulated-transcript (CART; Cowley et al., 1999). NPY is one of the most potent stimulators of food intake. It produces these effects through interaction with either the Y-1 or the Y-5 receptor. Mice that do not make NPY have no disturbances (phenotype) in food intake or body weight.

AGRP is the second peptide that is co-secreted with NPY into the paraventricular nucleus. This peptide antagonizes the inhibitory effect of α-MSH on food intake. Animals that overexpress AGRP overeat because the inhibitory effects of α-MSH are blocked.

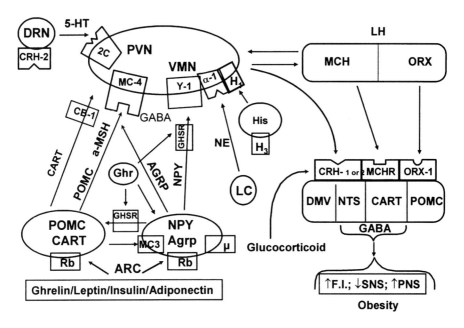

Fig. 17. Hypothalamic peptides that affect food intake.

The third peptide of interest in the arcuate nucleus is POMC, which is the precursor for several peptides, including α-MSH. α-MSH acts on the melanocortin 3/4 receptors in the medial hypothalamus to reduce feeding. When these receptors are knocked out by genetic engineering, the mice become grossly overweight. In recent human studies, genetic defects in the melanocortin receptors are associated with significant excess of body weight. Many genetic alterations have been identified in the MC4 receptor, some of which are in the coding region of the gene and others in the regulatory components (Farooqi et al., 2003). Some of these genetic changes profoundly affect feeding, whereas others have little or no effect (Appendix).

Another important peptide in the arcuate nucleus is CART. This peptide is co-localized with POMC, and, like α-MSH, CART inhibits feeding. Antagonists to these peptides or drugs that prevented them from being degraded would make sense as potential treatment strategies.

Two other peptide systems with neurons located in the lateral hypothalamus in the brain have also been linked to the control of feeding. The first of these is melanin-concentrating hormone (Ludwig et al., 2001b). This peptide increases food intake when injected into the ventricular system of the brain. It is found almost exclusively in the lateral hypothalamus. Animals that overexpress this peptide gain weight and animals that cannot produce this peptide are lean. These observations suggest an important physiological function for melanin-concentrating hormone.

The second peptide is orexin A (also called hypocretin). This peptide was identified in a search of G protein-linked peptides that affect food intake. It increases food intake, but its effects are less robust than those described previously. However, it does seem to play a role in sleep.

Another recent addition to the list of peptides involved in feeding is the arginine-phenylalanine-amide group, called RFa for short. The first of these peptides to be isolated from a mollusk had only four amino acids. The structure of the RFa peptides is highly conserved with nearly 80% homology between the frog, rat, cow, and man (Dockray, 2004). In mammals, there are five genes and five receptors for these peptides. The 26 and 43 amino acid members of the RFa peptide family stimulate feeding in mammals and are the ligands for two orphan G protein-coupled receptors located in the lateral hypothalamus and the ventromedial nucleus. This family of peptides have been involved in feeding from early phylogetic times, including *Caenorhabditis elegans*. The future of their role in human beings is yet to be established.

Neural and Hormonal Control of Metabolism

The motor system for acquisition of food and the endocrine and autonomic nervous systems provide the major information for control of the major efferent systems involved in acquiring food and regulating body fat stores. Among the endocrine controls are growth hormone, thyroid hormone, gonadal steroids (testosterone and estrogens), glucocorticoids, and insulin (Appendix).

During growth, growth hormone and thyroid hormone work together to increase the growth of the body. At puberty, gonadal steroids lead to shifts in the relationship of body fat to lean body mass in boys and girls. A distinctive role for growth hormone has been suggested from studies with transgenic mice overexpressing growth hormone in the central nervous system. These mice are hyerphagic and obese and show increased expression of NPY and agouti-related peptide as well as marked hyperinsulinemia and peripheral insulin resistance (Bohlooly et al., 2005). Testosterone increases lean mass relative to fat and reduces visceral fat. Estrogen has the opposite effect. Testosterone levels fall as human males grow older, and there is a corresponding increase in visceral and total body fat and a decrease in lean body mass in older men. This may be compounded by the decline in growth hormone that is also associated with an increase in fat relative to lean mass, particularly visceral fat.

One recent finding suggests that the activity of the enzyme 11-β-hydroxysteroid dehydrogenase type 1, which reversibly converts cortisone to cortisol, may be important in determining the quantity of visceral adipose tissue. Changes in this enzyme may contribute to the risk of women to develop more visceral fat after menopause. A high level of this enzyme keeps the quantity of cortisol in visceral fat high and provides a fertile ground for developing new fat cells.

This chapter provides a snapshot of the current understanding of the regulatory systems for factors that are etiological in obesity. Both epidemiological and metabolic feed back models have been reviewed in assembling this information. We have not reached the end of the story. However, it is clear that we have a much better glimpse into its operation—one that can provide us a better framework for thinking about the etiology of obesity and its possible treatments.

REFERENCES

(1999) Tobacco use—United States, 1900–1999. MMWR Morb Mortal Wkly Rep 48(43):980–983.
(2002). *Journal-Constitution*. Atlanta.
(2002). *Morning Herald*. Dallas.
Ailhaud, G. and Guesnet, P. (2004). Fatty acid composition of fats is an early determinant of childhood obesity: a short review and an opinion. Obes Rev 5(1):21–26.

Allison, D. B., et al. (1999). Antipsychotic-induced weight gain: a comprehensive research synthesis. Am J Psychiatry 156(11):1686–1696.

Arenz, S., et al. (2004). Breast-feeding and childhood obesity—a systematic review. Int J Obes Relat Metab Disord 28(10):1247–1256.

Astrup, A., et al. (2000). The role of low-fat diets in body weight control: a meta-analysis of ad libitum dietary intervention studies. Int J Obes Relat Metab Disord 24(12):1545–1552.

Barker, D. J., et al. (1993). Type 2 (non-insulin-dependent) diabetes mellitus, hypertension and hyperlipidaemia (syndrome X): relation to reduced fetal growth. Diabetologia 36(1):62–67.

Barth, S. W., et al. (2004). Peripheral amylin activates circumventricular organs expressing calcitonin receptor a/b subtypes and receptor-activity modifying proteins in the rat. Brain Res 997(1):97–102.

Barton, B. A., et al. (2005). The relationship of breakfast and cereal consumption to nutrient intake and body mass index: the National Heart, Lung, and Blood Institute Growth and Health Study. J Am Diet Assoc 105(9):1383–1389.

Bell, E. A., et al. (1998). Energy density of foods affects energy intake in normal-weight women. Am J Clin Nutr 67(3):412–420.

Berkey, C. S., et al. (2004). Sugar-added beverages and adolescent weight change. Obes Res 12(5): 778–788.

Berthoud, H. R. (2002). Multiple neural systems controlling food intake and body weight. Neurosci Biobehav Rev 26(4):393–428.

Blair, S. N. and Brodney, S. (1999). Effects of physical inactivity and obesity on morbidity and mortality: current evidence and research issues. Med Sci Sports Exerc 31(11 Suppl):S646–S662.

Blundell, J. E. and MacDiarmid, J. I. (1997). Fat as a risk factor for overconsumption: satiation, satiety, and patterns of eating. J Am Diet Assoc 97(7 Suppl):S63–S69.

Bohlooly, Y. M., et al. (2005). Growth hormone overexpression in the central nervous system results in hyperphagia-induced obesity associated with insulin resistance and dyslipidemia. Diabetes 54(1):51–62.

Bowman, S. A., et al. (2004). Effects of fast-food consumption on energy intake and diet quality among children in a national household survey. Pediatrics 113(1 Pt 1):112–118.

Bray, G. A. (1972). Lipogenesis in human adipose tissue: some effects of nibbling and gorging. J Clin Invest 51(3):537–548.

Bray, G. A. (1976). The Obese Patient: Major Problems in Internal Medicine. Philadelphia: WB Saunders.

Bray, G. A. (2003). Contemporary Diagnosis and Management of Obesity. Newtown, PA: Handbooks in Health Care.

Bray, G. A. and Greenway, F. L. (2007). Pharmacological treatment of the overweight patient. Pharm Rev 59(2):151–184.

Bray, G. A. and Popkin, B. M. (1998). Dietary fat intake does affect obesity! Am J Clin Nutr 68(6): 1157–1173.

Bray, G. A., et al. (2004). Consumption of high-fructose corn syrup in beverages may play a role in the epidemic of obesity. Am J Clin Nutr 79(4):537–543.

Campfield, L. A. and Smith, F. J. (2003). Blood glucose dynamics and control of meal initiation: a pattern detection and recognition theory. Physiol Rev 83(1):25–58.

Champagne, C. M., et al. (2002). Energy intake and energy expenditure: a controlled study comparing dietitians and non-dietitians. J Am Diet Assoc 102(10):1428–1432.

Cowley, M. A., et al. (1999). Integration of NPY, AGRP, and melanocortin signals in the hypothalamic paraventricular nucleus: evidence of a cellular basis for the adipostat. Neuron 24(1):155–163.

Crawley, H. and Summerbell, C. (1997). Feeding frequency and BMI among teenagers aged 16–17 years. Int J Obes Relat Metab Disord 21(2):159–161.

Cutler, D. M., et al. (2003). Why have Americans become more obese? J Econ Perspect 17:93–118.

Dabelea, D., et al. (1999). Birth weight, type 2 diabetes, and insulin resistance in Pima Indian children and young adults. Diabetes Care 22(6):944–950.

Davies, K. M., et al. (2000). Calcium intake and body weight. J Clin Endocrinol Metab 85(12):4635–4638.

Dietz, W. H. (2006). Sugar-sweetened beverages, milk intake, and obesity in children and adolescents. J Pediatr 148(2):152–154.

Dietz, W. H., Jr. and Gortmaker, S. L. (1985). Do we fatten our children at the television set? Obesity and television viewing in children and adolescents. Pediatrics 75(5):807–812.

Dockray, G. J. (2004). The expanding family of -RFamide peptides and their effects on feeding behaviour. Exp Physiol 89(3):229–235.

Drewnowski, A. and Darmon, N. (2005). The economics of obesity: dietary energy density and energy cost. Am J Clin Nutr 82(1 Suppl):265S–273S.

Drewnowski, A. and Specter, S. E. (2004). Poverty and obesity: the role of energy density and energy costs. Am J Clin Nutr 79(1):6–16.

Ebbeling, C. B., et al. (2004). Compensation for energy intake from fast food among overweight and lean adolescents. JAMA 291(23):2828–2833.

Edholm, O. G., et al. (1955). The energy expenditure and food intake of individual men. Br J Nutr 9(3):286–300.

Epstein, L. H., et al. (2005). Influence of changes in sedentary behavior on energy and macronutrient intake in youth. Am J Clin Nutr 81(2):361–366.

Farooqi, I. S., et al. (2003). Clinical spectrum of obesity and mutations in the melanocortin 4 receptor gene. N Engl J Med 348(12):1085–1095.

Finkelstein, E. A., et al. (2005). Economic causes and consequences of obesity. Annu Rev Public Health 26:239–257.

Flatt, J. P. (1995). Use and storage of carbohydrate and fat. Am J Clin Nutr 61(4 Suppl):952S–959S.

Flegal, K. M., et al. (1995). The influence of smoking cessation on the prevalence of overweight in the United States. N Engl J Med 333(18):1165–1170.

Frazao, E. and Allshouse, J. (2003). Strategies for intervention: commentary and debate. J Nutr 133(3): 844S–847S.

Fukuhara, A., et al. (2005). Visfatin: a protein secreted by visceral fat that mimics the effects of insulin. Science 307(5708):426–430.

Gangwisch, J. E., et al. (2005). Inadequate sleep as a risk factor for obesity: analyses of the NHANES I. Sleep 28(10):1289–1296.

Gilbertson, T. A., et al. (2005). Fatty acid responses in taste cells from obesity-prone and -resistant rats. Physiol Behav 86(5):681–690.

Gillman, M. W., et al. (2006). Breast-feeding and overweight in adolescence. Epidemiology 17(1): 112–114.

Gortmaker, S. L., et al. (1996). Television viewing as a cause of increasing obesity among children in the United States, 1986–1990. Arch Pediatr Adolesc Med 150(4):356–362.

Gupta, N. K., et al. (2002). Is obesity associated with poor sleep quality in adolescents? Am J Hum Biol 14(6):762–768.

Hancox, R. J., et al. (2004). Association between child and adolescent television viewing and adult health: a longitudinal birth cohort study. Lancet 364(9430):257–262.

Harder, T., et al. (2005). Duration of breastfeeding and risk of overweight: a meta-analysis. Am J Epidemiol 162(5):397–403.

Havel, P. J. (2002). Control of energy homeostasis and insulin action by adipocyte hormones: leptin, acylation stimulating protein, and adiponectin. Curr Opin Lipidol 13(1):51–59.

Hellerstein, M. K., et al. (1993). Model for measuring absolute rates of hepatic de novo lipogenesis and reesterification of free fatty acids. Am J Physiol 265(5 Pt 1):E814–E820.

Hida, K., et al. (2005). Visceral adipose tissue-derived serine protease inhibitor: a unique insulin-sensitizing adipocytokine in obesity. Proc Natl Acad Sci USA 102(30):10,610–10,615.

Hill, J. O. and Peters, J. C. (1998). Environmental contributions to the obesity epidemic. Science 280(5368):1371–1374.

Hu, F. B., et al. (2004). Adiposity as compared with physical activity in predicting mortality among women. N Engl J Med 351(26):2694–2703.

James, J., et al. (2004). Preventing childhood obesity by reducing consumption of carbonated drinks: cluster randomised controlled trial. BMJ 328(7450):1237.

Jeffery, R. W., et al. (2006). Are fast food restaurants an environmental risk factor for obesity? Int J Behav Nutr Phys Act 3:2.

Kral, T. V., et al. (2004). Combined effects of energy density and portion size on energy intake in women. Am J Clin Nutr 79(6):962–968.

Kripke, D. F., et al. (2002). Mortality associated with sleep duration and insomnia. Arch Gen Psychiatry 59(2):131–136.

Laugerette, F., et al. (2005). CD36 involvement in orosensory detection of dietary lipids, spontaneous fat preference, and digestive secretions. J Clin Invest 115(11):3177–3184.

Locard, E., et al. (1992). Risk factors of obesity in a five year old population. Parental versus environmental factors. Int J Obes Relat Metab Disord 16(10):721–729.

Ludwig, D. S., et al. (2001a). Relation between consumption of sugar-sweetened drinks and childhood obesity: a prospective, observational analysis. Lancet 357(9255):505–508.

Ludwig, D. S., et al. (2001b). Melanin-concentrating hormone overexpression in transgenic mice leads to obesity and insulin resistance. J Clin Invest 107(3):379–386.

Nakagawa, T., et al. (2006). A causal role for uric acid in fructose-induced metabolic syndrome. Am J Physiol Renal Physiol 290(3):F625–F631.

Newman, C. (2004). Why are we so fat? The heavy cost of fat. National Geographic 206(2):46–61.

Nielsen, S. J. and Popkin, B. M. (2003). Patterns and trends in food portion sizes, 1977–1998. JAMA 289(4):450–453.

Olney, J. W. (1969). Brain lesions, obesity, and other disturbances in mice treated with monosodium glutamate. Science 164(880):719–721.

Paeratakul, S., et al. (2003). Fast-food consumption among US adults and children: dietary and nutrient intake profile. J Am Diet Assoc 103(10):1332–1338.

Patti, M. E. and Kahn, B. B. (2004). Nutrient sensor links obesity with diabetes risk. Nat Med 10(10): 1049–1050.

Pereira, M. A., et al. (2002). Dairy consumption, obesity, and the insulin resistance syndrome in young adults: the CARDIA Study. JAMA 287(16):2081–2089.

Pereira, M. A., et al. (2005). Fast-food habits, weight gain, and insulin resistance (the CARDIA study): 15-year prospective analysis. Lancet 365(9453):36–42.

Perusse, L., et al. (2005). The human obesity gene map: the 2004 update. Obes Res 13(3):381–490.

Pijl, H. (2003). Reduced dopaminergic tone in hypothalamic neural circuits: expression of a "thrifty" genotype underlying the metabolic syndrome? Eur J Pharmacol 480(1–3):125–131.

Popkin, B. M., et al. (2006). A new proposed guidance system for beverage consumption in the United States. Am J Clin Nutr 83(3):529–542.

Power, C. and Jefferis, B. J. (2002). Fetal environment and subsequent obesity: a study of maternal smoking. Int J Epidemiol 31(2):413–419.

Putnam, J. and Allshouse, J. E. (1999). Food consumption, prices and expenditures, 1970–97. US Department of Agriculture Economic Research Service.

Raben, A., et al. (2003). Meals with similar energy densities but rich in protein, fat, carbohydrate, or alcohol have different effects on energy expenditure and substrate metabolism but not on appetite and energy intake. Am J Clin Nutr 77(1):91–100.

Ravelli, A. C., et al. (1999). Obesity at the age of 50 y in men and women exposed to famine prenatally. Am J Clin Nutr 70(5):811–816.

Reilly, J. J., et al. (2005). Early life risk factors for obesity in childhood: cohort study. BMJ 330(7504): 1357.

Rogers, I. (2003). The influence of birthweight and intrauterine environment on adiposity and fat distribution in later life. Int J Obes Relat Metab Disord 27(7):755–777.

Rolls, B. J., et al. (2002). Portion size of food affects energy intake in normal-weight and overweight men and women. Am J Clin Nutr 76(6):1207–1213.

Rolls, B. J., et al. (2004). Increasing the portion size of a packaged snack increases energy intake in men and women. Appetite 42(1):63–69.

Saelens, B. E., et al. (2003). Neighborhood-based differences in physical activity: an environment scale evaluation. Am J Public Health 93(9):1552–1558.

Schulze, M. B., et al. (2004). Sugar-sweetened beverages, weight gain, and incidence of type 2 diabetes in young and middle-aged women. JAMA 292(8):927–934.

Schwartz, M.B., Brownell, K.D./2007/97:667–675.

Seeley, R. J., et al. (1996). Behavioral, endocrine, and hypothalamic responses to involuntary overfeeding. Am J Physiol 271(3 Pt 2):R819–R823.

Sekine, M., et al. (2002). A dose–response relationship between short sleeping hours and childhood obesity: results of the Toyama Birth Cohort Study. Child Care Health Dev 28(2):163–170.

Smith, S. R., et al. (2000). Concurrent physical activity increases fat oxidation during the shift to a high-fat diet. Am J Clin Nutr 72(1):131–138.

Spiegel, K., et al. (2004). Brief communication: sleep curtailment in healthy young men is associated with decreased leptin levels, elevated ghrelin levels, and increased hunger and appetite. Ann Intern Med 141(11):846–850.

Stookey, J. D., et al. (2007). The altered fluid distribution in obesity may reflect plasma hypertonicity. Eur J Clin Nutr 61(2):190–199.

Striegel-Moore, R. H., et al. (2006). Correlates of beverage intake in adolescent girls: the National Heart, Lung, and Blood Institute Growth and Health Study. J Pediatr 148(2):183–187.

Stubbs, R. J., et al. (1998). Covert manipulation of energy density of high carbohydrate diets in "pseudo free-living" humans. Int J Obes Relat Metab Disord 22(9):885–892.

Taveras, E. M., et al. (2005). Family dinner and adolescent overweight. Obes Res 13(5):900–906.

Tillotson, J. E. (2004). Pandemic obesity: what is the solution? Nutr Today 39(1):6–9.

Tillotson, J. E. (2005). Wal-Mart and our food. Nutrition Today 40:234–237.

Toschke, A. M., et al. (2003). Maternal smoking during pregnancy and appetite control in offspring. J Perinat Med 31(3):251–256.

Tremblay, A., et al. (2004). Thermogenesis and weight loss in obese individuals: a primary association with organochlorine pollution. Int J Obes Relat Metab Disord 28(7):936–939.

Tremblay, A. and St-Pierre, S. (1996). The hyperphagic effect of a high-fat diet and alcohol intake persists after control for energy density. Am J Clin Nutr 63(4):479–482.

Tu, Y., et al. (2005). C75 alters central and peripheral gene expression to reduce food intake and increase energy expenditure. Endocrinology 146(1):486–493.

Ukropcova, B., et al. (2005). Dynamic changes in fat oxidation in human primary myocytes mirror metabolic characteristics of the donor. J Clin Invest 115(7):1934–1941.

US Department of Agriculture. (2006). ERS/USDA Data—Food Consumption (Per Capita) Data System. Retrieved 13 April 2006, from http://www.ers.usda.gov/Data/FoodConsumption/.

US Department of Agriculture. (1998). Food consumption through the 20th century. Retrieved September 2002, from http://www.barc.vsda.gov/bhnrc/foodsurvey/summary.

Vartanian, L. R., Schwartz, M. B., Brownell, K. D. (2007). Effects of soft-drink consumption on nutrition and health: a systematic review and meta-analysis. Am J Public Health 97:667–675.

Vioque, J., et al. (2000). Time spent watching television, sleep duration and obesity in adults living in Valencia, Spain. Int J Obes Relat Metab Disord 24(12):1683–1688.

von Kries, R., et al. (2002). Reduced risk for overweight and obesity in 5- and 6-y-old children by duration of sleep—a cross-sectional study. Int J Obes Relat Metab Disord 26(5):710–716.

Wansink, B. (1996). Can package size accelerate usage volume? J Market 60:1–14.

Wansink, B., et al. (2006). The office candy dish: proximity's influence on estimated and actual consumption. Int J Obes (Lond) 30(5):871–875.

Welsh, J. A., et al. (2005). Overweight among low-income preschool children associated with the consumption of sweet drinks: Missouri, 1999–2002. Pediatrics 115(2):e223–e229.

Williamson, D. F., et al. (1991). Smoking cessation and severity of weight gain in a national cohort. N Engl J Med 324(11):739–745.

Zemel, M. B., et al. (2000). Regulation of adiposity by dietary calcium. FASEB J 14(9):1132–1138.

Zhang, Y., et al. (1994). Positional cloning of the mouse obese gene and its human homologue. Nature 372(6505):425–432.

Zurlo, F., et al. (1990). Low ratio of fat to carbohydrate oxidation as predictor of weight gain: study of 24-h RQ. Am J Physiol 259(5 Pt 1):E650–E657.

APPENDIX

Glossary of Terms

Term	Definition and usage
Adiponectin	A protein produced in adipose tissue that circulates mainly in a hexameric form. It is inversely related to insulin resistance.
Amylin	A small peptide made in the beta-cell of the pancreas and co-released with insulin (*see* pramlintide).
Angiotensinogen	A protein precursor for angiotensin that stimulates blood vessels to contract and raise blood pressure. Angiotensinogen is produced in the liver and fat cells and is cleaved by renin to form angiotensin I, which is in turn cleaved by angiotensin-converting enzyme to form angiotensin II, the most active vasoconstrictor.
Acyl-stimulating protein	A complex of peptides produced by the fat cell that include adipsin (complement D).
Bariatric	"Barios" is the Greek word for weight. Batriatric surgery refers to surgery on people who are overweight. Bariatric medicine refers to medical treatment of people who are overweight.
Body mass index	Defined as body weight in kilograms divided by the height in square meters (kg/m^2). It can be calculated from pounds and inches as 703 multiplied by body weight in pounds divided by the height in inches squared. This is the usual measure for defining overweight and obesity (*see* "obesity").
Benzphetamine	One of the appetite suppressant drugs that has been approved for short-term use for more than 30 years but which is regulated by the Drug Enforcement Agency because its potential for addictive abuse.
Bombesin	A gastrointestinal peptide that can reduce body weight.
Bradykinin	A vasoconstrictor peptide that is produced from bradykinogen by angiotensin-converting enzyme
Calorie and kilocalorie	The amount of heat energy needed to raise the temperature of water from 14 to 15°C. Because this is a small unit, kilocalories (1000 calories) are typically used (*see* joule).
Cholecystokinin	A small gastrointestinal peptide that stimulates contraction of the gall bladder and reduces food intake.
Diabetes mellitus	A disease is defined by a high level of glucose in the blood, which often appears in the urine if it is high enough. There are two general types of diabetes mellitus. Type 1 refers to the disease in which the pancreas cannot produce enough insulin and thus there is not enough circulating insulin because of immunological damage. It usually occurs in younger individuals (<30 years of age). Type 2 refers to the disease in which there is more than enough circulating insulin but relatively poor response to this insulin. Type 2 diabetes usually occurs in older people who are most often overweight or obese.

Complement   Complement proteins are part of the blood clotting system.
                    Complement D produced in adipose tissue is also called
                    adipsin.

Diethylpropion   One of the appetite suppressant drugs that has been approved
                    for short-term use for more than 30 years but which is
                    regulated by the Drug Enforcement Agency because of
                    potential for addictive abuse.

Energy density   The amount of energy or calories in a food compared with
                    its weight. High energy-dense foods are usually high in fat.

Fatty acids   Organic molecules that form part of dietary fat and are stored in
                    fat cells. They are combined in ester linkage with glycerol, a
                    3-carbon molecule. Fatty acids and the triglycerides they make
                    can be solid or liquid at room temperature, depending on the
                    number of carbons in the fatty acid chain, and whether these
                    fatty acids have so-called double bonds. The most common
                    dietary fatty acids are palmitic acid (16 carbons), oleic acid
                    (18 carbons with 1 double-bond) and palmitoleic acid
                    (16 carbons with 1 double bond). Saturated fatty acids
                    (Carbons 14, 16, and 18) are associated with risk for heart
                    disease. Trans fatty acids (usually 18 carbons and 1 trans
                    located double bond) are also associated with heart disease.
                    Monounsaturated fatty acids, which have only one double
                    bond, are neutral for heart disease. Polyunsaturated fatty acids
                    have two or more double bonds, some of which are essential
                    for survival.

Ghrelin   A small peptide produced by the stomach that stimulates food
                    intake. Its active form has an octanoate on position 3.

Incidence   The number of new cases that develop of a particular condition
                    over time. If 10 people who were not overweight initially
                    become overweight in 1 year among 1000 people, the
                    incidence rate would be 10 cases per 1000 person-years.

Insulin   Hormone produced by the pancreas. This hormone lowers
                    blood glucose by enhancing its entry into cells.

Interleukins   A group of proteins involved in the immune response. They are
                    produced and released from many tissues and work
                    both locally and at a distance. They are markers of
                    and may cause inflammatory responses.

Joule   A unit of energy. The international nomenclature system uses
                    joules in place of calories to talk about food energy, and
                    most journals require its use instead of calories. 1 kcal =
                    4.18 kiloJoules (kJ). A 1000-kcal diet would be equivalent
                    to a 4180-kJ (4.18 megajoule = MJ) diet.

Leptin   A peptide of 167 amino acids that is produced primarily in fat
                    cells and released into the blood to circulate as a hormone to
                    the brain to tell the body about long-term regulation of body fat.

Linoleic acid and linolenic acid	These are 18 carbon fatty acids that have two and three double bonds, respectively. Linolenic acid is an essential fatty acid, meaning it, or some similar fatty acid, is essential for life.
Neuropeptide Y	A small peptide with 36 amino acids found in the intestine and brain. Among other things it stimulates food intake and modulates hormones involved in the menstrual cycle.
Orlistat	Drug that partially blocks pancreatic lipase, thus decreasing digestion of dietary fat. Available by prescription and over the counter. Its trade name is Xenical.
Obesity	An excess amount of body fat. Operationally, it is usually defined by the body mass index. The usual levels are:

- Normal weight = BMI 18.5–24.9 kg/m^2
- Overweight = BMI 25–29.9 kg/m^2
- Obesity = BMI >30 kg/m^2
    - Class 1 = BMI 30–34.9 kg/m^2
    - Class 2 = BMI 35–39.9 kg/m^2
    - Class 3 = BMI >40 kg/m^2

Overweight	A body weight above the upper limit of some arbitrarily set standard (*see* obesity).
Oxidative phosphorylation	Part of the metabolic process that put phosphates on adenosine that involves oxygen. The genes for this process—the so-called OX-PHOS genes—are reduced in diabetes, insulin resistance, and when eating a high-fat diet.
Pancreas	Gland located near the duodenum and small intestine. Its acinar cells secrete digestive enzymes into the intestine. The beta-cells produce and secrete insulin into the blood.
Pathology	Refers to the science of disease. Changes that reflect disease can be in organs (liver disease), tissues (skin disease), cells, or parts of cells.
Pathophysiological	Processes by which a disease develops.
Phendimetriazine	One of the appetite suppressant drugs that has been approved for short-term use for more than 30 years but which is regulated by the Drug Enforcement Agency because of potential for addictive abuse.
Peroxisome proliferator activator	A group of molecules that are nuclear transcription factors that initiate or inhibit part of the genetic coding system. There are three groups, α, γ and δ that have different tissue locations. The peroxisome proliferator activator-γ is activated by the group of glitazone drugs and improves insulin response (i.e., reduces insulin resistance).
Phentermine	One of the appetite suppressant drugs that has been approved for short-term use for more than 30 years but which is regulated by the Drug Enforcement Agency because of potential for addictive abuse.

Plasminogen activator inhibitor-1	A molecule produced by the liver or fat cells that acts to inhibit plasminogen activation, which is involved in slowing down blood coagulation. High levels of plasminogen activator inhibitor-1 are "pro-coagulant," meaning they tend to enhance coagulation risks.
Prediabetes (impaired glucose tolerance)	Defined as a fasting glucose between 100 and 126 mg/dL and a blood glucose 2 hours after ingesting 75 g of glucose that is between 140 and 199 mg/dL.
Prevalence	Relates the number of individuals with a particular condition at a particular time relative to the total number of people. If 10 people were overweight in a population of 1000 this would a prevalence of 1%.
Prostaglandins	A class of essential fatty acids that have 18, 20, or 22 fatty acids that can be metabolized to produce molecules involved in vascular contraction and relaxation, cell growth, inflammatory responses, and blood coagulation.
Resistin	A peptide produced in the liver that circulates to provide information for muscle and fat.
RQ	Ratio of carbon doxide produced to oxygen consumed.
Sibutramine	A newer appetite suppressant drug that has been approved for long-term use but which is still regulated by the Drug Enforcement Agency because of potential for addictive abuse.
Stigma	A mark or identification marking. In our case, it is an increased body fat that is obvious to the viewer and that elicits emotional feelings, which are usually negative.
Thermogenesis	Heat production. Usually used to refer to biological processes that generate heat rather than muscular movement. Thyroid hormone induces thermogenesis as does cold exposure.
Tumor necrosis factor-α	This peptide is produced by the liver and fat cells and acts locally or at a distance. It is an inflammatory peptide.
Uncoupling proteins	This is a group of membrane proteins that are involved in anion transport and can act as a "leak" for hydrogen in brown adipose, thus generating heat rather than coupling the flow of hydrogen molecules to adenosine triphosphate generation by the mitochondrion.

3 Costs, Pathology, and Health Risks of Obesity and the Metabolic Syndrome

*C*ONTENTS

KEY POINTS

- Overweight increases the risk of death.
- Underweight increases the risk of death.
- Detecting the levels of overweight that are clinically important requires either large epidemiological samples or smaller samples of subjects followed for an extended period of time.
- Early analysis of epidemiological studies has led to the conclusion that overweight is not a risk for early mortality, but this is controversial.
- The metabolic syndrome, as a collection of signs and clinical findings, predicts heart disease and diabetes.
- The pathological basis for overweight is an increase in the size of fat cells.
- Increased numbers of fat cells may also contribute in some individuals.
- Large fat cells secrete a variety of peptides that can be pathogenetic for various conditions associated with overweight.
- Diseases associated with overweight can be divided into those that cause these effects through enlarged fat cells and those that result from the increased mass of fat.
- The metabolic syndrome reflects the response to factors produced from fat cells.
- Weight loss reverses all of the associated risks.
- Only small amounts of weight loss are needed to significantly reduce the risk of developing diabetes in high-risk populations.
- Maintaining weight loss reduces the need for anti-hypertensive medication.
- Overweight increases hospitalization, use of the medical care system, and overall health care costs into old age.

From: *The Metabolic Syndrome and Obesity*
By: G. A. Bray © Humana Press Inc., Totowa, NJ

INTRODUCTION

We start with the premise that we all want to have a healthy weight, and that no one wants to be labeled obese. One reason for this ideal is self-image or cosmetic, and another is that excessive weight is a harbinger of ill health. This chapter develops the historical context for this understanding and provides ideas about how fatness produces these problems. In this chapter, overweight refers to any individual whose body weight is above 25 kg/m^2 (*see* Chapter 1). Some individuals who are overweight are not at risk from this weight, such as athletes and naturally muscular people. However, for most of the population, the rise in body weight with age is associated with increased fatness and the ill health it produces.

HISTORICAL CONTEXT FOR THE RISKS OF OVERWEIGHT AS A DISEASE

More than 2500 years ago a physician named Hippocrates, often called the father of medicine, recognized that people who were overweight had increased risk for sudden death. Closer to modern times, Dr. Malcolm Flemyng, a physician from the 18th century who wrote one of the two earliest books on overweight in the English language, said the following:

> *Corpulency, when in an extraordinary degree, may be reckoned a disease, as it in some measure obstructs the free exercise of the animal functions; and hath a tendency to shorten life, by paving the way to dangerous distempers (1760).*

To Flemyng, just as to Hippocrates, excess fat obstructs the free or normal functions of the body and tends to shorten life through a variety of diseases. Just over a half century after Flemyng, similar sentiments were articulated by a surgeon named William Wadd:

> *Fat is, of all the humours or substances forming part of the human body, the most diffused; a certain proportion of it is indicative of health, and denotes being in good condition—nay, is even conducive to beauty; but when in excess—amounting to what may be termed OBESITY—it is not only in itself a disease, but may be the cause of many fatal effects, particularly in acute disorders (1810).*

This concern for overweight as a health problem attracted the attention of the life insurance industry, because they pay money when people die. If excess weight carries increased health risks, then overweight people purchasing their own insurance policies might expect to pay higher premiums. Beginning in 1913, the life insurance industry identified overweight as a risk for factor ill health and then published tables of ideal or desirable weights—those weights associated with the lowest risks of mortality from overweight (*see* Chapter 1).

Although the life insurance companies repeated their messages throughout the 20th century, not everyone was convinced. Information developed from life insurance statistics did not represent the population as a whole—most insured people were men (90%) and most were white. To determine the truth of the assertion that "overweight is risking fate," a number of other epidemiological studies began, some of which continue today.

One challenge for all of these trials was how to assess body weight in relation to height. The life insurance tables provided a range of weights for each height based on small, medium, and large frame sizes. However, frame sizes were not measured when life insurance policies were sold, and there were no clear criteria for assessing an individual's frame size. The earliest epidemiological studies, such as the famous Framingham study, related the weight of individuals in Framingham, MA, to the weights of people in the Metropolitan Life Insurance tables (Metropolitan relative weight).

Interest in overweight has taken a sharp up-turn in recent years as the prevalence of excess body weight has increased rapidly. Overweight can be viewed as a chronic, stigmatized, neurochemical disease (Bray, 2004b). In this context, the goal is to return weight to a healthy level and to remove the stigma associated with the use of the word obesity. To consider it in the context of a neurochemical derangement has the advantage of focusing on the underlying mechanisms that produce the distortion in energy balance that produces the unhealthy state (Bray and Champagne, 2005). The neurochemical basis for this problem is developed in Chapter 2.

COSTS OF OVERWEIGHT

Overweight is expensive. Various estimates have placed the annual costs between 5.3 and 7.0% of annual medical expenditures (Table 1; Finkelstein et al., 2003; Finkelstein et al., 2004; Wolf and Colditz, 1994; Wolf and Colditz, 1998). The overall expenditure estimated in 2004 was $75 billion or 5.7% of the health care budget. For Medicare, it was 6.8% (17.7 billion) and for Medicaid 10.6% (21.3 billion; Finkelstein et al., 2004). A similar pattern of increased disability was reported in a study of adult Finns. Overweight men and women 20 to 64 years of age had 0.63 years of disability at work, 0.36 years of coronary heart disease (CHD), and 1.68 years more of long-term use of medication than their normal weight counterparts (Visscher et al., 2004).

Hospital costs and use of medication increase with increasing body mass index (BMI). In a large health maintenance organization, mean annual costs were 25% higher in participants with a BMI between 30 and 35 kg/m^2 and 44% higher in those with a BMI higher than 35 kg/m^2 compared with individuals with a BMI between 20 and 25 kg/m^2 (Quesenberry et al., 1998). Costs for lifetime treatment of hypertension, hypercholesterolemia, type 2 diabetes, heart disease, and stroke in men and women with a BMI of 37.5 kg/m^2 was $10,000 higher than for men and women with a BMI of 22.5 kg/m^2, according to data from the National Center for Health Statistics (NCHS) and the Framingham Heart Study (N. A., 2005; Thompson et al., 1999).

The expenditures by Medicare for health care from ages 65 to 83 (or death) were related to BMI in 1967 to 1973 nearly 40 years earlier. There was a graded increase in total costs related to overweight with each higher category of BMI from normal (BMI 18.5–25) to overweight (BMI 25–30) and grades I and II overweight (BMI 30–34.9 and BMI >35; Daviglus et al., 2004; Fig. 1). A second examination of mid-life weight status on mortality and hospitalization later in life from cardiovascular disease (CVD) used the Chicago Heart Association Detection Project in Industry study (Yan et al., 2006). In this predominantly white cohort, risk of hospitalization and mortality was higher in all overweight people who survived to age 65 and older than in those with normal weight who had a similar cardiovascular risk profile at ages 31 to 64. Allison et al. (1999) estimates that lifetime costs associated with grade I overweight were 4.3%.

In addition to the health care costs, there is increased use of medical services. Sturm, using the Healthcare for Communities Survey from 1998, found that annual medical

Table 1
Cost of Obesity in the United States, 1995

Disease	Direct cost in billions
Diabetes mellitus	$32.4
Coronary heart disease	$7.0
Osteoarthritis	$4.3
Hypertension	$3.2
Gallbladder disease	$2.6
Colon cancer	$1.0
Breast cancer	$0.84
Endometrial cancer	$0.29

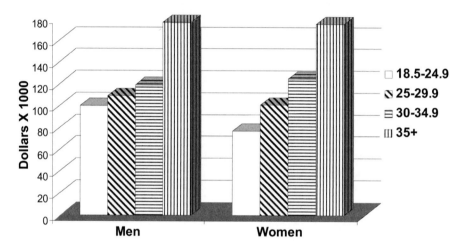

Fig. 1. Relation of Medicare costs between ages 65 and 83 (or death) and body mass index determined at age 45. (Adapted from Daviglus et al., 2004.)

expenditures were 36% higher in the grade I overweight individual (BMI > 30 kg/m^2) than for normal weight individuals (2002). Finkelstein et al., using the Medical Expenditure Panel Survey, also found increased costs ranging from 26% for Medicare recipients to 39% for Medicaid recipients (2003). Both Quesenberry et al. (1998) and Thompson et al. (2001) have found that obese adults (BMI > 30 kg/m^2) have more physician visits and use more health-related resources, such as medication (particularly diabetic medications), than normal weight individuals.

THE PATHOLOGY

Big Fat Cells

The etiology or cause of overweight is an imbalance between the energy ingested in food and the energy expended. The excess energy is stored in fat cells that enlarge in size and/or increase in number. It is this hyperplasia and hypertrophy of fat cells that is the pathological lesion of the overweight patient. Enlarged fat cells produce the clinical problems associated with overweight either because of the weight or mass of the extra fat or because of the increased secretion of free fatty acids and numerous peptides from enlarged fat cells (*see* Chapter 2). Fat cells store and release fatty acids that flow to the liver and can modulate hepatic metabolism of insulin. They also secrete a variety of adipokines (adiponectin and visfatin) and cytokines (tumor necrosis factor-α and interleukin-6) that also flow to the liver and may provide part of the inflammatory environment related to overweight. Finally, the secretion of leptin from fat cells provides a signal to the brain about the size of fat stores in the body. The fat cell, then, is an endocrine cell and adipose tissue is an endocrine organ. It is the hypertrophy and/or hyperplasia of this organ that is the pathological lesion in overweight.

Visceral Fat Cells and Central Adiposity

Visceral fat cells are an important unit in the production of endocrine products that produce the pathological features resulting from being overweight. Visceral adipocytes are located strategically because they empty their products into the portal vein that flows initially through the liver. Thus, adipokines from visceral fat cells reach the liver in higher concentrations from these cells than from peripheral fat cells. Visceral fat cells also respond differentially to some drugs, particularly thiazolidinediones (glitazones), which increase subcutaneous fat without a change in visceral fat (Smith et al., 2005). The visceral fat cells also produce adipokines, such as visfatin, that are not produced in similar amounts in peripheral fat cells.

The accumulation of fat in visceral fat cells is modulated by a number of factors. Androgens and estrogen produced by the gonads and adrenals, as well as peripheral conversion of Δ^4-androstenedione to estrone in stromal cells in fat, are pivotal in regulating fat distribution and the estrogen levels of post-menopausal women. Male or android fat distribution, and female or gynoid fat distribution, develop during adolescence. The increasing accumulation of visceral fat in adult life is also related to gender, but the effects of cortisol, decreasing growth hormone, and decreasing testosterone levels are important in age-related fat deposition. Increased visceral fat enhances the degree of insulin resistance associated with overweight and hyperinsulinemia. Together, hyperinsulinemia and insulin resistance enhance the risk of the co-morbidities described later.

Increased Fat Mass

In addition to the pathology produced by enlarged fat, additional pathology results from extra mass of tissue and the effort that it requires for the overweight individual to move this extra mass. The consequences of these two mechanisms, increased fat cell size and increased fat mass, are other diseases, such as diabetes mellitus, gallbladder disease, osteoarthritis, heart disease, and some forms of cancer. The spectrum of medical, social, and psychological disabilities includes a range of medical and behavioral problems. One way of viewing these two mechanisms are shown in Fig. 2. A similar approach to the pathology of obesity was suggested by Visscher and Seidell (2001).

Lipodystrophy

Lipodystrophy is a loss of body fat, and in one sense is the opposite of the excess fat associated with being overweight. However, both lipodystrophy and overweight have one feature in common: insulin resistance. Depending on the pattern of fat loss, lipodystrophies are classified as either partial or total. The partial lipodystrophies have

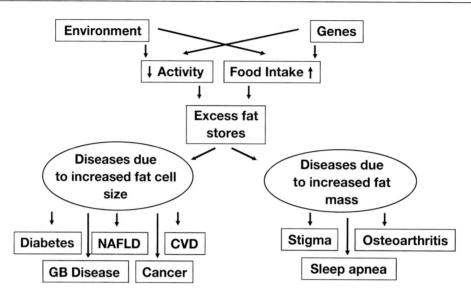

Fig. 2. A model for the pathological changes associated with overweight. The effects are divided into those related to the metabolic changes associated with increased fat cell size and those related to the increased mass of fat. NAFLD, Non-alcoholic fatty liver diease, CVD, cardiovascular diease.

a decrease in the quantity of subcutaneous fat. In some individuals, it is the upper half of the body; in some, the lower half. When total subcutaneous fat is absent, the condition is called total lipodystrophy. There is also an acquired lipodystrophy seen in patients with human immunodeficiency virus who are treated with the protease drugs (Table 2; Garg, 2004).

THE PATHOPHYSIOLOGY OF CENTRAL AND TOTAL FAT

As noted previously, each disease whose risk is increased by overweight can be classified into one of two pathophysiological categories (Bray, 2004a). The first category includes the risks that result from the metabolic changes associated with the products secreted from the enlarged fat cells. These include diabetes mellitus, gallbladder disease, hypertension, CVD, and some forms of cancer. The second category of disabilities arises from the increased mass of fat itself. These include osteoarthritis, sleep apnea, and the stigma of obesity and the behavioral responses it produces.

Risks Related to Enlarged Fat Cells and Central Adiposity

EXCESS MORTALITY

The net effect of increased fat mass and enlarged fat cells is a decrease in life expectancy, which has been shown in many studies beginning with the life insurance data described earlier. One of the largest studies to examine the influence of ethnic differences used the Cancer Prevention Study II database, which enrolled more than 1 million people with nearly equal numbers of men and women. Among healthy people who never smoked, the nadir in BMI for longevity was between 23.5 and 24.9 in men and 22.0 and 23.4 in women. Among the heaviest individuals, relative risk of death increased by 2.58 for white men and 2.0 for white women. Black men and women

Table 2
A Summary of Some of the Features of Lipodystrophy

Type	Gene	Chromo-some	Product	Clinical	Laboratory
Total lipodystro-phy Berardinelli-Seip syndrome)				Poor infant feeding, failure to thrive, hepatomegaly, hirsutism, acanthosis nigricans rapid growth, hollowed cheeks, early puberty	High trigly-cerides (TG)
Type 1	BSCL-1	9q34	Acylglycerol-phosphacyl transferase 2		
Type II	GNG3LG1	11q13	Seipin		
Partial lipodystro-phy (Dunnigan type)				Profound insulin resistance, diabetes, acanthosis nigricans, high TG, low leptin and adiponectin	High TG, low leptin, low adiponectin
Type I					
Type II		1q21	Lamin A		
Type III			PPAR-γ		
Acquired immune deficiency syndrome lipodystrophy					

Source: Garg, 2004.

had a lower relative risk with increasing BMI. These authors concluded that over the range of BMI, there was an increased risk of death from all causes, from CVD to cancer, as BMI increased.

More deaths occurred during the 14 years of follow-up in the Framingham study. Using data from this study, Peeters et al. (2003) estimated that nonsmoking women who were overweight (BMI 25 to 30 kg/m^2) at age 40 lost 3.3 years and nonsmoking men lost 3.1 years compared with normal weight men and women. If overweight was grade I (BMI > 30 kg/m^2), nonsmoking women lost 7.1 years and nonsmoking men lost 5.8 years compared with those with a BMI lower than 25 kg/m^2. Fontaine et al. (2003), using data from the Third Health and Nutrition Examination Survey, found that the optimal BMI for longevity was a BMI between 23 and 25 kg/m^2 in whites and a BMI between 23 and 30 kg/m^2 in blacks. Thirteen years of life were lost with a BMI higher than 45 kg/m^2 for white men and 8 years for white women. The effect on years of life lost in black women was considerably less, suggesting important ethnic differences in the health manifestations of overweight. Indeed Olshansky et al. (2005) even concluded that there might be decline in longevity in the United States related to the burgeoning epidemic of overweight.

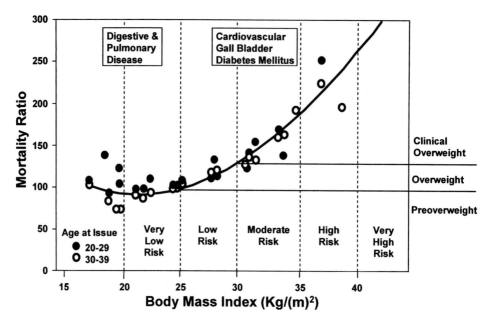

Fig. 3. Body mass index has a curvilinear relationship to all-cause mortality.

The mortality associated with excess weight increases as the degree of overweight increases. One study estimated that between 280,000 and 325,000 deaths could be attributed to overweight annually in the United States (Allison et al., 1999). More than 80% of these deaths occur among people with a BMI higher than 30 kg/m². When the impact of a sedentary lifestyle is coupled with poor diet, the Centers for Disease Control and Prevention estimated that an extra 365,000 lives may be lost per year, putting these lifestyle issues just behind smoking as a leading cause of death in the United States (N. A., 2005). A more recent estimate decreased the number of excess deaths to 112,000 (Flegal et al., 2005). Because all of these studies used the same data sources (NHANES I, II, III), but with different assumptions, there remains uncertainty about the actual number of the excess deaths.

As the BMI increases, there is a curvilinear rise in excess mortality (Bray, 2003; Fig. 3). This excess mortality rises more rapidly when the BMI is above 30 kg/m². A BMI higher than 40 kg/m² is associated with a further increase in overall risk and for the risk of sudden death. The principal causes of the excess mortality associated with over-weight are hypertension, stroke and other CVDs, diabetes mellitus, certain cancers, reproductive disorders, gallbladder disease, and sudden death. Whichever assumptions are used, excess deaths are associated with being overweight.

There are at least three important reasons for the differences in estimates of excess mortality associated with overweight. The first is the way in which the comparison group is selected, the second is the size of the sample, and the third is the duration of follow-up. In large population studies (Calle et al., 1999; Manson et al., 1995; Waaler and Lund, 1983), the lowest mortality is associated with a BMI of 22–23 kg/m². As BMI rises on either side of this lowest mortality, there is an increase in mortality. When desirable body weights were obtained from life insurance tables, the normal body weight range was from a BMI of about 20 to 25 kg/m² for men and 19 to 24 kg/m² for women (Metropolitan 1959 table). When the BMI was adopted by the National Heart, Lung, and Blood Institute and the World Health Organization in 1998, they selected a lower limit of 18.5 for BMI with the normal range of 18.5 to 25 kg/m². As seen in Fig. 3, including this lower limit increases the number of people in the normal range. It also raises the overall mortality within the normal range because the risk of death rises when the BMI either falls below or rises above the minimal death rate, which is a BMI of about 22 to 23 kg/m². When the relative risk of mortality for those with a BMI of 25 to 30 kg/m² is compared with the reference, it depends on what the reference number is as to the result you get. Within the range of BMIs from 18.5 kg/m² to 25 kg/m², there are more deaths in the short-term NCHS follow-up (Flegal et al., 2005) than among those with a BMI between 25 and 30 kg/m², suggesting, erroneously in my view, that it is better to be overweight than normal weight. If the comparison range were 20 to 25 kg/m², the relative difference within the 25 to 30 kg/m² category would be reduced. If the comparison were from 22 kg/m², the minimal death rate, the relative risk for a BMI of 25 to 30 kg/m² would be higher. Furthermore, if the study were of longer duration, we could be more confident of the death rates. Thus the selection of BMI values becomes an important consideration in the conclusion that is reached when reading the paper by Flegal et al. (2005). Because few Americans or Europeans have BMI values below 20, including the range from 18.5 to 20 kg/m² makes the slightly overweight group look better.

A second consideration in evaluating studies dealing with overweight and mortality is the duration of follow-up (Fig. 4). Short-term follow-up tends to bias the results. As Sjostrom noted in his review of BMI and mortality (1992), the BMI predicted increased mortality with large population groups followed for a short time or with smaller groups followed for a much longer time. The NCHS data samples range from 9000 to 14,000 people and are thus relatively small in epidemiological terms, compared with the Nurses' Health Study with more than 100,000 participants, the American Cancer Society Follow-up Study with nearly 1 million participants (Calle et al., 1999; Stevens et al., 1998), The Norwegian Population Study with 2 million participants (Waaler and Lund, 1983) and the Life Insurance Follow-Up with 5 million participants (Lew et al., 1979). It may thus be unreasonable to conclude, as a recent NHANES study and others have concluded, that there is no danger to being overweight with a BMI between 25 and 30 kg/m² because, as in the NHANES study, of the small number of participants (compared with those described earlier) and the short follow-up period (Flegal et al., 2005).

A recent study from China shows a similar curvilinear relationship between BMI and mortality. Using a BMI of 24 to 24.9 kg/m² as the reference level, a higher or lower BMI in both men and women in this study of 154,736 Chinese showed an increase in the relative risk of mortality. The "U"-shaped relationship persisted even after excluding participants who were current or former smokers, heavy alcohol drinkers, or had chronic illnesses. This association was observed between BMI and mortality from CVD, cancer, and other causes (Gu et al., 2006).

Diabetes Mellitus, Insulin Resistance, and the Metabolic Syndrome

Type 2 diabetes mellitus is strongly associated with overweight in both genders and in all ethnic groups (Chan et al., 1994; Colditz et al., 1995). One estimate from the

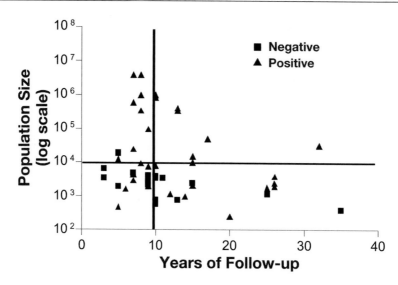

Fig. 4. Relationship between size and duration of follow-up for cohort studies and whether they find a relationship between body mass index and mortality. (Adapted from Sjostrom, 1992.)

NCHS (NHANES III) reported that 78.5% of diabetics were overweight and 45.7% had a BMI higher than 30 kg/m². In the 1999 to 2002 survey, these numbers had risen slightly to 82.7% of diabetics being overweight and 54.8% having a BMI higher than 30 kg/m² (N. A., 2004).

The risk of type 2 diabetes increases with the degree and duration of overweight, and with a more central distribution of body fat. The relationship between increasing BMI and the risk of diabetes in the Nurses' Health Study is shown in Fig. 5 (Chan et al., 1994; Colditz et al., 1995). The risk of diabetes was lowest in individuals with a BMI below 22 kg/m². As BMI increased, the relative risk increased such that at a BMI of higher than 35 kg/m², the relative risk increased 40-fold, or 4000%. A similar strong curvilinear relationship was observed in men in the Health Professionals Follow-Up Study. The lowest risk in men was associated with a BMI below 24 kg/m², slightly higher than for the women in the Nurses' Health Study. At a BMI above 35 kg/m², the age-adjusted relative risk for diabetes in nurses increased to 60.9, or more than 6000%. The risks of diabetes among a cohort of 37,878 women in the Women's Health Study were related to both BMI and level of physical activity, but BMI predominated. Compared with the normal weight active group, the hazard ratio was 1.15 for normal-weight inactive women, 3.68 for overweight active women, 4.16 for overweight inactive women, and 11.5 for very overweight (BMI > 30 kg/m²) active women, and 11.8 for very overweight inactive women (Weinstein et al., 2004).

Weight gain also increases the risk of diabetes. Up to 65% of the cases of type 2 diabetes mellitus are associated with overweight. Using the BMI at age 18, a 20-kg weight gain increased the risk for diabetes 15-fold, whereas a weight reduction of 20 kg reduced the risk for diabetes to almost zero. In the Health Professionals Follow-Up Study, weight gain was also associated with an increasing risk of type 2 diabetes, whereas a 3-kg weight loss was associated with a reduction in relative risk (Chan et al., 1994; Colditz et al., 1995). The National Health and Examination Survey showed an

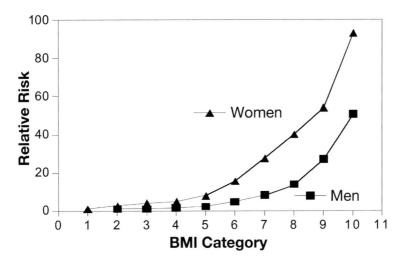

Fig. 5. Relationship of body mass index and risk of diabetes in the Nurses Health Study of Women and the Health Professionals Follow-up Study of Men. (Composite drawn from Chan et al., 1994 and Colditz et al., 1995.)

increase in diagnosed cases of diabetes as BMI categories increased in each of the national surveys from 1960 to 1961 to 1999 to 2000 (Gregg et al., 2005). In the group with a BMI 30 kg/m^2 or higher, the prevalence increased from 2.9% in 1960 to 1961 to 6.3% in 1976 to 1980 and to 10.1% in the 1999 to 2000 survey. In contrast, hypertension and abnormal cholesterol values declined over the same time interval, reflecting improved diagnostic and therapeutic intervention for cholesterol and blood pressure. For any given BMI, the risk of developing impaired glucose tolerance is higher with greater weight gain since age 20 (Black et al., 2005). Obese men maintaining their weight since age 20 had lower risk of impaired glucose tolerance than non-obese men who became similarly obese by age 51.

Weight gain appears to precede the onset of diabetes. Among the Pima Indians, body weight steadily and slowly increased by 30 kg (from 60 to 90 kg) in the years preceding the diagnosis of diabetes (Ravussin, 1993). After the diagnosis of diabetes, body weight slightly decreased. In the Health Professionals Follow-Up Study, the relative risk of developing diabetes increased with weight gain, as well as with increased BMI. In long-term follow-up studies, the duration of overweight and the change in plasma glucose during an oral glucose tolerance test also were strongly related. When overweight was present for less than 10 years, plasma glucose was not increased. With longer durations, of up to 45 years, a nearly linear increase in plasma glucose occurred after an oral glucose tolerance test. Risk of diabetes is increased in hypertensive individuals treated with diuretics or β-blocking drugs, and this risk was increased further in the overweight.

Weight loss or moderating weight gain reduces the risk of developing diabetes. In the Swedish Obese Subjects Study, Sjostrom et al. observed that diabetes was present in 13 to 16% of obese subjects at baseline (2004). Of those who underwent gastric bypass and subsequently lost weight, 69% who initially had diabetes went into remission, and only 0.5% of those who did not have diabetes at baseline developed it during the first 2 years of follow-up. In contrast, in the obese control group that lost no weight, the cure rate was low, with only 16%, going into remission. The incidence of new cases of diabetes was 7.8% in 2 years. The benefit of weight loss is also clearly shown in the Health Professionals Follow-Up Study, in which the relative risk of developing diabetes declined by nearly 50% with a weight loss of 5 to 11 kg. Type 2 diabetes was almost nonexistent with a weight loss of more than 20 kg or a BMI below 20 kg/m^2 (Colditz et al., 1995).

Both increased insulin secretion and insulin resistance result from overweight. The relationship of insulin secretion to BMI has already been noted. A greater BMI correlates with greater insulin secretion. Overweight develops in more than 50% of nonhuman primates as they age (Hansen et al., 1999). Nearly half of these obese animals subsequently develop diabetes. The time course for the development of obesity in nonhuman primates, and in the Pima Indians, is spread over a number of years. After the animals gain weight, the next demonstrable effects are impaired glucose removal and increased insulin resistance as measured by impaired glucose clearance with a euglycemic hyperinsulinemic clamp. The hyperinsulinemia in turn increases hepatic very low-density lipoprotein (VLDL) triglyceride synthesis and secretion, plasminogen activator inhibitor-1 synthesis, sympathetic nervous system activity, and renal sodium reabsorption.

Insulin resistance is the hallmark of the metabolic syndrome, which is also called the dysmetabolic syndrome. However, there are few clinically useful ways to measure insulin resistance. Thus, the National Cholesterol Education Program Adult Treatment Panel III has provided defining values for this syndrome without having to measure insulin resistance directly. When three of the five criteria listed in Chapter 1, Table 7 (left column) are abnormal, the patient is defined as having the metabolic syndrome. A major feature of this syndrome is central adiposity, measured as a high waist circumference, which is a requirement for the diagnosis of the metabolic syndrome using the criteria of the International Diabetes Federation. The increased release of free fatty acids from visceral fat impairs insulin clearance by the liver and alters peripheral metabolism. The reduced production of adiponectin by the fat cell is another potential player in the development of insulin resistance.

GALLBLADDER DISEASE

Cholelithiasis is the primary hepatobiliary pathology associated with overweight (Ko and Lee, 2002). The old clinical adage "fat, female, fertile, and forty" describes the epidemiological factors often associated with the development of gallbladder disease. This is admirably demonstrated in the Nurses' Health Study (Stampfer et al., 1992). When BMI was lower than 24 kg/m^2, the incidence of clinically symptomatic gallstones was approximately 250 per 100,000 person-years of follow-up. The incidence of gallstones gradually increases with increasing BMI to the level of 30 kg/m^2, and increases very steeply when BMI exceeds 30 kg/m^2.

Part of the explanation for the increased risk of gallstones is the increased cholesterol turnover related to total body fat (Caroli-Bosc et al., 1999). Cholesterol production is linearly related to body fat; approximately 20 mg of additional cholesterol is synthesized for each kilogram of extra body fat. Thus, a 10-kg increase in body fat leads to the daily synthesis of as much cholesterol as is contained in the yolk of one egg. The increased cholesterol is in turn excreted in the bile. High cholesterol concentrations relative to bile acids and phospholipids in bile increase the likelihood of precipitation of cholesterol gallstones in the gallbladder. Additional factors, such as nidation conditions, are also involved in whether gallstones do or do not form (Caroli-Bosc et al., 1999).

During weight loss, the likelihood of gallstones increases because the flux of cholesterol mobilized from fat is increased through the biliary system. Diets with moderate levels of fat that trigger gallbladder contraction, and thus empty its cholesterol content, may reduce this risk. Similarly, the use of bile acids, such as ursodeoxycholic acid, may be advisable if the risk of gallstone formation is thought to be increased.

NONALCOHOLIC FATTY LIVER DISEASE, NON-ALCOHOLIC STEATOHEPATITIS, AND GASTROINTESTINAL DISEASES

Increased fat in the liver is a feature in many overweight patients (Caroli-Bosc et al., 1999). Nonalcoholic fatty liver disease is the term given to describe a constellation of liver abnormalities associated with overweight, including hepatomegaly, elevated liver enzymes, and abnormal liver histology, such as steatosis, steatohepatitis, fibrosis, and cirrhosis (Matteoni et al., 1999). It may reflect increased VLDL production associated with hyperinsulinemia. The accumulation of lipid in the liver suggests that the secretion of VLDL in response to hyperinsulinemia is inadequate to keep up with the high rate of triglyceride turnover. A retrospective analysis of liver biopsy specimens obtained from overweight and obese patients with abnormal liver biochemistries but without evidence of acquired, autoimmune, or genetic liver disease demonstrated a 30% prevalence of septal fibrosis and a 10% prevalence of cirrhosis (Matteoni et al., 1999). Another study utilizing a cross-sectional analysis of liver biopsies suggests that the prevalence of steatosis, steatohepatitis, and cirrhosis are approximately 75, 20, and 2% in overweight patients, respectively (Bellentani et al., 2000). The level with more marked insulin resistance as determined from the homeostasis assessment model had a higher prevalence of severe steatosis (Angelico et al., 2005). Using ultrasound as a criterion for diagnosing increased liver fat, Hamaguchi et al. (2005) found that there was a 10% incidence of new cases of nonalcoholic fatty liver disease after a mean follow-up of 414 days in a Japanese population, which was predicted by the metabolic syndrome. If increased fat in the liver is suspected, an ultrasound of the liver can provide a quantitative estimate that is much better than serum liver enzymes (aspartate transaminase; alanine transaminase).

Overweight may also be a contributing factor in gastroesophageal reflux disease (GERD). A total of nine studies have examined the association of GERD with BMI (Hampel et al., 2005). In six of these studies, a statistically significant association between GERD and BMI was reported. Erosive esophagitis and esophageal adenocarinoma were more common. The odds ratio for GERD was 1.43 in the overweight group (BMI 25–29.9 kg/m^2) compared with the normal weight group and rose to 1.94 when the BMI was greater than 30 kg/m^2.

HYPERTENSION

Blood pressure is often increased in overweight individuals (Rocchini 2002). In the Swedish Obese Subjects Study, hypertension was present at baseline in 44 to 51% of subjects. One estimate suggests that control of overweight would eliminate 48% of the hypertension in whites and 28% in blacks. For each decline of 1 mmHg in diastolic blood pressure, the risk of myocardial infarction decreases an estimated 2 to 3%.

Overweight and hypertension interact with cardiac function. Hypertension in normal-weight people produces concentric hypertrophy of the heart with thickening of the ventricular walls. In overweight individuals, eccentric dilatation occurs. Increased preload and stroke work are associated with hypertension. The combination of over-weight and hypertension leads to thickening of the ventricular wall and larger heart volume, and thus to a greater likelihood of cardiac failure.

The hypertension of overweight people appears strongly related to altered sympathetic activity. During insulin infusion, overweight subjects have a much greater increase in muscle sympathetic nerve firing rate than do normal-weight subjects, but the altered activity is associated with a lesser change in the vascular resistance of calf muscles.

Hypertension is strongly associated with type 2 diabetes, impaired glucose tolerance, hypertriglyceridemia, and hypercholesterolemia, as noted earlier in the discussion of the metabolic syndrome. Hyperinsulinemia in overweight and in hypertensive patients suggests insulin resistance and the metabolic syndrome. An analysis of the factors that predict blood pressure and changes in peripheral vascular resistance in response to body weight gain showed that a key determinant of the weight-induced increases in blood pressure was a disproportionate increase in cardiac output that could not be fully accounted for by the hemodynamic contribution of new tissue. This hemodynamic change may be attributable to a disproportionate increase in cardiac output related to an increase in sympathetic activity.

KIDNEY DISEASE

Overweight may also affect the kidney. An obesity-related glomerulopathy characterized as focal segmental glomerulosclerosis has increased significantly from 0.2% of biopsies of pathological specimens between 1986 and1990 to 2.0% in biopsies taken between 1996 and 2000 (Kambham et al., 2001). Kidney stones are also an increased risk of overweight patients (Taylor et al., 2005).

BMI is related to the risk of end-stage renal disease, in which dialysis is essential to maintain life. In a study from the Kaiser Permanente Group of Northern California, Hsu et al. (2006) found that a higher BMI was a progressively greater risk factor for end-stage renal disease that persisted even after correcting for multiple potential confounding factors including baseline blood pressure or diabetes mellitus. Compared with normal-weight individuals, those who were overweight (BMI 25–29.9 kg/m^2) had an 87% greater relative risk (1.87; 95% confidence interval [CI] 1.64 to 2.14). This risk increased to 3.51 (95% CI 3.05 to 4.18) with a BMI between 30 and 34.9 kg/m^2 and rose further to 7.07 (95% CI 5.37 to 9.31) when the BMI was above 40 kg/m^2.

HEART DISEASE

Many studies show that as BMI increases there is an increased risk for heart disease (Kenchaiah et al., 2002). Data from the Nurses' Health Study indicate that the risk for US women developing coronary artery disease is increased 3.3-fold with a BMI higher than 29 kg/m^2, compared with women with a BMI less than 21 kg/m^2 (Colditz et al., 1995). A BMI of 27 to 29 kg/m^2 increases the relative risk to 1.8. Weight gain also strongly affects this risk at any initial BMI (Meigs et al., 1997). That is, at all levels of initial BMI, weight gain was associated with a graded increase in risk of heart disease. This was particularly evident in the highest quintile in which weight gain was more than 20 kg. Similar effects are seen in men. Major risk of CVD was increased 6% for each 1.1 kg/m^2 increase in BMI among 6452 British men (Emberson et al., 2005). In contrast to these studies reporting detrimental effects of increasing weight on cardiovascular end points, there is one paper that shows that overweight individuals survive better after coronary bypass surgery. Among 16,218 individuals who had a coronary artery bypass in the Providence Health System between 1997 and 2003, body size was not a significant factor for mortality, but, the authors note, the lowest mortality is found in the high-normal and overweight subgroups compared with the obese or underweight (Jin et al., 2005).

Both atrial fibrillation (Wang et al., 2004) and congestive heart failure (Kenchaiah et al., 2002) have a higher risk in overweight subjects. During a mean 13.7 years of follow-up in the Framingham study, there was a 4% increase in the risk of new onset atrial fibrillation for each unit of BMI increase in men and women.

Dyslipidemia may be important in the relationship of BMI to increased risk of heart disease (Despres and Krauss, 2002). A positive correlation between BMI and triglycerides has been demonstrated repeatedly. However, the inverse relationship between high-density lipoprotein (HDL) cholesterol and BMI may be even more important because a low HDL cholesterol carries a greater relative risk than do elevated triglycerides. Central fat distribution is also important in lipid abnormalities. Waist circumference alone accounted for as much as or more of the variance in triglycerides and HDL cholesterol as either waist-to-hip ratio or sagittal diameter, two other measures of central fat. A positive correlation for central fat and triglycerides and the inverse relationship for HDL cholesterol is evident for all measures.

Dyslipidemia, however, is only part of the story. Inflammation is another part. Using C-reactive protein (CRP) as a marker of inflammatory status, Ridker and his colleagues (2002) have shown that the risk of myocardial infarction is predicted by CRP and by lipids. They operate independently and the worst risk is in individuals with high CRP and high LDL cholesterol and the best outcome is seen in those with low CRP and low LDL (Ridker et al., 2002).

Increased body weight is associated with a number of cardiovascular abnormalities. Cardiac weight increases with increasing body weight, consistent with increased cardiac work. Heart weight as a percentage of body weight, however, is lower than in a normal-weight control group. The increased cardiac work associated with overweight may produce cardiomyopathy and heart failure in the absence of diabetes, hypertension, or atherosclerosis (Kenchaiah et al., 2002). Weight loss decreases heart weight; this decrease was linearly related to the degree of weight loss in both men and women. An echocardiographic study of left ventricular midwall function showed that obese individuals compensated by using cardiac reserve, especially in the presence of hypertension. Interestingly, heart rate was well within normal limits.

Central fat distribution is associated with small dense LDLs as opposed to large fluffy LDL particles (Despres and Krauss, 2002). For a similar level of cholesterol, the risk of CHD is significantly higher in individuals with small dense LDL than with large fluffy LDL. Because each LDL particle has a single molecule of apo B protein, the concentration of apo B can be used to estimate the number of LDL particles. Despres and Krauss (2002) demonstrated that the level of apo B is a strong predictor of the risk for CHD. Based on a study of French Canadians, these researchers proposed that estimating apo B, the levels of fasting insulin, the concentration of triglycerides, the concentration of HDL cholesterol, and waist circumference could help identify individuals at high risk for the metabolic syndrome and CHD.

Central adiposity, as reflected in the waist circumference, is a strong predictor of the risk for CVD. When increased central adiposity is added to other components of the metabolic syndrome, the prediction is even higher. Using the National Health and Examination Survey Data, Janssen et al. (2004) showed that body mass predicted the risk of the metabolic syndrome in men, but when BMI is adjusted for waist circumference as a continuous variable, waist circumference accounts for essentially all of the risk for the metabolic syndrome. The importance of the waist circumference was also shown by Yusuf et al. (2005) in the INTERHEART study of myocardial infarction among 27,000 participants from 52 countries. The odds ratio of developing a myocardial infarction increased with each increasing quintile. The population attributable risks of myocardial infarction for increased waist-to-hip circumference ratio in the top two quintiles was 24.3% compared with only 7.7% for the top two quintiles of BMI, making waist circumference a more robust predictor.

Overweight children may be at higher risk for future CVD. Longitudinal studies from the Bogulasa Heart Study, the Muscatine Study, the Harvard Growth Study, and the Boyd Orr cohort have all shed light on several dimensions of the problem (Berenson et al., 1998; Gunnell et al., 1998; Mahoney et al., 1996; Must et al., 1992). LDL cholesterol and triglycerides both increase in children above the 80th percentile (Freedman, 2002). Blood pressure rises in children above the 90th percentile. Finally, carotid intima-medial thickness in children rises as the weight status rises (Freedman et al., 2004).

CANCER

Certain forms of cancer are significantly increased in overweight individuals (Calle et al., 2003 ; Lew, 1985; Manson et al., 1995; Table 3). Males face increased risk for neoplasms of the colon, rectum, and prostate. In women, cancers of the reproductive system and gallbladder are more common. One explanation for the increased risk of endometrial cancer in overweight women is the increased production of estrogens by stromal cells in adipose tissue. This increased production is related to the degree of excess body fat that accounts for a major source of estrogen production in post-menopausal women. Breast cancer is not only related to total body fat, but also may have a more important relationship to central body fat (Schapira et al., 1994). It may also help explain why breast cancer risk is increased at age 75 in women in the highest versus the lowest quartile of BMI (Sweeney et al., 2004). The increased visceral fat measured by computed tomography shows an important relationship to the risk of breast cancer.

ENDOCRINE CHANGES IN THE OVERWEIGHT PATIENT

A variety of endocrine changes are associated with being overweight and these are summarized in Table 4. First are the effects of increasing body weight on reproductive function and pregnancy. Polycystic ovary syndrome, which is one of these reproductive changes, is discussed in Chapter 4 as a clinical type of obesity. Even more than effects on pregnancy and reproductive function, overweight may be associated with insulin resistance. The diagnosis of Cushing's disease is also discussed in more detail in Chapter 4. Hyperparathyroidism is associated with a clear increase in body weight.

Table 3
Relation of Cancer and Mortality Among
Overweight Men and Women

Men	Women
• Liver	• Uterus
• Pancreas	• Kidney
• Stomach/esophagus	• Cervix
• Colon/rectum	• Pancreas/esophagus
• Gallbladder	• Gallbladder
• Multiple myeloma	• Breast
• Kidney	• Non-Hodgkin's
• Non-Hodgkin's	• Liver
• Prostate	• Ovary
	• Colon/rectum

Source: Calle et al., 2003.

Table 4
Endocrine Abnormalities Associated With Overweight

Endocrine gland	Changes noted
Hypothalamus	
Pituitary–adrenal axis	Normal 24-hour cortisol secretion
	Increased stress-induced adrenocorticotropic hormone
	Increased cortisol secretion
	Flat diurnal cortisol profile
	Increased cortisol clearance
	Reduced morning cortisol peak
	Impaired dexamethasone suppression
	Decreased cortisol-binding protein
	Increased adrenal androgens production
Pituitary–growth hormone axis	Decreased growth hormone (GH) secretion
	Increased GH-binding protein
	Decreased insulin-like growth factor (IGF)-binding protein-1
	Decreased IGF-binding protein-3 Low or normal total IGF-1
	Decreased ghrelin secretion
Pituitary–thyroid axis	Increased thyrotropin
	Normal thyroid hormones
	Reduced thyroid-stimulating hormone response to thyrotropin-releasing hormone (TRH)
	Reduced prolactin response to thyrotropin-releasing hormone
Pituitary–gonadal axis	Early menarche in obese girls
	Reduced sex-hormone-binding globulin
Pancreatic–visceral fat	Increased insulin secretion
	Reduced hepatic insulin clearance
	Reduced aciponectin
	Insulin resistance

Problems With Pregnancy in the Overweight Woman

The changes in the reproductive system are among the most important endocrine effects of excess weight. Irregular menses and frequent anovular cycles are common, and the rate of fertility may be reduced (Grodstein et al., 1994). In the Nurses' Health Study, as BMI increased the relative risk of infertility rose. Compared with the reference group (BMI 20–21.9 kg/m^2), the relative risk of infertility was 1.7 for a BMI of 26 to 27.9 kg/m^2 and 2.7 for a BMI above 30 kg/m^2 (Rich-Edwards et al., 1994). Some reports describe increased risks of toxemia during pregnancy. Hypertension and cesarean section may also be more frequent. Women with a BMI higher than 30 kg/m^2 have abnormalities in secretion of hypothalamic gonadotropin-releasing hormone, pituitary luteinizing hormone, and follicle-stimulating hormone, which results in anovulation (Yen, 1999). Increasing pre-pregnancy body weight produces a significant and weight-related increase in the likelihood of Caesarean delivery. Pre-term birth was higher in the smallest women, but heavier women had no increased risk of a low-birth-weight infant. Weight gain of more than 18.6 kg (41 pounds) also increases risk of Caesarean delivery. Low-birth-weight infants were less likely in heavier women and in those who gained more weight (Rosenberg et al., 2005). The risk of postpartum urinary tract infection also appears to be increased in overweight women based on an observational study of 60,167 women (Usha Kiran et al., 2005).

PNEUMONIA

Community-acquired pneumonia may be an additional risk related to being overweight. In both the Health Professionals Follow-Up Study and the Nurses' Health Study II, the risk of pneumonia was increased as BMI increased (Baik et al., 2000). In addition, significant weight gain in women after age 18 also increased the risk of pneumonia.

Diseases Associated With Increased Fat Mass

OBSTRUCTIVE SLEEP APNEA

Alterations in pulmonary function have been described in overweight subjects, but subjects were free of other potential chronic pulmonary diseases in only a few studies. When underlying pulmonary disease was absent, only major degrees of increased body weight significantly affected pulmonary function. The chief effect is a decrease in residual lung volume associated with increased abdominal pressure on the diaphragm (Strohl et al., 2004). Fat distribution, independent of total fat, also influences ventilatory capacity in men, possibly through effects of visceral fat level.

In contrast to the relatively benign effects of excess weight on respiratory function, overweight is often associated with sleep apnea, which can be severe and need clinical care (Strohl et al., 2004; Young et al., 2005). Overweight subjects with obstructive sleep apnea show a number of significant differences from overweight subjects without sleep apnea. Sleep apnea was considerably more common in men than women and, as a group, subjects were significantly taller than individuals without sleep apnea. People with sleep apnea have an increased snoring index and increased maximal nocturnal sound intensity. Nocturnal oxygen saturation also was significantly reduced. One interesting hypothesis is that the increased neck circumference and fat deposits in the pharyngeal area may lead to the obstructive sleep apnea of overweight.

DISEASES OF THE BONES, JOINTS, MUSCLES, CONNECTIVE TISSUE, AND SKIN

Osteoarthritis is significantly increased in overweight individuals. The osteoarthritis that develops in the knees and ankles may be directly related to the trauma associated with the degree of excess body weight (Felson et al., 1988). However, the increased osteoarthritis in other non-weight-bearing joints suggests that some components of the overweight syndrome alter cartilage and bone metabolism, independent of weight bearing. Increased osteoarthritis accounts for a significant component of the cost of overweight. Increased body weight also produces disability from joint disease (Okoro et al., 2004). Using the Behavioral Risk Factor Surveillance System telephone survey data on individuals over 45 years of age, Okoro et al. found that class 3 overweight (BMI > 40 kg/m2) was associated with disability among individuals who reported arthritis as well as those who did not report arthritis. Even lighter individuals had increased likelihood of disability compared with those of normal weight respondents.

Rheumatoid arthritis and BMI have a paradoxical relationship. In a study of rheumatoid arthritis that accrued 123 deaths in 3460 patient-years of observation the BMI was found to be inversely related to mortality. The study was conducted between 1996 and 2000 and is thus relatively short term with a small number of subjects and may not have a long enough follow-up (Escalante et al., 2005).

Several skin changes are associated with excess weight (Garcia Hidalgo, 2002). Stretch marks, or striae, are common and reflect the pressures on the skin from expanding lobular deposits of fat. Acanthosis nigricans with deepening pigmentation in the folds of the neck, knuckles, and extensor surfaces occurs in many overweight individuals, but is not associated with increased risk of malignancy. Hirsutism in women may reflect the altered reproductive status in these individuals (Bray, 2003).

PSYCHOSOCIAL DYSFUNCTION

Psychosocial Problems for Children

Overweight is stigmatized (Gortmaker et al., 1993; Strauss and Pollack, 2003; Williams et al., 2005), that is, overweight individuals are exposed to the consequences of public disapproval of their fatness. This was recognized more than 40 years ago in a study of disabilities in children. Children were given six pictures of children of the same sex with different disabilities. One of the pictures was of an overweight child. They were asked to pick out the child that it would be easiest to play with until they had ranked all six pictures. In almost all settings, urban, rural, suburban, inner city, and affluent or poor, the children ranked the overweight child at the bottom or next to the bottom. This occurred in both pre-school as well as 11-year-old children. Latner and Stunkard (2003) repeated the study with the same technology to re-examine the issue of stigma. They found that if anything, the stigma against the overweight child had worsened in the 40 years since the original studies by Richardson et al. (Goodman et al., 1963; Latner and Stunkard, 2003; Richardson et al., 1961). Self-image is also negative for overweight children and their parents are aware of this problem. Quality of life for children has been evaluated in several other studies. In one report, children who were severely overweight had a quality of life similar to children diagnosed as having cancer, both of which were substantially lower than normal-weight children (Schwimmer et al., 2003). This study was based on a hospital population and had somewhat worse prognosis than a cohort study based on a two-stage sampling design of primary school children in

Australia (Williams et al., 2005). In this study, 4.3% were described as overweight and 20.2% as at risk for overweight. The decreases in physical and social functioning for the overweight children were significant when compared with normal-weight children, but not as severe as in the hospital-based population.

Stigma From Overweight in Adults

Stigma against overweight people occurs in education, employment, health care, and elsewhere. One group that used the Medical Outcomes Study Short-Form Health Survey demonstrated that overweight people presenting for treatment at a weight management center had profound abnormalities in health-related quality of life (Fontaine et al., 1996). Higher BMI values were associated with greater adverse effects. Overweight women appear to be at greater risk of psychological dysfunction, when compared with overweight men, potentially resulting from increased societal pressures on women to be thin (Carpenter et al., 2000). Intentional weight loss improves the quality of life (Williamson and O'Neil, 1998). Severely overweight patients who lost an average of 43 kg through gastric bypass demonstrated improvements on all domains of the Medical Outcomes Study Short-Form Health Survey to such an extent that their post-weight loss scores were equal to or better than population norms (Choban et al., 1999). An increasing BMI may lead to psychological distress (Istvan et al., 1992). Central adiposity has also been associated with the risk of a depressive mood (Lee et al., 2005). In a large study of 497 patients with BMI higher than 40 kg/m^2 who were preparing for bariatric surgery, the Beck Depression Inventory assessment of depression was above 16 (depressed) in 53% of the subjects with an average value of 17.7. Higher scores were found in those women, young patients, and those with poor self-image (Dixon et al., 2003). After weight loss, their depression scores improved significantly, averaging 7.8 1 year after surgery and 9.6 4 years after surgery.

BENEFITS AND POTENTIAL RISKS OF WEIGHT LOSS

A considerable body of data documents that weight loss improves a number of the intermediate risk factors for disease states (Douketis et al., 2005; N. A., 1998; N. A., 2000). Documentation that intentional weight loss benefits mortality is scantier. In one study of intentional versus unintentional weight loss, Williamson et al. reported a 20% reduction in all-cause mortality rate among 15,069 women with health-related conditions who were followed from 1959/1960 to 1972. Most of this reduction was related to reduction in cancer-related deaths. Mortality related to diabetes was reduced 30 to 40%. In women with no pre-existing illness ($N = 28,388$), intentional weight loss of 20 lb. or more (9.1 kg), in the previous year was associated with a 25% reduction in all cause mortality (Williamson et al., 1995). Using a different data set, Williamson et al. (2000) carried out a prospective analysis of 12-year mortality among 4970 overweight individuals with diabetes aged 40 to 64 enrolled in the American Cancer Society Prevention Study I. Intentional weight loss was reported by 34% of the cohort and resulted in a 25% decrease in total mortality and a 28% reduction in CVD and diabetes mortality. A weight loss of 20 to 29 lbs. was associated with the largest reductions in mortality. Similar results came from a follow-up of the National Health Interview Survey that included enough subjects to link 20,439 to the National Death Index. In this group with a 9 year follow-up, those reporting intentional weight loss had a 24% lower overall mortality rate when compared with individuals not trying to lose weight (Gregg et al., 2003). In the follow-up of individuals who underwent bariatric gastric bypass surgery, Flum and Dellinger (2004) noted a modest overall survival benefit associated with the procedure, suggesting again that "intentional" weight loss can reduce mortality.

Weight loss is also beneficial in reducing the risk of diabetes, hypertension, CVD, and sleep disorders, but primarily in high-risk individuals. In the Framingham cohort, the effect on blood pressure of weight loss was examined in middle aged (30–49 years) and older (50–65 years) adults. After adjusting the confounding variables, they found that a 6.8% weight loss over 4 years was associated with a 21 to 29% decrease in risk of hypertension. After adjusting for cancer and cardiovascular risk, these percentages increased further with middle-aged individuals reducing their risk of hypertension by 28% and older adults reducing their risk of hypertension by 37%. Thus, a modest weight loss significantly reduced the risk of hypertension (Moore et al., 2005).

The risk of diabetes is also reduced by modest weight loss. The Diabetes Prevention Program showed that, after 3.2 years in an intensive lifestyle program with an initial weight loss of 7% of body weight, the conversion rate was reduced by 55% compared with the placebo-treated control group (Knowler et al., 2002). Similarly, hypertensive individuals who maintained their weight loss following a weight loss intervention were able to maintain lower blood pressure compared with the individuals who regained weight, in whom blood pressure returned to baseline levels (Stevens et al., 2001). Blood lipids and sleep disturbances also improve with weight loss (Peppard et al., 2000). Indeed, effective weight loss would be the first order to treatment for individuals with the metabolic syndrome, because it can reverse all of the components of this syndrome, including insulin resistance. In a systematic review of long-term weight loss studies and their applicability to clinical practice, Douketis et al. (2005) found that dietary and lifestyle therapy provided less than 5 kg weight loss after 2 to 4 years, whereas pharmacological therapy could produce 5 to 10 kg weight loss over 1 to 2 years. Weight loss of 5% or more from baseline is not consistently associated with improvements in cardiovascular risk factors and these benefits appear primarily in the individuals with concomitant cardiovascular risk factors.

This discussion could not be ended without noting the possibility that weight reduction may have detrimental effects. In a study of older men, bone mineral density (BMD) declined with weight loss (Ensrud et al., 2005). In this study, the BMD at the hip increased 0.1% per year in men who gained weight over an average of 1.8 years of follow-up. In the men whose weight was stable, BMD declined −0.3% per year and in men who lost weight the decline was −1.4% per year. The initial BMI, body composition, or intention to lose weight did not affect these changes. Among men with a BMI of 30 kg/m^2 or higher who intentionally lost weight, there was a decrease in BMD of the hip.

In summary, this chapter deals with the costs and risks associated with being overweight. From the time that life insurance statistics became available, there has been a growing body of information showing that overweight is dangerous to one's health. The effects are the result of enlarging fat cells and increased total fat mass, each of which relates to one or more of the problems associated with being overweight. Diabetes, liver disease, high blood pressure, heart disease, and some forms of cancer are among the most important. There is also data arguing that weight loss is beneficial.

REFERENCES

Allison, D. B., et al. (1999). Annual deaths attributable to obesity in the United States. JAMA 282(16): 1530–1538.

Angelico, F., et al. (2005). Insulin resistance, the metabolic syndrome, and nonalcoholic fatty liver disease. J Clin Endocrinol Metab 90(3):1578–1582.

Baik, I., et al. (2000). A prospective study of age and lifestyle factors in relation to community-acquired pneumonia in US men and women. Arch Intern Med 160(20):3082–3088.

Bellentani, S., et al. (2000). Prevalence of and risk factors for hepatic steatosis in Northern Italy. Ann Intern Med 132(2):112–117.

Berenson, G. S., et al. (1998). Association between multiple cardiovascular risk factors and atherosclerosis in children and young adults. The Bogalusa Heart Study. N Engl J Med 338(23):1650–1656.

Black, E., et al. (2005). Long-term influences of body-weight changes, independent of the attained weight, on risk of impaired glucose tolerance and Type 2 diabetes. Diabet Med 22(9):1199–1205.

Bray, G. (2003). Contemporary Diagnosis and Management of Obesity. Newtown, PA: Handbooks in Health Care.

Bray, G. A. (2004a). Medical consequences of obesity. J Clin Endocrinol Metab 89(6):2583–2589.

Bray, G. A. (2004b). Obesity is a chronic, relapsing neurochemical disease. Int J Obes Relat Metab Disord 28(1):34–38.

Bray, G. A. and Champagne, C. M. (2005). Beyond energy balance: there is more to obesity than kilocalories. J Am Diet Assoc 105(5 Pt 2):17–23.

Calle, E. E., et al. (2003). Overweight, obesity, and mortality from cancer in a prospectively studied cohort of U.S. adults. N Engl J Med 348(17):1625–1638.

Calle, E. E., et al. (1999). Body-mass index and mortality in a prospective cohort of U.S. adults. N Engl J Med 341(15):1097–1105.

Caroli-Bosc, F. X., et al. (1999). Gallbladder volume in adults and its relationship to age, sex, body mass index, body surface area and gallstones. An epidemiologic study in a nonselected population in France. Digestion 60(4):344–348.

Carpenter, K. M., et al. (2000). Relationships between obesity and DSM-IV major depressive disorder, suicide ideation, and suicide attempts: results from a general population study. Am J Public Health 90(2):251–257.

Chan, J. M., et al. (1994). Obesity, fat distribution, and weight gain as risk factors for clinical diabetes in men. Diabetes Care 17(9):961–969.

Choban, P. S., et al. (1999). A health status assessment of the impact of weight loss following Roux-en-Y gastric bypass for clinically severe obesity. J Am Coll Surg 188(5):491–497.

Colditz, G. A., et al. (1995). Weight gain as a risk factor for clinical diabetes mellitus in women. Ann Intern Med 122(7):481–486.

Daviglus, M. L., et al. (2004). Relation of body mass index in young adulthood and middle age to Medicare expenditures in older age. JAMA 292(22):2743–2749.

Despres, J. P. and Krauss, R. M. (2002). Obesity and lipoprotein metabolism. In: Handbook of Obesity, edited by G. Bray and C. Bouchard. New York: Marcel Dekker; pp. 845–871.

Dixon, J. B., et al. (2003). Depression in association with severe obesity: changes with weight loss. Arch Intern Med 163(17):2058–2065.

Douketis, J. D., et al. (2005). Systematic review of long-term weight loss studies in obese adults: clinical significance and applicability to clinical practice. Int J Obes (Lond) 29(10):1153–1167.

Emberson, J. R., et al. (2005). Lifestyle and cardiovascular disease in middle-aged British men: the effect of adjusting for within-person variation. Eur Heart J 26(17):1774–1782.

Ensrud, K. E., et al. (2005). Voluntary weight reduction in older men increases hip bone loss: the osteoporotic fractures in men study. J Clin Endocrinol Metab 90(4):1998–2004.

Escalante, A., et al. (2005). Paradoxical effect of body mass index on survival in rheumatoid arthritis: role of comorbidity and systemic inflammation. Arch Intern Med 165(14):1624–1629.

Felson, D. T., et al. (1988). Obesity and knee osteoarthritis. The Framingham Study. Ann Intern Med 109(1):18–24.

Finkelstein, E. A., et al. (2003). National medical spending attributable to overweight and obesity: how much, and who's paying? Health Aff (Millwood) Suppl Web Exclusives:W3-219–W3-226.

Finkelstein, E. A., et al. (2004). State-level estimates of annual medical expenditures attributable to obesity. Obes Res 12(1):18–24.

Flegal, K. M., et al. (2005). Excess deaths associated with underweight, overweight, and obesity. JAMA 293(15):1861–1867.

Flemyng, M. (1760). A discourse on the nature, causes, and cure of corpulency. Illustrated by a remarkable case. Read before the Royal Society November 1757. London: L. Davis and C. Reymers.

Flum, D. R. and Dellinger, E. P. (2004). Impact of gastric bypass operation on survival: a population-based analysis. J Am Coll Surg 199(4):543–551.

Fontaine, K. R., et al. (1996). Health-related quality of life in obese persons seeking treatment. J Fam Pract 43(3):265–270.

Fontaine, K. R., et al. (2003). Years of life lost due to obesity. JAMA 289(2):187–193.

Freedman, D. S. (2002). Risk of CVD Complications. In: Child and Adolescent Obesity Cambridge (Burniat, W., ed.): Cambridge University Press; pp. 221–239.

Freedman, D. S., et al. (2004). The relation of obesity throughout life to carotid intima-media thickness in adulthood: the Bogalusa Heart Study. Int J Obes Relat Metab Disord 28(1):159–166.

Garcia Hidalgo, L. (2002). Dermatological complications of obesity. Am J Clin Dermatol 3(7):497–506.

Garg, A. (2004). Acquired and inherited lipodystrophies. N Engl J Med 350(12):1220–1234.

Goodman, N., et al. (1963). Variant reactions to physical disabilities. Am Sociol Rev 28:429–435.

Gortmaker, S. L., et al. (1993). Social and economic consequences of overweight in adolescence and young adulthood. N Engl J Med 329(14):1008–1012.

Gregg, E. W., et al. (2005). Secular trends in cardiovascular disease risk factors according to body mass index in US adults. JAMA 293(15):1868–1874.

Gregg, E. W., et al. (2003). Intentional weight loss and death in overweight and obese U.S. adults 35 years of age and older. Ann Intern Med 138(5):383–389.

Grodstein, F., et al. (1994). Body mass index and ovulatory infertility. Epidemiology 5(2):247–250.

Gu, D., et al. (2006). Body weight and mortality among men and women in China. JAMA 295(7):776–783.

Gunnell, D. J., et al. (1998). Childhood obesity and adult cardiovascular mortality: a 57-y follow-up study based on the Boyd Orr cohort. Am J Clin Nutr 67(6):1111–1118.

Hamaguchi, M., et al. (2005). The metabolic syndrome as a predictor of nonalcoholic fatty liver disease. Ann Intern Med 143(10):722–728.

Hampel, H., et al. (2005). Meta-analysis: obesity and the risk for gastroesophageal reflux disease and its complications. Ann Intern Med 143(3):199–211.

Hansen, B. C., et al. (1999). Calorie restriction in nonhuman primates: mechanisms of reduced morbidity and mortality. Toxicol Sci 52(2 Suppl):56–60.

Hsu, C. Y., et al. (2006). Body mass index and risk for end-stage renal disease. Ann Intern Med 144(1): 21–28.

Istvan, J., et al. (1992). Body weight and psychological distress in NHANES I. Int J Obes Relat Metab Disord 16(12):999–1003.

Janssen, I., et al. (2004). Waist circumference and not body mass index explains obesity-related health risk. Am J Clin Nutr 79(3):379–384.

Jin, R., et al. (2005). Is obesity a risk factor for mortality in coronary artery bypass surgery? Circulation 111(25):3359–3365.

Kambham, N., et al. (2001). Obesity-related glomerulopathy: an emerging epidemic. Kidney Int 59(4): 1498–1509.

Kenchaiah, S., et al. (2002). Obesity and the risk of heart failure. N Engl J Med 347(5):305–313.

Knowler, W. C., et al. (2002). Reduction in the incidence of type 2 diabetes with lifestyle intervention or metformin. N Engl J Med 346(6):393–403.

Ko, C. W. and Lee, S. P. (2002). Obesity and gallbladder disease. In: Handbook of Obesity: Etiology and Pathophysiology, edited by G. A. Bray and C. Bouchard. New York: Marcel Dekker; pp. 919–934.

Latner, J. D. and Stunkard, A. J. (2003). Getting worse: the stigmatization of obese children. Obes Res 11(3):452–456.

Lee, E. S., et al. (2005). Depressive mood and abdominal fat distribution in overweight premenopausal women. Obes Res 13(2):320–325.

Lew, E., et al. (1979). The new build and blood pressure study. Trans Assoc Life Insur Med Dir Am 62:154–174.

Lew, E. A. (1985). Mortality and weight: insured lives and the American Cancer Society studies. Ann Intern Med 103(6 Pt 2):1024–1029.

Mahoney, L. T., et al. (1996). Coronary risk factors measured in childhood and young adult life are associated with coronary artery calcification in young adults: the Muscatine Study. J Am Coll Cardiol 27(2):277–284.

Manson, J. E., et al. (1995). Body weight and mortality among women. N Engl J Med 333(11):677–685.

Matteoni, C. A., et al. (1999). Nonalcoholic fatty liver disease: a spectrum of clinical and pathological severity. Gastroenterology 116(6):1413–1419.

Meigs, J. B., et al. (1997). Risk variable clustering in the insulin resistance syndrome. The Framingham Offspring Study. Diabetes 46(10):1594–1600.

Moore, L. L., et al. (2005). Weight loss in overweight adults and the long-term risk of hypertension: the Framingham study. Arch Intern Med 165(11):1298–1303.

Must, A., et al. (1992). Long-term morbidity and mortality of overweight adolescents. A follow-up of the Harvard Growth Study of 1922 to 1935. N Engl J Med 327(19):1350–1355.

N. A. (1998). Clinical guidelines on the identification, evaluation, and treatment of overweight and obesity in adults—the evidence report. National Institutes of Health. Obes Res 6 (Suppl 2):51S–209S.

N. A. (2000). Obesity: preventing and managing the global epidemic. Report of a WHO consultation. World Health Organ Tech Rep Ser 894:i–xii, 1–253.

N. A. (2004). Prevalence of overweight and obesity among adults with diagnosed diabetes—United States, 1988–1994 and 1999–2000. MMWR CDC Surveillance Summaries 53:1066–1068.

N. A. (2005). National Center for Health Statistics. Retrieved March 2005 from http://www.cdc.gov/nchs/.

Okoro, C. A., et al. (2004). Disability, arthritis, and body weight among adults 45 years and older. Obes Res 12(5):854–861.

Olshansky, S. J., et al. (2005). A potential decline in life expectancy in the United States in the 21st century. N Engl J Med 352(11):1138–1145.

Peeters, A., et al. (2003). Obesity in adulthood and its consequences for life expectancy: a life-table analysis. Ann Intern Med 138(1):24–32.

Peppard, P. E., et al. (2000). Longitudinal study of moderate weight change and sleep-disordered breathing. JAMA 284(23):3015–3021.

Quesenberry, C. P., et al. (1998). Obesity, health services use, and health care costs among members of a health maintenance organization. Arch Intern Med 158(5):466–472.

Ravussin, E. (1993). Energy metabolism in obesity. Studies in the Pima Indians. Diabetes Care 16:232–238.

Rich-Edwards, J. W., et al. (1994). Adolescent body mass index and infertility caused by ovulatory disorder. Am J Obstet Gynecol 171(1):171–177.

Richardson, S. A., et al. (1961). Cultural uniformity in reaction of physical disabilities. American Sociological Review 26:241–247.

Ridker, P. M., et al. (2002). Comparison of C-reactive protein and low-density lipoprotein cholesterol levels in the prediction of first cardiovascular events. N Engl J Med 347(20):1557–1565.

Rocchini, A. P. (2002). Obesity and blood pressure regulation. In: Handbook of Obesity, edited by G. Bray and C. Bouchard. New York: Marcel Dekker; pp. 873–897.

Rosenberg, T. J., et al. (2005). Maternal obesity and diabetes as risk factors for adverse pregnancy outcomes: differences among 4 racial/ethnic groups. Am J Public Health 95(9):1545–1551.

Schapira, D. V., et al. (1994). Visceral obesity and breast cancer risk. Cancer 74(2):632–639.

Schwimmer, J. B., et al. (2003). Health-related quality of life of severely obese children and adolescents. JAMA 289(14):1813–1819.

Sjostrom, C. D., et al. (1997). Relationships between changes in body composition and changes in cardiovascular risk factors: the SOS Intervention Study. Swedish Obese Subjects. Obes Res 5(6):519–530.

Sjostrom, L., et al. (2004). Lifestyle, diabetes, and cardiovascular risk factors 10 years after bariatric surgery. N Engl J Med 351(26):2683–2693.

Sjostrom, L. V. (1992). Mortality of severely obese subjects. Am J Clin Nutr 55(2 Suppl):516S–523S.

Smith, S. R., et al. (2005). Effect of pioglitazone on body composition and energy expenditure: a randomized controlled trial. Metabolism 54(1):24–32.

Stampfer, M. J., et al. (1992). Risk of symptomatic gallstones in women with severe obesity. Am J Clin Nutr 55(3):652–658.

Stevens, J., et al. (1998). The effect of age on the association between body-mass index and mortality. N Engl J Med 338(1):1–7.

Stevens, V. J., et al. (2001). Long-term weight loss and changes in blood pressure: results of the Trials of Hypertension Prevention, phase II. Ann Intern Med 134(1):1–11.

Strauss, R. S. and Pollack, H. A. (2003). Social marginalization of overweight children. Arch Pediatr Adolesc Med 157(8):746–752.

Strohl, K. P., et al. (2004). Obesity and pulmonary function. In: Handbook of Obesity: Evaluation and Treatment, edited by G. Bray and C. Bouchard. New York: Marcel Dekker; pp. 935–952.

Sturm, R. (2002). The effects of obesity, smoking, and drinking on medical problems and costs. Health Aff (Millwood) 21(2):245–253.

Sweeney, C., et al. (2004). Risk factors for breast cancer in elderly women. Am J Epidemiol 160(9): 868–875.

Taylor, E. N., et al. (2005). Obesity, weight gain, and the risk of kidney stones. JAMA 293(4):455–462.

Thompson, D., et al. (2001). Body mass index and future healthcare costs: a retrospective cohort study. Obes Res 9(3):210–218.

Thompson, D., et al. (1999). Lifetime health and economic consequences of obesity. Arch Intern Med 159(18):2177–2183.

Usha Kiran, T. S., et al. (2005). Outcome of pregnancy in a woman with an increased body mass index. BJOG 112(6):768–772.

Visscher, T. L., et al. (2004). Obesity and unhealthy life-years in adult Finns: an empirical approach. Arch Intern Med 164(13):1413–1420.

Visscher, T. L. and Seidell, J. C. (2001). The public health impact of obesity. Annu Rev Public Health 22:355–375.

Waaler, H. T. and Lund, E. (1983). Association between body height and death from breast cancer. Br J Cancer 48(1):149–150.

Wadd, W. (1810). Cursory remarks on corpulence: by a member of the Royal College of Surgeons. London: J. Callow.

Wang, T. J., et al. (2004). Obesity and the risk of new-onset atrial fibrillation. JAMA 292(20):2471–2477.

Weinstein, A. R., et al. (2004). Relationship of physical activity vs body mass index with type 2 diabetes in women. JAMA 292(10):1188–1194.

Williams, J., et al. (2005). Health-related quality of life of overweight and obese children. JAMA 293(1): 70–76.

Williamson, D. A. and O'Neil, P. M. (1998). Obesity and quality of life. In: Handbook of Obesity: Evaluation and Treatment, edited by G. Bray and C. Bouchard. New York: Marcel Dekker; pp. 1005–1022.

Williamson, D. F., et al. (1995). Prospective study of intentional weight loss and mortality in never-smoking overweight US white women aged 40–64 years. Am J Epidemiol 141(12):1128–1141.

Williamson, D. F., et al. (2000). Intentional weight loss and mortality among overweight individuals with diabetes. Diabetes Care 23(10):1499–1504.

Wolf, A. M. and Colditz, G. A. (1994). The cost of obesity: the US perspective. Pharmacoeconomics 5(Suppl 1):34–37.

Wolf, A. M. and Colditz, G. A. (1998). Current estimates of the economic cost of obesity in the United States. Obes Res 6(2):97–106.

Yan, L. L., et al. (2006). Midlife body mass index and hospitalization and mortality in older age. JAMA 295(2):190–198.

Yen, S., S., C. (1999). Chronic anovluation due to CNS–hypothalamic–pituitary dysfunction. In: Reproductive endocrinology: physiology, pathophysiology and clinical management, edited by S. S. C. Yen, R. B. Jaffee, and R. L. Barbieri. Philadelphia: Saunders; p. 516.

Young, T., et al. (2005). Excess weight and sleep-disordered breathing. J Appl Physiol 99(4):1592–1599.

Yusuf, S., et al. (2005). Obesity and the risk of myocardial infarction in 27,000 participants from 52 countries: a case–control study. Lancet 366(9497):1640–1649.

4 Natural History of Obesity

Differential Diagnosis, Clinical Types,
and Age-Related Changes

KEY POINTS

- Genetic factors can be a primary cause of overweight.
- In most cases, the genetic background is more subtle and less well described.
- Very high birth weights are predictive of later overweight.
- Infants who are small for their dates of birth are at high risk of diabetes.
- Infants of mothers who smoke are at higher risk for later overweight.
- Infants of mothers with diabetes are at higher risk for later overweight.
- Early weight gain in childhood increases risk of later overweight.
- Prediction of overweight in adults is better at later ages of childhood and adolescence.
- Weight gain can follow cessation of smoking or use of some drugs.
- Weight gain in different times of life often has different causes.
- Pregnancy increases overweight.
- Androgenization in early life may increase risk of polycystic ovary syndrome and overweight in adolescence.
- Hypothalamic diseases, such as tumors, inflammatory diseases, and trauma can damage critical brain areas and produce overweight.
- Endocrine diseases, such as Cushing's disease and parathyroidism, can affect body weight.

INTRODUCTION

The previous three chapters defined overweight and provided a graded classification system; described the mechanisms by which the body regulates body fat stores and how these mechanisms can fail from an epidemiological, biological, or hedonic point of view; and enumerated the health risks that can result from carrying too much body

From: *The Metabolic Syndrome and Obesity*
By: G. A. Bray © Humana Press Inc., Totowa, NJ

fat, particularly fat that is located in visceral fat cells that drain their products of secretion into the hepatic–portal system.

This chapter is a transition from these basic concepts to a discussion of the types of clinical settings that are associated with increasing body fat. We begin with genetic factors as part of the discussion of the differential diagnosis; that is, the decision-making process that determines if a person is too fat and, when possible, why. One goal is to identify those clinical problems that can be treated now. Another is to identify other problems for which solutions may become available in the future.

Finally, this chapter looks at the age-related events that can precipitate increasing rates of fat deposition. The first group discusses the pre-pubertal individual in whom genetic and epigenetic factors are so important. However, as we noted earlier, more than 50% of overweight adults become so after age 20. Thus, factors contributing to this weight gain need to be identified, and, if possible, treated specifically or by more general treatments that are outlined in Chapters 6–11. The final part of this chapter deals with excess fat seen in older individuals and whether and when this is a problem. A number of specific settings that are associated with and may cause overweight are described in the following sections.

CLASSIFICATION OF OVERWEIGHT

Overweight has been classified in a number of ways. These approaches can be subdivided into a descriptive classification, an anatomic classification, a functional classification, and an etiological or mechanistic classification. During much of the 20th century, the use of "exogenous" and "endogenous" as descriptors proposed by von Noorden was one of the most common ways to classify overweight individuals. The exogenously overweight were those who ate too much, for what ever reason. In contrast, endogenous causes of overweight included genetic and endocrine factors. In a later classification, endogenous and exogenous were subdivided into 13 categories plus those who had localized fat deposits.

Because the base for understanding the mechanisms for excess fat accumulation have expanded, largely from the study of experimental animals, newer classifications have been proposed. One of these was based on the number and size of fat cells. As noted in Chapter 3, the large and possibly more numerous fat cells are the pathological basis for the problems associated with overweight. In the discussion that follows, an etiologic classification is used, as shown in Table 1.

CLINICAL CAUSES FOR OVERWEIGHT

Genetic Factors for Overweight

MONOGENIC CAUSES OF EXCESS BODY FAT

The rare syndromes causing massive weight gain are listed in Table 2. These include leptin deficiency, leptin receptor defect, defects in the melanocortin-4 receptor, a defect in the processing of pro-opiomelanocortin, a defect in pro-convertase 1, a defect in thyroid-stimulating hormone (TSH)-β and a defect in peroxisome proferator-activated receptor (PPAR)-γ. Although these defects, except the melanocortin-4 receptor defect are relatively rare, they show the powerful effects that some genes have on the deposition of body fat. More important, they show that the information obtained from the study of

Table 1
Classification of the Overweight Patient

Genetic
Neuroendocrine
Drug-induced
Sedentary lifestyle
Diet

genetic defects in animals can be directly applied to human beings. Discovery of the basis for the single-gene defects that produce overweight in animals was followed by the recognition that these same defects, although rare, also produce overweight in human beings.

There are several forms of the melanocortin receptor that transmit signals for the activation of the adrenal gland by adrenocorticotropic hormone (melanocortin 1-receptor), activation of the melanocyte (melanocortin 2-receptor), and suppression of food intake by α-melanocyte-stimulating hormone (melanocortin 3-receptor and melanocortin 4-receptor). Genetic engineering to eliminate the melanocortin-4 receptor in the mouse brain produces massive weight gain. Several reports show that defects in this receptor produce overweight in human beings (Hinney et al., 1999; Vaisse et al., 1998; Yeo et al., 1998; Farooqi et al., 2000). These individuals are of either sex and are massively obese. The effect on food intake of two different mutations in the melanocortin-4 receptor is shown in Fig. 1.

A much rarer form of overweight in human beings has been reported when production of proopiomelanocortin, the precursor for peptides that act on the melanocortin receptors, is defective (Krude et al., 1998). These people usually have red hair (lack of α-melanocyte-stimulating hormone to stimulate MC-1 receptor), endocrine defects, and are moderately overweight.

The rare humans with leptin deficiency correspond to the obese (ob/ob) mouse animal model (Montague et al., 1997; Ozata et al., 1999; Strobel et al., 1998). Leptin is a 167-amino-acid protein produced in adipose tissue, the placenta, and possibly other tissues. It signals the brain through leptin receptors about the size of fat stores. In several families, consanguineous marriages led to expression of the genetically recessive leptin-deficient gene. These very fat children are hypogonadal, but are not hypothalamic. They lose weight dramatically when treated with leptin. The growth pattern for two children is shown in Fig. 2. During treatment of these and other children with leptin deficiency, several important responses besides reduced food intake, reduced appetite, reduced fat mass, and lowered insulin have been noted. There was a rapid increase in TSH, free thyroxine, and triiodothyronine. Pubertal development resumed, and there was improvement in function and number of CD4+ T-cells (Farooqi et al., 2002). In 13 heterozygotes from 3 families with the frameshift mutation (deletion of a glycine residue at position 133), leptin levels were significantly lower than in controls. In contrast to all other populations so far studied in which leptin is related to body fatness, there was no correlation in the heterozygotes of leptin with body mass index (BMI). However, 76% of the heterozygotes had a BMI higher than 30 kg/m^2, compared with only 26% of the controls. Thus, the effects of leptin on body weight are gene-dose-dependent (Farooqi et al., 2001).

Table 2
Monogenic Human Obesities

	Melanocortin-4 receptor deficiency	Leptin deficiency	Leptin receptor deficiency	Proopiomelanocortin deficiency	Prohormone convertase-1
Frequency	0.5–1% of adults, up to 6% of severely overweight children. Prevalence 1:2000	$N = 9$	$N = 11$	$N = 7$	$N = 2$ (adult and child)
Appearance	Normal but fat	Short and fat	Not as fat as leptin deficiency	Pale skin, reddish hair	Normal but fat
Growth	Accelerated	Normal	Retarded, ↓ IGF-1		
Lean body mass	↑				
Bone Density	↑				
Food intake	Normal to ↑↑	↑↑↑	↑↑↑ (aggressive when food deprived)	↑↑	
Metabolic rate	Normal	Normal	Normal		
Insulin	↑↑	↑↑↑	SI ↑		↑ Proinsulin
Immune function		T-cells abnormal			
Thyrotropin		Slightly low	Hypothalamic hypothyroidism		
Cortisol	Normal		Normal	Low adrenocorticotropic hormone	Low
Reproduction		Impaired	Impaired		Impaired
Growth hormone	Normal		Low basal and stimulation ↓ IGF-1, ↓ IGFBP3		
Heterozygotes	Overweight but less than homozygotes	Overweight			

Adapted from Farooqi and O'Rahilly, 2005.
IGF, insulin-like growth factor; SI, insulin sensitivity.

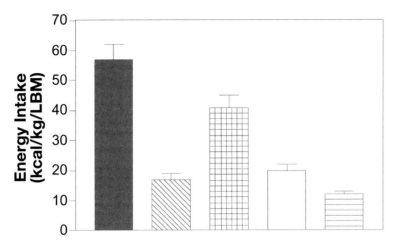

Fig. 1. Food intake in malenocortin-4 receptor- and leptin-deficient individuals. (Redrawn from Farooqi et al., 2000.)

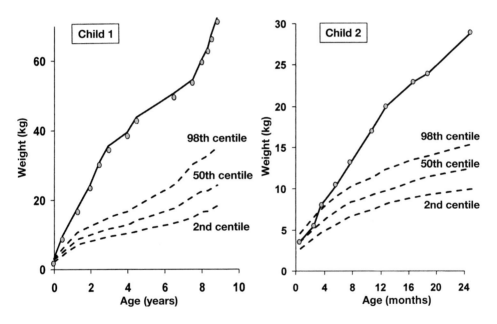

Fig. 2. Growth charts for two leptin-deficient children. (From Montague et al., 1997.)

A defect in the leptin receptor (Clement et al., 1998; Farooqi et al., 2007) has also been described, and these patients are fat, but not as fat as the children with leptin deficiency. They do not respond to leptin because they lack the leptin receptor. In experimental animals, the replacement of the leptin receptor using gene transfer technologies reverses the obesity by restoring sensitivity to leptin (Kalra and Kalra, 2005).

The PPAR-γ is important in the control of fat cell differentiation (Ristow et al., 1998). Defects in the PPAR-γ receptor in humans have been reported to produce modest degrees of overweight that begin later in life. The activation of this receptor by thiazo-lidinediones, a class of anti-diabetic drugs, is also a cause for an increase in body fat.

The final human defect that has been described is in prohormone convertase 1 (Jackson et al., 1997; Snyder et al., 2004). In one family, a defect in this gene and in a second gene were associated with overweight. Members of the family with only the PC-1 defect were not overweight, suggesting that it was the interaction of two genes that led to overweight.

POLYGENIC CAUSES OF EXCESS BODY FAT

The more common genetic factors are involved in accumulation of excess fat, regulation of body fat distribution, the metabolic rate and its response to exercise and diet, and the control of feeding and food preferences. Several approaches are being used to identify these genes, such as studies of genetic linkage of families in which overweight people are prevalent, screening the genome with genetic markers in conditions in which there are clear-cut phenotypes related to overweight, using animal models that can be examined by breeding to pinpoint areas of the human genome in which defects are likely to be found, and the candidate gene approach, which uses physiological clues to regulatory steps in control of energy balance to examine possible genetic relationships. It is with the candidate gene approach that the defects in the melanocortin receptor described earlier were identified. Presently, there are more than 25 sites on the genome that have been identified as possible links in the development of excess body fat. One interesting example is the angiotensinogen gene with substitution of a methionine for threonine at position 235 (M235T). In the Heritage Family Study, a study of the response to physical activity in two generations (parents and children), the angiotensinogen M235T polymorphism was associated with body fatness in women.

One of the areas of greatest progress in the past few years has been through the development of animals that express or fail to express genes that may be important for controlling energy intake or expenditure. The list of these so-called "transgenic" animals is outside the scope of this chapter. However, a few general points may be made. Alteration in any one of three genes can produce massive obesity in animals. Two of these are the leptin gene and the melanocortin-4 receptor gene, both discussed previously. The third gene is one involved with control of brain levels of γ-aminobutyric acid (GABA). Like other neurotransmitters, GABA can be taken up into neuronal cells. When the transporter that controls this process is overly active, the animals become very fat, suggesting that GABA plays a role in energy balance.

Congenital Disorders/Genetic Syndromes Causing Excess Fat

Several congenital syndromes of overweight exist (Table 3). Prader-Willi syndrome results from an abnormality on chromosome 15q11.2 that is usually transmitted paternally (Gunay-Aygun et al., 1997). This chromosomal defect produces a "floppy" baby who usually has trouble feeding. Overweight in these children begins at about age two and is associated with overeating, hypogonadism, and mental retardation (Gunay-Aygun et al., 1997). The levels of plasma ghrelin, a peptide that stimulates food intake, are very high in children with Prader-Willi syndrome (Cummings et al., 2002). (*See* Table 4 for features of this syndrome.)

Bardet-Biedl syndrome (BBS; Grace, 2001; Green et al., 1989) is a rare variety of congenital overweight. It is named after the two physicians who described it in separate publications in the 1920s. It is a recessively inherited disorder that can be diagnosed

Table 3
Congenital Syndromes of Overweight

Pleitrophic syndromes of human obesity	
Bardet-Biedl syndrome	*BBS-1*
	BBS-2
	BBS-3 (ARL6)
	BBS-4
	BBS-5
	BBS-6
	BBS-7
	BBS-8
Albright hereditary osteodystrophy	*GNAS1*
Fragile X syndrome	*FMR1*
Cohen syndrome	*COH1*
Alstrom syndrome	*ALMS1*
Ulnar mammary syndrome	
Syndromes with chromosomal deletions or rearrangement	
Prader-Willi syndrome	*IPW, MKRN3,*
	PWCR1, SNRP,
	MAGEL2, NDN
Single-minded	*SIM1*
WAGR with obesity	*WT1, PAX6*
Borjeson-Forssman-Lehman syndrome (X-linked)	*PHF-6*

Adapted from Farooqi and O'Rahilly, 2005.

Table 4
Prader-Willi Syndrome

- 2/3 Chromosome 15 defect
- Short stature
- Generalized obesity (onset 1–3 years)
- Primary hypogonadism
- Mental retardation
- Craniofacial abnormalities

when four of six cardinal features are present. These features are progressive tapeto-retinal degeneration, distal limb abnormalities, overweight, renal involvement (O'Dea et al., 1996), hypogenitalism in men, and mental retardation. Eight different genes can produce this syndrome, so-called BBS-1 through BBS-8. The protein for BBS-4 is involved as a subunit in transport machinery that recruits pericentrolar material-1 to the satellites during cell division. Loss of this protein produces mislocation of the protein with cell death (Kim et al., 2004). The genetic defect in BBS-6 has been identified on chromosome 20q12 as a "chaperonin-like" protein that is involved in folding proteins (Katsanis et al., 2000). It is allelic with McKusick-Kaplan syndrome. This latter syndrome is characterized by polydactyly, hydrometrocolpus, and heart problems, but without overweight.

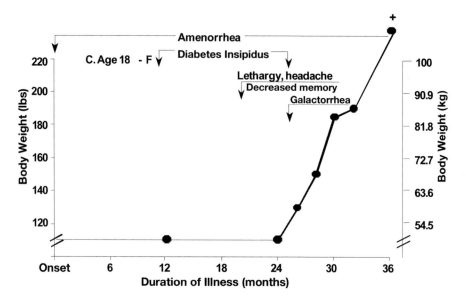

Fig. 3. Weight gain associated with hypothalamic injury (King et al., 1985).

Neuroendocrine Causes of Overweight

HYPOTHALAMIC CAUSES OF OVERWEIGHT

Overweight resulting from hypothalamic injury is rare in humans (Bray and Gallagher, 1975; Muller et al., 2001; Srinivasan et al., 2004), but it can be regularly produced in animals by injuring the ventromedial or paraventricular region of the hypothalamus or the amygdala (Bray and York, 1998; King 2006). These brain regions are responsible for integrating metabolic information on nutrient stores provided by leptin with afferent sensory information on food availability. When the ventromedial hypothalamus is damaged, hyperphagia develops, the response to leptin is eliminated, and overweight follows. Hypothalamic overweight in humans may be caused by trauma, tumor, inflammatory disease, surgery in the posterior fossa, or increased intracranial pressure (Bray and Gallagher, 1975). The symptoms usually present in one or more of three patterns: headache, vomiting, and diminished vision resulting from increased intracranial pressure; impaired endocrine function affecting the reproductive system with amenorrhea or impotence, diabetes insipidus, and thyroid or adrenal insufficiency; or neurological and physiological derangements, including convulsions, coma, somnolence, and hypothermia or hyperthermia. As noted earlier, ghrelin, a peptide released from the stomach that can stimulate food intake is low in overweight individuals and increased in people with Prader-Willi syndrome. In a group of 16 adolescents with hypothalamic obesity, most because of craniopharyngioma, ghrelin averaged 1345 pg/mL, which was similar to that in 16 overweight adolescents (1399 pg/mL), both of which were significantly lower than in 16 normal weight controls (1759 pg/mL; Kanumakala et al., 2005).

CUSHING'S SYNDROME

Overweight is one of the cardinal features of Cushing's syndrome (Findling, 2006). Thus, the differential diagnosis of overweight from Cushing's syndrome and pseudo-Cushing's syndrome is clinically important for therapeutic decisions (Orth, 1995; Findling et al., 2006). Pseudo-Cushing's is a name used for a variety of conditions that distort the dynamics of the hypothalamic–pituitary–adrenal axis and can confuse the interpretations of biochemical tests for Cushing's syndrome. Pseudo-Cushing's includes such things as depression, anxiety disorder, obsessive–compulsive disorder, poorly controlled diabetes mellitus, and alcoholism.

POLYCYSTIC OVARY SYNDROME

Polycystic ovary syndrome (PCOS) was originally described in the first half of the 20th century by Stein and Levinthal and bore their name for many years. It is characterized by polycystic ovaries and thus its name. The criteria for establishing the diagnosis of this syndrome comes from a conference at the National Institutes of Health in 1990 and one in Rotterdam in 2003. The diagnosis can be made if two of the following three features are present, and other causes are eliminated. Those features are: 1) polycystic ovaries on ultrasound examination; 2) elevated testosterone; and 3) chronic anovulation manifested as prolonged menstrual periods (oligomenorrhea). Clinical studies show that 80 to 90% of women with oligomenorrhea have PCOS. The syndrome has a prevalence in the population of 6 to 8%.

Better understanding of this syndrome has come from studies of families in which more than one woman has PCOS. In these families, the presence of hyperandrogenemia appears to be the central feature. In some women there is the additional presence of polycystic ovaries. Overweight appears in about half of the women and seems to exaggerate the appearance of the other features, including the insulin resistance that is so characteristic of the syndrome. Insulin resistance and overweight make diabetes a common association (Palmert et al., 2002).

The mechanism for the abnormalities seems to be an increase in the normal pulsatile release of luteinizing hormone (LH) from the pituitary resulting from high androgens. LH is normally released in a pulsatile fashion responsive to the gonadotrophin-releasing hormone released from the hypothalamus and is inhibited by estrogen from the ovary. The high androgen levels block this feedback of estrogen and thus allow the excessive secretion of LH. An animal model in non-human primates occurs when androgens are given to young female monkeys. One concept for the human condition is that there is early exposure to androgens by the mothers with subsequent impairment of the androgen-feedback system.

Insulin resistance is a characteristic feature of the PCOS. In the family study noted earlier, it occurred even when the individuals were not overweight, and it too probably reflects the influence of increased androgen on the responses of the insulin signaling system.

From the pathophysiology of the syndrome, effective treatment might result from inhibiting androgen production or action or enhancing insulin sensitivity. Metformin, an insulin-sensitizing drug, improves ovulation. A similar result of reduced insulin resistance is produced by blocking androgen production with spironolactone, flutamide, or buserelin (Gambineri et al., 2004).

GROWTH HORMONE DEFICIENCY

Lean body mass is decreased and fat mass is increased in adults and children who are deficient in growth hormone, compared with those who have normal growth hormone secretion. However, the increase in fat does not produce clinically significant over-weight. Growth hormone replacement reduces body fat and visceral fat (Lonn et al., 1996). The high growth hormone secretion in acromegaly also reduces body fat, particularly visceral fat. Treatment of people with acromegaly, which lowers growth hormone, increases body fat and visceral fat. The gradual decline in growth hormone with age may be one reason for the increase in visceral fat as people age.

HYPOTHYROIDISM

Patients with hypothyroidism frequently gain weight because of a generalized slowing of metabolic activity. Some of this weight gain is fat. However, the weight gain is usually modest, and marked overweight is uncommon. Hypothyroidism is common, particularly in older women.

HYPERPARATHYROIDISM

Hyperparathyroidism is a disease with increased secretion of parathyroid hormone that mobilizes calcium from bone, increases renal reabsorption of calcium, and indirectly increases intestinal calcium absorption by increasing production of 1,25 dihydroxy-vitamin D2. In a meta-analysis of 13 studies, patients with hyperparathyroidism were found to be 3.34 kg (95% confidence interval 1.97 to 4.71 kg) heavier than controls. One explanation is that overweight may increase parathyroid hormone and vitamin D or vice versa (Bolland et al., 2005).

Drug-Induced Weight Gain

Several drugs can cause weight gain, including a variety of psychoactive agents (Allison et al., 1999) and hormones (Table 5). The degree of weight gain is usually limited to 10 kg or less, but occasionally patients treated with high-dose corticosteroid, psychoactive drugs, or valproate may gain more.

Some phenothiazines and many of the "atypical" antipsychotics are particularly prone to cause weight gain. This weight gain is primarily fat and is associated with an increase in respiratory quotient, suggesting that there is an increase in carbohydrate utilization, which might stimulate food intake. Metabolic rates do not change (Graham et al., 2005). A recent multi-center trial compared changes in body weight among other outcomes during treatment of schizophrenia with anti-psychotics. Olanzapine produced the most weight gain (4.3 ± 0.4 kg [9.4 ± 0.9 lb.]) compared with smaller weight gains from newer anti-psychotics, such as quietapine (0.5 ± 0.4 kg [1.1 ± 0.9 lb.]), respiridone (0.36 ± 0.4 kg [0.8 ± 0.9 lb.]), and ziprasidone (0.73 ± 0.5 kg [−1.6 ± 1.1 lb.]) compared with the older perphenazine (−0.91 ± 0.5 kg [−2.0 ± 1.1 lb.]; Lieberman et al., 2005). The change in body weight in one study of olanzapine and haloperidol is shown in Fig. 4. Body weight increased to a plateau that was about 10% above baseline and then remained there.

Some antidepressants also can cause weight gain. The tricyclic antidepressant amitriptyline is a common culprit and may also increase the preference for carbo-hydrates. Lithium has also been implicated in weight gain. Two antiepileptic drugs, valproate and carbamazepine, which act on the N-methyl-D-aspartate (glutamate) receptor, cause weight gain in up to 50% of patients.

Glucocorticoids cause weight gain and fat accumulation on the neck and trunk, similar to that seen in patients with Cushing's syndrome. These changes occur mostly in

Table 5
Drugs That Produce Weight Gain and Alternative Choices for Similar Problems

Category	Drugs that cause weight gain	Possible alternatives
Neuroleptics	Thioridazine, olanzepine quetiapine, resperidone clozapine, ziprasodone	Molindone, haloperidol, aripiprazole
Antidepressants		
Tricyclics	Amitriptyline, nortriptyline	Protriptyline
Monoamine oxidase inhibitors	Imipramine, mitrazapine	Bupropion, nefazadone
Selective serotonin reuptake inhibitors	Paroxetine	Fluoxetine, sertraline
Anti-convulsants	Valproate, carbamazepine gabapentin	Topiramate, lamotrigine, zonisamide
Anti-diabetic drugs	Insulin, sulfonylureas thiazolidinediones	Acarbose, miglitol, metformin, sibutramine
Anti-Serotonin	Pizotifen	
Antihistamines	Cyproheptidine	Inhalers, decongestants
β-adrenergic blockers	Propranolol, terazosin	Angiotensin-converting enzyme inhibitors, calcium channel blockers
Steroid hormones	Contraceptives, glucocorticoids, progestational steroids	Barrier methods, nonsteroidal anti-inflammatory agents

© 2001 George A. Bray.

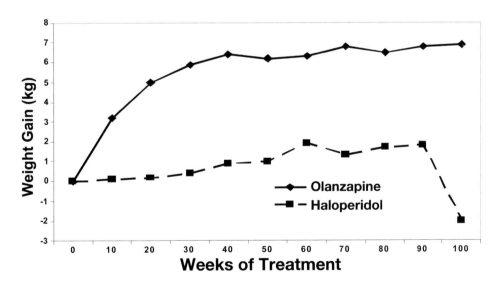

Fig. 4. Features of patients with overweight resulting from Prader-Willi syndrome. (From Kinon et al., 2001.)

patients taking more than 10 mg per day of prednisone or its equivalent. Megestrol acetate is a progestin used to increase appetite and induce weight gain in women with breast cancer and in patients with AIDS. The increase in weight is fat. The serotonin antagonist cyproheptadine is also associated with weight gain.

Many anti-diabetic drugs produce weight gain. Insulin probably produces weight gain by stimulating appetite, with intermittent hypoglycemia as the most likely mechanism. Weight gain occurs in diabetes treated with sulfonylureas, which enhance endogenous insulin release. Glitazones such as pioglitazone and rosiglitazone act on the PPAR-γ receptor to increase insulin sensitivity (Smith et al., 2005). In one clinical trial, 48 adults with diabetes not being treated with thiazolidinediones were randomized to receive either placebo or pioglitazone and 42 completed the trial. The average age was close to 54 years and the subjects averaged a weight of 92 kg with 35% body fat. Body weight decreased by 0.7 kg in the placebo group and increased by 3.6 kg in the glitazone group ($p < 0.0001$). Essentially all of the weight gain was fat (3.5 kg; $p < 0.0001$). Using multi-slice measurements of visceral fat to measure the volume of visceral fat showed no significant change from baseline to 12 weeks of treatment (5.7 $\pm$ 2.2 to 5.5 $\pm$ 2.3 kg in the glitazone group [$p = 0.058$]; 5.9 $\pm$ 1.9 to 5.8 $\pm$ 2.0 kg in the placebo group [$p = 0.075$]). After 6 months, the visceral fat mass for both placebo and glitazone-treated groups were not different from baseline or each other. Stratifying the group into those who received sulfonylurea treatment and those who did not had no effect on the response to pioglitazone. Thus, glitazones cause significant increases in body fat, almost all of which is subcutaneous (Smith et al., 2005).

Several antidiabetic drugs, including metformin, pramlintide, exenatide, sitagliptin, and vildagliptin do not cause weight gain, and may actually cause weight loss. In the large United King Prospective Diabetes Study, patients with diabetes who received conventional treatment with metformin gained 3.1 kg in 10 years, not significantly different than what would be expected in the population as a whole. In contrast, those treated with chlorpropamide gained 5.7 kg, those treated with glibenclamide gained 4.8 kg, and the patients treated with insulin gained 7.1 kg during the trial. The effect of insulin was dose-dependent. Patients with type 1 diabetes who were treated intensively in the Diabetes Control and Complications Trial (Lasker, 1993) gained 5.1 kg in contrast to the lower weight gain of 2.4 kg in those receiving insulin in a conventional manner (N. A., 1988; N. A., 1998).

Cessation of Smoking

Weight gain is very common when people stop smoking and is at least partly mediated by nicotine withdrawal. Weight gain of 1 to 2 kg in the first few weeks is often followed by an additional 2- to 3-kg weight gain over the next 4 to 6 months. Average weight gain is 4 to 5 kg, but can be much greater (Flegal et al., 1995). Researchers have estimated that smoking cessation increases the odds ratio of overweight to 2.4-fold in men and 2.0-fold in women, compared with nonsmokers. The weight gain after cessation of smoking is shown in Fig. 5. This weight gain is the result of increased food intake and reduced energy expenditure.

Sedentary Lifestyle

A sedentary lifestyle lowers energy expenditure and promotes weight gain in both animals and humans. Restriction of physical activity in rats causes weight gain, and animals in zoos tend to be heavier than those in the wild. In an affluent society, energy-sparing

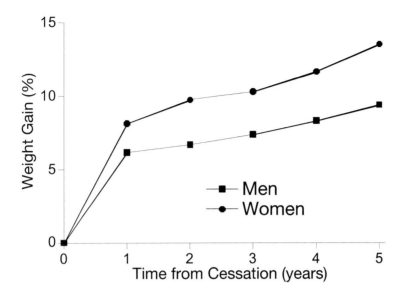

Fig. 5. Effect of smoking cessation on weight gain. (From O'Hara et al., 1998.)

devices in the workplace and at home reduce energy expenditure and may enhance the tendency to gain weight (Prentice and Jebb, 1995). In children, there is a graded increase in BMI as the number of hours of television watching increases (Crespo et al., 2001).

A number of additional observations illustrate the importance of decreased energy expenditure in the pathogenesis of weight gain. The highest frequency of overweight occurs in men in sedentary occupations. Estimates of energy intake and energy expenditure in Great Britain suggest that reduced energy expenditure is more important than increased food intake in causing overweight (Prentice and Jebb, 1995). A study of middle-aged men in the Netherlands found that the decline in energy expenditure accounted for almost all the weight gain (Kromhout, 1983). According to the Surgeon General's Report on Physical Activity (N. A., 1996), the percentage of adult Americans participating in physical activity decreases steadily with age, and reduced energy expenditure in adults and children predicts weight gain. In the United States, and possibly other countries, the amount of time spent watching television is related to the degree of overweight in children (Crespo et al., 2001) and the number of automobiles is related to the degree of overweight in adults. Finally, the fatness of men in several affluent countries (The Seven Countries Study) was inversely related to levels of physical activity (Kromhout et al., 2001).

Diet

The amount of energy intake relative to energy expenditure is the central reason for the development of overweight. Dietary factors can be influenced in a variety of ways and when the total energy intake is above what is needed for daily energy expenditure for an extended period of time excess body fat results.

OVEREATING

Voluntary overeating (repeated ingestion of energy exceeding daily energy needs) can increase body weight in normal-weight men and women. This has been demonstrated

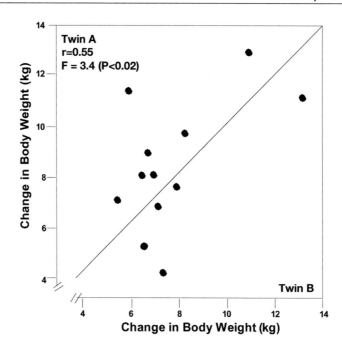

Fig. 6. Weight gain in 12 pairs of identical twins who voluntarily overate 1000 kcal per day for 84 out of 100 consecutive days.

repeatedly in the experimental setting (Levitsky et al., 2005; McDevitt et al., 2001; Redden and Allison, 2004; Schutz, 2000; Tappy, 2004; Teran-Garcia et al., 2004). The most convincing study, however, is the one by Bouchard et al. (1990) in which identical twins were given an extra 1000 kcal per day for 84 out of 100 days under observed conditions. The pattern of weight gain is shown in Fig. 6. The similarity of weight gain for each pair was closer than for weight gain between pairs of twins. This study shows two important things. First, there is a significant difference in weight gain between individuals, and second, an individual's genetic make-up influences the amount of weight gained, keeping the twins relatively close together. When these men stopped overeating, they lost most or all of the excess weight. The use of overeating protocols to study the consequences of food ingestion has shown the importance of genetic factors in the pattern of weight gain (Bouchard et al., 1990; Fig. 6).

Overfeeding has also been practiced culturally among both women and men before marriage. Pasquet and Apfelbaum reported data on nine young men who participated in the traditional fattening ceremony called Guru Walla in the northern Cameroon. These men overate during a 5-month period, gaining 19 kg of body weight and 11.8 kg of body fat. Before fattening, these men ate on average 12.9 MJ (3086 kcal) per day increasing to 28.2 MJ (6746 kcal) per day during the fattening period. Over the 2.5 years following the overfeeding time, the men returned to their pre-fattening body weight (Pasquet and Apfelbaum, 1994).

Progressive Hyperphagic Overweight

A second form of overeating with clinical implications is called progressive hyperphagic overweight (Bray, 1976). A number of patients who begin to be overweight in childhood have unrelenting weight gain. This can only mean that month by month and year by year their intake is exceeding their energy expenditure. Because it takes more energy to exceed energy expenditure as weight is gained, this must mean that they have steadily increasing intakes of food. These individuals usually surpass 140 kg (300 lb.) by 30 years of age for a weight gain of about 4.5 kg (10 lb.) per year. The recent death of a 13 year old weighing 310 kg (680 lb.) illustrates a nearly maximal rate of weight gain of 25 kg per year. These patients gain about the same amount of weight year after year. Because approximately 22 kcal/kg is required to maintain an extra kilogram of body weight in an overweight individual, the energy requirements in these patients must increase year by year, with the weight gain being driven by excess energy intake.

Japanese sumo wrestlers are another example of conscious overeating. During their training, they eat large quantities of food twice a day for many years. While in training they have a very active training schedule and low visceral fat relative to total body weight. When their active career ends, however, the wrestlers tend to remain overweight and have a high probability of developing diabetes mellitus (Nishizawa et al., 1976).

Fat Cravers

Epidemiologic data suggest that a high-fat diet is associated with overweight. The relative weight in several populations, for example, is directly related to the percentage of dietary fat in the diet (Astrup et al., 2000; Bray and Popkin, 1998; Yu-Poth et al., 1999). A study in England (Blundell and MacDiarmid, 1997) compared fat-preferring and non-fat preferring individuals. The striking feature of these two groups is that most people in each of them have body weights in the normal range. However, among the fat cravers, the distribution of body weight was tilted toward the high end, where there were almost no people in the non-fat craving group.

A high-fat diet introduces palatable foods into the diet, with a corresponding increase in energy density (i.e., lesser weight of food for the same number of calories). This makes overconsumption of food energy more likely. Differences in the storage capacity for various macronutrients may also be involved. The capacity to store glucose as glycogen in liver and muscle is limited and needs to be replenished frequently. This contrasts with fat stores, which are more than 100 times the daily intake of fat. This difference in storage capacity makes eating carbohydrates a more important physiological priority that may lead to overeating when dietary carbohydrate is limited and carbohydrate oxidation cannot be reduced sufficiently.

Carbohydrate Cravers

Consumption of sugar-sweetened beverages in children may enhance the risk of more rapid weight gain, which could be favored by the sweet taste for which they clamor. As noted in Chapter 2, both the baseline consumption of soft drinks and the change in consumption over 2 years were positively related to an increase in BMI over 2 years. That is, children who drank more sugar-sweetened beverages gained more weight and those who increased their beverage consumption had an even greater increase (Ludwig et al., 2001). The sugar and high-fructose corn syrup that make soft drinks sweet both have "fructose" either combined with glucose in sucrose or free as in high-fructose corn syrup. In evolution, nature rejected fructose as the primary sugar for metabolism and selected glucose. The reason is the higher chemical reactivity of fructose. Infants and children, before the advent of sugar, had very little, if any, fructose in their diet. Following the cultivation of sugar in the West Indies and elsewhere, sugar became plentiful, and we have overcome nature's rejection of fructose by putting it into our diet every day with potentially serious consequences (*see* Chapter 2).

A second relationship between overweight and carbohydrate intake may be through the glycemic index, which is a way of describing the ease with which starches are digested in the intestine with the release of glucose, which can be readily absorbed. A high glycemic index food is one that is readily digested and produces a large and rapid rise in plasma glucose. In contrast, a low glycemic index food is more slowly digested and associated with a slower and lower rise in glucose. Comparative studies show that eating high glycemic index foods suppresses food intake less than low glycemic index foods. Fruits and vegetables are low glycemic index foods, which tend to have fiber. Potatoes, white rice, and white bread are high glycemic index foods. Legumes and whole wheat are low glycemic index foods.

In a review of six studies, Roberts documented that the consumption of higher glycemic index foods was associated with higher energy intake than the consumption of lower glycemic index foods, meaning that higher fiber foods that release carbohydrates more slowly stimulate food intake less than the food in which glucose is rapidly released, as it is in high-glycemic-index foods (Roberts et al., 1998).

FREQUENCY OF EATING: GRAZERS AND GORGERS

The relationship between the frequency of meals and the development of overweight is unsettled. Many anecdotal reports argue that overweight persons eat less often than normal-weight persons, but documentation is scanty. However, frequency of eating does change lipid and glucose metabolism. When normal subjects eat several small meals a day, serum cholesterol concentrations are lower than when they eat a few large meals a day. Similarly, mean blood glucose concentrations are lower when meals are frequent (Jenkins et al., 1989). One explanation for the effects of frequent small meals compared with a few large meals could be the greater insulin secretion associated with larger meals.

Behavioral, Psychological, and Social Factors

PSYCHOLOGICAL FACTORS

Psychological factors are widely recognized as related to the development of over-weight, although attempts to define a specific personality type that causes overweight have not been successful. One condition linked to weight gain is seasonal affective disorder, which refers to depression that occurs during the winter season in some people living in the north, where days are short. People with this disorder tend to increase body weight in winter. This disorder can be effectively treated by providing higher-intensity artificial lighting in the winter (Partonen and Lonnqvist, 1998).

RESTRAINED EATING

A pattern of conscious limitation of food intake is called "restrained" eating (Lawson et al., 1995). It is common in many, if not most, middle-age women of "normal weight." It also may account for the inverse relationship of body weight to social class: women of upper socioeconomic status (SES) often use restrained eating to maintain their weight. In a weight-loss clinic, higher restraint scores were associated with lower body weights (Williamson et al., 1995). Weight loss was associated with a significant increase in restraint, indicating that higher levels of conscious control can maintain lower weight. Greater increases in restraint correlate with greater weight loss, but also with higher risk of "lapse" or loss of control and overeating.

BINGE-EATING DISORDER

Binge-eating disorder is a psychiatric illness characterized by uncontrolled episodes of eating, usually in the evening (Yanovski, 1994). The patient may respond to treatment with drugs that modulate serotonin. Individuals with binge-eating disorder showed more objective bulimic and overeating episodes, more concerns about their shape and body weight, and were disinhibited on the three-factor eating inventory when compared with patients with night-eating syndrome (Allison et al., 2005).

NIGHT-EATING SYNDROME

Night-eating syndrome is the consumption of at least 25% of energy between the evening meal and the next morning and awakening to eat three or more times per week (Stunkard, 1955; Stunkard, 2000). In a study of 399 patients in psychiatric outpatient clinics, 12.5% met the criteria for the night-eating syndrome (Lundgren et al., 2006). In a comparison of overweight individuals (average BMI 36.1 kg/m^2) with night-eating syndrome who ate on average 35.9% of their food after the evening meal and who awakened to eat an average 1.5 times per night with comparably overweight individuals (BMI 38.7 kg/m^2) who did not have these features, Allison et al. showed that glucose and insulin were higher at night (as expected from the eating pattern) and that ghrelin was lower. Plasma cortisol, melatonin, leptin, and prolactin did not differ, but there was a trend toward higher TSH. Patients with night-eating syndrome were also more depressed (Allison et al., 2005).

SOCIOECONOMIC AND ETHNIC FACTORS

Overweight, particularly in women, is more prevalent in those with less education in the United States and elsewhere. The inverse relationship of SES and overweight is found in both adults and children. In the Minnesota Heart Study (Jeffery et al., 1989), for example, SES and BMI were inversely related. People of higher SES were more concerned with healthy weight-control practices, including exercise, and tended to eat less fat. In the National Heart, Lung and Blood Institute Growth and Health Study (Obarzanek et al., 1994), SES and overweight were strongly associated in Caucasian 9- and 10-year-old girls and their mothers, but not in African-American girls. The association of SES and overweight is much stronger in Caucasian women than in African-American women. African-American women of all ages are more overweight than are Caucasian women (*see* Chapter 1). African-American men are less overweight than white men, and socioeconomic factors are much less evident in men. The prevalence of overweight in Hispanic men and women is higher than in Caucasians. The basis for these ethnic differences is unclear. In men, the socioeconomic effects of overweight are weak or absent. This gender difference, and the higher prevalence of overweight in women, suggests important interactions of gender with many factors that influence body fat and fat distribution. The reason for this association is not known.

AGE-RELATED FACTORS IN THE DEVELOPMENT OF OVERWEIGHT

Individuals can become overweight at any age, but it is more common at certain ages. At birth, whether one will become overweight later in life can rarely be distinguished

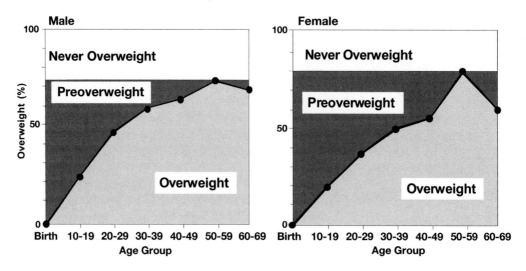

Fig. 7. Pre-overweight, overweight, and clinical overweight.

by weight, except for the infants whose mothers have diabetes, for whom the likelihood of overweight later in life is increased. Thus, at birth, a large pool of individuals will eventually become overweight, and a smaller group will never become overweight. I have labeled these pools "pre-overweight" (Fig. 7) and "never overweight," using the National Center for Health Statistics data for prevalence of BMI higher than 25 kg/m^2 as the solid line. Several surveys suggest that one-third of overweight adults become overweight before age 20, and two-thirds do so after that (Bray, 1976). Thus, 75 to 80% of adults will become overweight at some time in their lives. Between 20 and 25% of the population will become overweight before age 20, and 50% will do so after age 20. Some of these overweight individuals will develop clinically significant problems, such as diabetes, hypertension, gallbladder disease, or the metabolic syndrome. These individuals are referred to as "clinically overweight."

The lifetime risk of developing overweight in the United States is significant. Using data from the Framingham Heart Study, Vasan et al. (2005) have calculated the 4-year risk and the long-term (10- to 30-year) risk of becoming overweight. They examined the effects for men and women at ages 30, 40, and 50 who had a normal BMI at each age. The 4-year risk of becoming overweight (developing a BMI > 25 kg/m^2) was 14 to 19% in women and 26 to 30% in men in these three age groups. The 4-year risk for developing a BMI higher than 30 kg/m^2 (if BMI was normal) was 5 to 7% for women and 7 to 9% for men. Over the longer 30-year interval, the risks were similar in men and women, and varied somewhat with age, being lower for those younger than 50. The 30-year risk was 1 in 2 (50%) for developing a BMI higher than 25 kg/m^2, 1 in 4 (25%) for developing a BMI higher than 30 kg/m^2, and 1 in 10 (10%) for developing a BMI higher than 35 kg/m^2.

Because most pre-overweight people will become overweight, it is important to have as much insight as possible into the risk factors (Vasan et al., 2005). These predictors fall into two broad groups: demographic and metabolic. When an individual becomes overweight (i.e., BMI > 25 kg/m^2) without clinically significant problems, they manifest "overweight" or "preclinical overweight." With the passage of time or a further increase

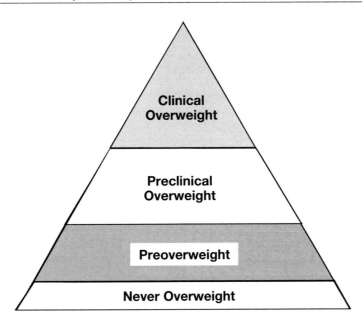

Fig. 8. Weight gain pyramid.

in weight, they may show clinical signs of diabetes, hypertension, gallbladder disease, or dyslipidemia, thus becoming "clinically overweight." The relationship of one to the other may be depicted as a pyramid (Fig. 8).

At the base of this pyramid is the reservoir of never overweight and pre-overweight individuals, many of whom will become overweight in their adult life. Some of these individuals will in turn show signs of clinical disease and become clinically overweight.

Overweight Developing Before Age 10

A number of factors are related to the risk of developing overweight later in life. Table 6 summarizes a number of these.

PRENATAL FACTORS

Caloric intake by the mother may influence body size, shape, and later body composition of their babies. Birth weights of identical and fraternal twins have the same correlation ($r = 0.63$), indicating that birth weight is a poor predictor of future overweight. In the first years of life, the correlation of body weight among identical twins begins to converge, rapidly becoming much closer together ($r = 0.9$), whereas dizygotic twins diverge during this same period ($r = 0.5$). Infants born to mothers with diabetes have a higher risk of being overweight as children and adults (Barker et al., 1993). Infants who are small for their age, short, or have a small head circumference are at higher risk of developing abdominal fatness and other comorbidities associated with overweight later in life (Barker et al., 1993).

Maternal smoking is discussed in Chapter 2. It is clear from the data that infants of mothers who smoke during pregnancy, whether for the first trimester only or for the entire pregnancy, have infants who are at higher risk for increased body weight than infants from mothers who do not smoke during pregnancy. Thus, advising women not to smoke during pregnancy has a particularly important potential future impact on the infant.

Table 6
Predictors of Weight Gain

Infant of mother with diabetes or mother who smoked
Overweight parents
Overweight in childhood
Lower education or income group
Cessation of smoking
Sedentary lifestyle
Low metabolic rate
Lack of maternal knowledge of child's sweet-eating habits
Recent marriage
Multiple births.

INFANCY THROUGH AGE 3

Genetic Defects

Infancy and early childhood are important times to identify genetic defects in which obesity is a primary component. These defects are discussed in detail earlier in this chapter.

Breastfeeding

Several papers have suggested that breastfeeding may reduce the prevalence of overweight in later life. In a large German study of more than 11,000 children, von Kries et al. (1999) showed that the duration of breastfeeding as the sole source of nutrition was inversely related to the incidence of overweight, defined as a weight above the 95th percentile when children entered the first grade. In this study, the incidence was 4.8% in children with no breastfeeding, falling in a graded fashion to 0.8% in children who were solely breastfed for 12 months or more. A second large report (Gillman et al., 2001) also showed that breastfeeding reduced the incidence of overweight, but not obese adolescents. The third report, with fewer subjects and more ethnic heterogeneity, failed to show this effect (Hediger et al., 2001). However, the potential that breastfeeding can reduce the future risk of overweight is another reason to recommend breastfeeding for at least 6 to 12 months (Table 7; Bergmann et al., 2003; Rogers, 2003). In a study of breastfeeding by mothers with diabetes, Rodekamp et al. concluded that the first week of life that has the most influence on subsequent changes in weight (2005).

The composition of human breast milk changed over the last 50 years of the 20th century (Ailhaud and Guesnet, 2004), with an increasing proportion of linoleic acid derived largely from vegetable fats relative to a stable amount of the ω-3 fatty acid α-linolenic acid, which suggest the possibility that this changing proportion of n-6 and n-3 fatty acid may affect prostacyclin production, which in turn could influence the proliferation of new fat cells in the early months of life.

Normally, body weight triples and body fat doubles in the first year of life. This increase in body fat and how long the infant was breastfed in the first year of life are important predictors of overweight later in life. Birth weight and weight gain over the first 6 months of life are positively associated with being overweight and ages 5 and 14 (Mamun et al., 2005). In infants and young children with overweight parents, an infant

Table 7
Effect of Breastfeeding on the Prevalence
of Overweight Children Ages 5 to 6

Duration of breastfeeding	Prevalence of obesity
None	4.5%
3 months	3.8%
3–5 months	2.3%
6–12 months	1.7%
<12 months	0.8%

Reprinted from Von Kries, et al. 1999.

above the 85th percentile at ages 1 to 3 has a fourfold increased risk of adult overweight if either parent is overweight, compared with non-overweight infants. If neither parent is overweight, infantile overweight does not predict overweight in early adult life (Whitaker et al., 1997). These observations are similar to older observations suggesting that the risk for overweight in adults was 80% for children with two overweight parents, 40% for those with one overweight parent, and less than 10% if neither parent were overweight (Bray, 1976).

Low Metabolic Rate

A low metabolic rate has been proposed as a predictor of weight gain. In two studies published nearly simultaneously, Roberts et al. (1988) and Ravussin et al. (1988) provided information suggesting that a low metabolic rate might predict future weight gain. The study by Roberts et al. was done in new born infants using doubly labeled water. They reported that the infants with a lower metabolic rate gained more weight over the next year. The study by Ravussin et al. was done in Pima Indians, whose metabolic rate was measured in a respiration calorimeter. Subjects were divided into tertiles of initial metabolic rate. Those in the lowest tertile gained more weight over the next 3 years. A more recent study by DeLany that studied children at the transition into puberty also found that those with a lower metabolic rate had more fat gain over 2 years than those that did not. Several measures of energy metabolism, including total daily energy expenditure by doubly labeled water, resting metabolic rate, and substrate oxidation during a test meal, predicted up to 7% of the variance in changes in percent body fat over the 2-year interval in the whole group (DeLany et al., 2006). Thus some data suggest that a lower metabolic rate may be predictive of future weight gain.

CHILDHOOD OVERWEIGHT FROM AGES 3 TO 10

Genetic factors that influence body weight can be manifested in the 3- to 10-year age group as well as earlier. Pediatricians need to keep these factors in mind. This is also the age in which the children with Prader-Willi syndrome may first manifest increasing body weight.

Between the ages 3 and 10 are high-risk years for developing overweight, but body weight can increase or decrease. At this age, as at earlier ages, parental weight status is a strong predictor of which children will increase to overweight between ages 5 and 14 (Mamun et al., 2005).

Adiposity rebound describes the inflection point between a declining BMI from birth to ages 5 to 7 and an increasing BMI that occurs between ages 5 and 7 years and later. The earlier this rebound occurs, the greater the risk of overweight later in life.

About half of overweight grade school children remain overweight as adults. Moreover, the risk of overweight in adulthood is at least twice as great for overweight children as for non-overweight children. The risk is 3 to 10 times higher if the child's weight is above the 95th percentile for their age. Parental overweight plays a strong role in this group as well. Nearly 75% of overweight children ages 3 to 10 remained overweight in early adulthood if they had at least one overweight parent, compared with 25 to 50% if neither parent was overweight. Overweight in a 3- to 10-year-old child with an overweight parent thus constitutes an ideal group for behavioral therapy. When body weight progressively deviates from the upper limits of normal in this age group, it is labeled "progressive overweight" (Bray, 1976), which is usually severe, lifelong, and associated with an increase in the number of fat cells.

Overweight Developing in Adolescence and Adult Life

ADOLESCENCE

Weight in adolescence becomes a progressively better predictor of adult weight status. In a 55-year follow-up of adolescents, the weight status in adolescence predicted later adverse health events (Must et al., 1992). Adolescents above the 95th percentile had a 5- to 20-fold greater likelihood of overweight in adulthood. In contrast with younger ages, parental overweight is less important, or has already had its effect. Although 70 to 80% of overweight adolescents with an overweight parent were overweight as young adults, the numbers were only modestly lower (54–60%) for overweight adolescents without overweight parents. Despite the importance of childhood and adolescent weight status, however, it remains clear that most overweight individuals develop their problem in adult life (Bray, 1976).

ADULT WOMEN

Most overweight women gain their excess weight after puberty. This weight gain may be precipitated by a number of events, including pregnancy, oral contraceptive therapy, and menopause.

Pregnancy. Weight gain during pregnancy and the effect of pregnancy on subsequent weight gain are important events in the weight gain history of women (Williamson et al., 1994). A few women gain a considerable amount of weight during pregnancy, occasionally more than 50 kg. The pregnancy itself may leave a legacy of increased weight, as suggested by one study that evaluated women prospectively between the ages of 18 and 30 years (Smith et al., 1994). Women who were nulliparous ($n = 925$) were compared with women who had a single pregnancy of 28 weeks' duration during that period and who were at least 12 months postpartum. The primiparas gained 2 to 3 kg more weight and had a greater increase in waist-to-hip ratio (WHR) compared with the nulliparous women during this period. The overall risk of weight gain associated with pregnancy after age 25, however, is quite modest for most American women (Williamson et al., 1994).

Oral Contraceptives. Oral contraceptive use may initiate weight gain in some women, although this effect is diminished with low-dose estrogen pills. One study evaluated 49 healthy women initiating treatment with a low-dose oral contraceptive (30 mg ethinyl estradiol plus 75 mg gestodene). Anthropometric measurements before and after the initiation of this formulation were used to compare 31 age- and weight-matched women (Reubinoff et al., 1995). Baseline BMI, percent fat, percent water, and WHR did not change significantly after six cycles in the birth control pill users. A similar number of women gained weight in both groups (30.6% of users, 35.4% of controls). The typical weight gain in the pill user group was only 0.5 kg, but the small weight gain in these women was attributable to the accumulation of fat, not body water. Approximately 20% of women in both groups lost weight.

Menopause. Weight gain and changes in fat distribution occur after menopause. The decline in estrogen and progesterone secretion alters fat cell biology so that central fat deposition increases. Estrogen replacement therapy does not prevent weight gain, although it may minimize fat redistribution (Aloia et al., 1995). A prospective study of 63 early postmenopausal women compared 34 women who initiated continuous estrogen and progesterone therapy with the remaining women who refused it. Body weight and fat mass increased significantly in both the treatment (73.2–75.6 kg) and control groups (71.5–73.5 kg). However, WHR increased significantly only in the control group (0.80–0.85). Caloric and macronutrient intake did not change in either group. A 2-year trial with estrogen in postmenopausal women also showed an increase in body fat (Haarbo and Christiansen, 1992).

ADULT MEN

The transition from an active lifestyle during the teens and early 20s to a more sedentary lifestyle thereafter is associated with weight gain in many men. The rise in body weight continues through the adult years until the sixth decade. After ages 55 to 64, relative weight remains stable and then begins to decline. Evidence from the Framingham Study and studies of men in the armed services suggests that men have become progressively heavier for height during the 20th century.

Weight Stability and Weight Cycling

Weight cycling associated with dieting is popularly known as yo-yo dieting (N. A., 1994). Weight cycling refers to the downs and ups in weight that often happen to people who diet, lose weight, stop dieting, and regain the weight they lost and sometimes more. The possibility that loss and regain is more detrimental than staying heavy has been debated. In a review of the literature between 1964 and 1994, a group of experts concluded that most studies did not support any adverse effects on metabolism associated with weight cycling. Also, little or no data supported the contention that it is more difficult to lose weight a second time after regaining weight from a previous therapeutic approach. Most researchers agree that weight cycling neither necessarily increases body fat, nor adversely affects blood pressure, glucose metabolism, or lipid concentrations.

FROM THE PROBLEM TO ITS SOLUTIONS

This chapter has set the clinical stage for the next steps, which include evaluation of the overweight patient and the selection and administration of appropriate therapies.

REFERENCES

Ailhaud, G. and Guesnet, P. (2004). Fatty acid composition of fats is an early determinant of childhood obesity: a short review and an opinion. Obes Rev 5(1):21–26.

Allison, D. B., et al. (1999). Antipsychotic-induced weight gain: a comprehensive research synthesis. Am J Psychiatry 156(11):1686–1696.

Allison, K. C., et al. (2005). Neuroendocrine profiles associated with energy intake, sleep, and stress in the night eating syndrome. J Clin Endocrinol Metab 90(11):6214–6217.

Allison, K. C., et al. (2005). Binge eating disorder and night eating syndrome: a comparative study of disordered eating. J Consult Clin Psychol 73(6):1107–1115.

Aloia, J. F., et al. (1995). The influence of menopause and hormonal replacement therapy on body cell mass and body fat mass. Am J Obstet Gynecol 172(3):896–900.

Astrup, A., et al. (2000). The role of dietary fat in body fatness: evidence from a preliminary meta-analysis of ad libitum low-fat dietary intervention studies. Br J Nutr 83(Suppl 1):S25–S32.

Barker, D. J., et al. (1993). Type 2 (non-insulin-dependent) diabetes mellitus, hypertension and hyperlipidaemia (syndrome X): relation to reduced fetal growth. Diabetologia 36(1):62–67.

Bergmann, K. E., et al. (2003). Early determinants of childhood overweight and adiposity in a birth cohort study: role of breast-feeding. Int J Obes Relat Metab Disord 27(2):162–172.

Blundell, J. E. and MacDiarmid, J. I. (1997). Fat as a risk factor for overconsumption: satiation, satiety, and patterns of eating. J Am Diet Assoc 97(7 Suppl):S63–S69.

Bolland, M. J., et al. (2005). Association between primary hyperparathyroidism and increased body weight: a meta-analysis. J Clin Endocrinol Metab 90(3):1525–1530.

Bouchard, C., et al. (1990). The response to long-term overfeeding in identical twins. N Engl J Med 322(21):1477–1482.

Bray, G. A. (1976). The Obese Patient: Major Problems in Internal Medicine. Philadelphia: WB Saunders.

Bray, G. A. and Gallagher, T. F., Jr. (1975). Manifestations of hypothalamic obesity in man: a comprehensive investigation of eight patients and a reveiw of the literature. Medicine (Baltimore) 54(4): 301–330.

Bray, G. A. and Popkin, B. M. (1998). Dietary fat intake does affect obesity! Am J Clin Nutr 68(6): 1157–1173.

Bray, G. A. and York, D. A. (1998). The MONA LISA hypothesis in the time of leptin. Recent Prog Horm Res 53:95–117; discussion 117–118.

Clement, K., et al. (1998). A mutation in the human leptin receptor gene causes obesity and pituitary dysfunction. Nature 392(6674):398–401.

Crespo, C. J., et al. (2001). Television watching, energy intake, and obesity in US children: results from the third National Health and Nutrition Examination Survey, 1988–1994. Arch Pediatr Adolesc Med 155(3): 360–365.

Cummings, D. E., et al. (2002). Elevated plasma ghrelin levels in Prader Willi syndrome. Nat Med 8(7): 643–644.

De Lany, J. P., et al. (2006). Energy expenditure and substrate oxidation predict changes in body fat in children. Am J Clin Nutr 84(4):862–870.

Farooqi, I. S., Yeo, G. S., Keogh, J. M., et al. (2000). Dominant and recessive inheritance of morbid obesity associated with melanocortin 4 receptor deficiency. J Clin invest 106:271–279.

Farooqi, I. S., et al. (2001). Partial leptin deficiency and human adiposity. Nature 414(6859):34–35.

Farooqi, I. S., et al. (2002). Beneficial effects of leptin on obesity, T cell hyporesponsiveness, and neuroendocrine/metabolic dysfunction of human congenital leptin deficiency. J Clin Invest 110(8): 1093–1103.

Farooqi, I. S., Wangensteen, T., Collins, S., et al. (2007). Clinical and molecular genetic spectrum of congenital deficiency of the leptin recetor. N Engl J Med 356:237–247.

Findling, J. W., et al. (2006). Cushing's syndrome: important issues in diagnosis and management. J Clin Endocrinal Metab 91(10):3746–3753.

Flegal, K. M., et al. (1995). The influence of smoking cessation on the prevalence of overweight in the United States. N Engl J Med 333(18):1165–1170.

Gambineri, A., et al. (2004). Effect of flutamide and metformin administered alone or in combination in dieting obese women with polycystic ovary syndrome. Clin Endocrinol (Oxf) 60(2):241–249.

Gillman, M. W., et al. (2001). Risk of overweight among adolescents who were breastfed as infants. JAMA 285(19):2461–2467.

Grace, C., et al. (2001). The effect of Bardet-Biedl syndrome in the components on energy balance. Int J Obes Relat Metab Disord 25(Suppl 2):S42.

Graham, K. A., et al. (2005). Effect of olanzapine on body composition and energy expenditure in adults with first-episode psychosis. Am J Psychiatry 162(1):118–123.

Green, J. S., et al. (1989). The cardinal manifestations of Bardet-Biedl syndrome, a form of Laurence-Moon-Biedl syndrome. N Engl J Med 321(15):1002–1009.

Gunay-Aygun, M., et al. (1997). Prader-Willi and other syndromes associated with obesity and mental retardation. Behav Genet 27(4):307–324.

Haarbo, J. and Christiansen, C. (1992). Treatment-induced cyclic variations in serum lipids, lipoproteins, and apolipoproteins after 2 years of combined hormone replacement therapy: exaggerated cyclic variations in smokers. Obstet Gynecol 80(4):639–644.

Hediger, M. L., et al. (2001). Association between infant breastfeeding and overweight in young children. JAMA 285(19):2453–2460.

Hinney, A., et al. (1999). Several mutations in the melanocortin-4 receptor gene including a nonsense and a frameshift mutation associated with dominantly inherited obesity in humans. J Clin Endocrinol Metab 84(4):1483–1486.

Jackson, R. S., et al. (1997). Obesity and impaired prohormone processing associated with mutations in the human prohormone convertase 1 gene. Nat Genet 16(3):303–306.

Jeffery, R. W., et al. (1989). The relationship between social status and body mass index in the Minnesota Heart Health Program. Int J Obes 13(1):59–67.

Jenkins, D. J., et al. (1989). Nibbling versus gorging: metabolic advantages of increased meal frequency. N Engl J Med 321(14):929–934.

Kalra, S. P. and Kalra, P. S. (2005). Gene-transfer technology: a preventive neurotherapy to curb obesity, ameliorate metabolic syndrome and extend life expectancy. Trends Pharmacol Sci 26(10):488–495.

Kanumakala, S., et al. (2005). Fasting ghrelin levels are not elevated in children with hypothalamic obesity. J Clin Endocrinol Metab 90(5):2691–2695.

Katsanis, N., et al. (2000). Mutations in MKKS cause obesity, retinal dystrophy and renal malformations associated with Bardet-Biedl syndrome. Nat Genet 26(1):67–70.

Kim, J. C., et al. (2004). The Bardet-Biedl protein BBS4 targets cargo to the pericentriolar region and is required for microtubule anchoring and cell cycle progression. Nat Genet 36(5):462–470.

King, B. M., et al. (1985). Nonirritative lesions of VMI effects on plasma insulin, obesity and hyper-reactivity. Am J Physiol 248(6 pt 1):E669–E675.

King, B. M. (2006). The rise, fall, and resurrection of the ventromedial hypothalamus in the regulation of feeding behavior and body weight. Physiol Behav 54:2664–2670.

Kinon, B. J., et al. (2001). Long-term olanzepine treatment: weight change and weight relatedhealth factors in schizophrenia. J Clin Psychiatry 62(2):92–100.

Kromhout, D. (1983). Changes in energy and macronutrients in 871 middle-aged men during 10 years of follow-up (the Zutphen study). Am J Clin Nutr 37(2):287–294.

Kromhout, D., et al. (2001). Physical activity and dietary fiber determine population body fat levels: the Seven Countries Study. Int J Obes Relat Metab Disord 25(3):301–306.

Krude, H., et al. (1998). Severe early-onset obesity, adrenal insufficiency and red hair pigmentation caused by POMC mutations in humans. Nat Genet 19(2):155–157.

Lasker, R. D. (1993). The diabetes control and complications trial. Implications for policy and practice. N Engl J Med 329(14):1035–1036.

Lawson, O. J., et al. (1995). The association of body weight, dietary intake, and energy expenditure with dietary restraint and disinhibition. Obes Res 3(2):153–161.

Levitsky, D. A., et al. (2005). Imprecise control of energy intake: absence of a reduction in food intake following overfeeding in young adults. Physiol Behav 84(5):669–675.

Lieberman, J. A., et al. (2005). Effectiveness of antipsychotic drugs in patients with chronic schizophrenia. N Engl J Med 353(12):1209–1223.

Lonn, L., et al. (1996). Body composition and tissue distributions in growth hormone deficient adults before and after growth hormone treatment. Obes Res 4(1):45–54.

Ludwig, D. S., et al. (2001). Relation between consumption of sugar-sweetened drinks and childhood obesity: a prospective, observational analysis. Lancet 357(9255):505–508.

Lundgren, J. D., et al. (2006). Prevalence of the night eating syndrome in a psychiatric population. Am J Psychiatry 163(1):156–158.

Mamun, A. A., et al. (2005). Family and early life factors associated with changes in overweight status between ages 5 and 14 years: findings from the Mater University Study of Pregnancy and its outcomes. Int J Obes (Lond) 29(5):475–482.

McDevitt, R. M., et al. (2001). De novo lipogenesis during controlled overfeeding with sucrose or glucose in lean and obese women. Am J Clin Nutr 74(6):737–746.

Montague, C. T., et al. (1997). Congenital leptin deficiency is associated with severe early-onset obesity in humans. Nature 387(6636):903–908.

Muller, H. L., et al. (2001). Obesity after childhood craniopharyngioma—German multicenter study on pre-operative risk factors and quality of life. Klin Padiatr 213(4):244–249.

Must, A., et al. (1992). Long-term morbidity and mortality of overweight adolescents. A follow-up of the Harvard Growth Study of 1922 to 1935. N Engl J Med 327(19):1350–1355.

N. A. (1988). Weight gain associated with intensive therapy in the diabetes control and complications trial. The DCCT Research Group. Diabetes Care 11(7):567–573.

N. A. (1994). Weight cycling. National Task Force on the Prevention and Treatment of Obesity. JAMA 272(15):1196–1202.

N. A. (1996). Surgeon General's report on physical activity and health. From the Centers for Disease Control and Prevention. JAMA 276(7):522.

N. A. (1998). Intensive blood-glucose control with sulphonylureas or insulin compared with conventional treatment and risk of complications in patients with type 2 diabetes (UKPDS 33). UK Prospective Diabetes Study (UKPDS) Group. Lancet 352(9131):837–853.

Nishizawa, T., et al. (1976). Some factors related to obesity in the Japanese sumo wrestler. Am J Clin Nutr 29(10):1167–1174.

O'Dea, D., et al. (1996). The importance of renal impairment in the natural history of Bardet-Biedl syndrome. Am J Kidney Dis 27(6):776–783.

Obarzanek, E., et al. (1994). Energy intake and physical activity in relation to indexes of body fat: the National Heart, Lung, and Blood Institute Growth and Health Study. Am J Clin Nutr 60(1): 15–22.

O'Hara, P., et al. (1998). Early and late weight gain following smoking cessation in the Lung Health Study. Am J Epidemiol 148(9):821–830.

Orth, D. N. (1995). Cushing's syndrome. N Engl J Med 332(12):791–803.

Ozata, M., et al. (1999). Human leptin deficiency caused by a missense mutation: multiple endocrine defects, decreased sympathetic tone, and immune system dysfunction indicate new targets for leptin action, greater central than peripheral resistance to the effects of leptin, and spontaneous correction of leptin-mediated defects. J Clin Endocrinol Metab 84(10):3686–3695.

Palmert, M. R., et al. (2002). Screening for abnormal glucose tolerance in adolescents with polycystic ovary syndrome. J Clin Endocrinol Metab 87(3):1017–1023.

Partonen, T. and Lonnqvist, J. (1998). Seasonal affective disorder. Lancet 352(9137):1369–1374.

Pasquet, P. and Apfelbaum, M. (1994). Recovery of initial body weight and composition after long-term massive overfeeding in men. Am J Clin Nutr 60(6):861–863.

Prentice, A. M. and Jebb, S. A. (1995). Obesity in Britain: gluttony or sloth? BMJ 311(7002):437–439.

Ravussin, E., et al. (1988). Reduced rate of energy expenditure as a risk factor for body-weight gain. N Engl J Med 318(8):467–472.

Redden, D. T. and Allison, D. B. (2004). The Quebec Overfeeding Study: a catalyst for new hypothesis generation. Obes Rev 5(1):1–2.

Reubinoff, B. E., et al. (1995). Effects of low-dose estrogen oral contraceptives on weight, body composition, and fat distribution in young women. Fertil Steril 63(3):516–521.

Ristow, M., et al. (1998). Obesity associated with a mutation in a genetic regulator of adipocyte differentiation. N Engl J Med 339(14):953–959.

Roberts, S. B., et al. (1998). Physiology of fat replacement and fat reduction: effects of dietary fat and fat substitutes on energy regulation. Nutr Rev 56(5 Pt 2):S29–S41; discussion S41–S49.

Roberts, S. B., et al. (1988). Energy expenditure and intake in infants born to lean and overweight mothers. N Engl J Med 318(8):461–466.

Rodekamp, E., et al. (2005). Long-term impact of breast-feeding on body weight and glucose tolerance in children of diabetic mothers: role of the late neonatal period and early infancy. Diabetes Care 28(6):1457–1462.

Rogers, I. (2003). The influence of birthweight and intrauterine environment on adiposity and fat distribution in later life. Int J Obes Relat Metab Disord 27(7):755–777.

Schutz, Y. (2000). Human overfeeding experiments: potentials and limitations in obesity research. Br J Nutr 84(2):135–137.

Smith, D. E., et al. (1994). Longitudinal changes in adiposity associated with pregnancy. The CARDIA Study. Coronary Artery Risk Development in Young Adults Study. JAMA 271(22):1747–1751.

Smith, S. R., et al. (2005). Effect of pioglitazone on body composition and energy expenditure: a randomized controlled trial. Metabolism 54(1):24–32.

Snyder, E. E., et al. (2004). The human obesity gene map: the 2003 update. Obes Res 12(3):369–439.

Srinivasan, S., et al. (2004). Features of the metabolic syndrome after childhood craniopharyngioma. J Clin Endocrinol Metab 89(1):81–86.

Strobel, A., et al. (1998). A leptin missense mutation associated with hypogonadism and morbid obesity. Nat Genet 18(3):213–215.

Stunkard, A. (2000). Two eating disorders: binge eating disorder and the night eating syndrome. Appetite 34(3):333–334.

Stunkard, A. J. (1955). The night eating syndrome: a pattern of food intake among certain obese patients. Am J Med 19:78–86.

Tappy, L. (2004). Metabolic consequences of overfeeding in humans. Curr Opin Clin Nutr Metab Care 7(6):623–628.

Teran-Garcia, M., et al. (2004). Effects of long-term overfeeding on plasma lipoprotein levels in identical twins. Atherosclerosis 173(2):277–283.

Vaisse, C., et al. (1998). A frameshift mutation in human MC4R is associated with a dominant form of obesity. Nat Genet 20(2):113–114.

Vasan, R. S., et al. (2005). Estimated risks for developing obesity in the Framingham Heart Study. Ann Intern Med 143(7):473–480.

von Kries, R., et al. (1999). Breast feeding and obesity: cross sectional study. BMJ 319(7203):147–150.

Whitaker, R. C., et al. (1997). Predicting obesity in young adulthood from childhood and parental obesity. N Engl J Med 337(13):869–873.

Williamson, D. A., et al. (1995). Association of body mass with dietary restraint and disinhibition. Appetite 25(1):31–41.

Williamson, D. F., et al. (1994). A prospective study of childbearing and 10-year weight gain in US white women 25 to 45 years of age. Int J Obes Relat Metab Disord 18(8):561–569.

Yanovski, S. Z. (1994). Binge eating disorder affects outcome of comprehensive very-low-calorie diet treatment. Obes Res 2:205–212.

Yeo, G. S., et al. (1998). A frameshift mutation in MC4R associated with dominantly inherited human obesity. Nat Genet 20(2):111–112.

Yu-Poth, S., et al. (1999). Effects of the National Cholesterol Education Program's Step I and Step II dietary intervention programs on cardiovascular disease risk factors: a meta-analysis. Am J Clin Nutr 69(4):632–646.

II THE SOLUTIONS

5   Evaluation, Prevention, and Introduction to Treatment

CONTENTS

KEY POINTS

- Careful evaluation of the overweight patient is the initial step before treatment.
- Setting realistic goals is important for the physician and patient.
- Body mass index and waist circumference are vital signs in evaluating an overweight patient.
- Prevention is the most important objective. Prevention is the preferred strategy, but when it fails, treatment options based on age, degree of excess weight, and the components of the metabolic syndrome should be considered.
- Treatment strategies can be grouped by age of the patient.
- Choices of treatment should be based on the degree of overweight and the presence of components of the metabolic syndrome.
- Reducing body weight will reduce the prevalence of the metabolic syndrome.
- Reducing body weight will correct most abnormalities associated with excess levels of body weight.
- Cognitive strategies—those that require individual effort—have been tried with limited success.
- Non-cognitive strategies—changes that don't require individual effort—may offer more promise (changing basis for economic decisions).

INTRODUCTION

Weight loss is the big American game. At any one time millions of people are trying to lose weight. One approach to quantifying this craze is the behavioral risk factor surveillance system, which contacts a random sample of American homes through a telephone survey conducted by state health departments in collaboration with the US

From: *The Metabolic Syndrome and Obeslty*
By: G. A. Bray © Humana Press Inc., Totowa, NJ

Centers for Disease Control and Prevention (Bish et al., 2005). In the 2000 survey, 46% of women and 33% of men were trying to lose weight. Women reported trying to lose weight at a lower body mass index (BMI) than did men. Among the women who admitted to being overweight, 60% were trying to lose weight, but men did not reach this level until their BMI exceeded 30 kg/m². The likelihood of trying to lose weight increased with the amount of education the respondent had. Nearly 20% of the men and women reported using fewer calories and trying to exercise more than 150 minutes per week as their strategy to accomplish their goal. With this degree of interest in the problem of losing weight, it is important for the physician to have a plan of how to approach the issues that are raised by prevention and treatment of overweight.

EVALUATION

The first step, before deciding on diet, behavior modification, or any other therapy for the overweight patient, is to evaluate the risk of overweight to the individual. Selection of treatment can then be made using a risk–benefit assessment. A summary of this strategy using the BMI as a guideline is presented in Table 1. Once the evaluation is complete and both the physician and patient wish to engage in an effort to lose weight, the potential treatment options can be discussed. The choice of therapy depends on several factors, including the degree of risk associated with the overweight, patient preference, and whether the patient is ready to make the changes needed to lose weight. This chapter focuses on evaluating the overweight patient and preventing overweight. Subsequent chapters review the treatment modalities for those people whose overweight could not be prevented. The use of medications and surgery will be dealt with in separate chapters as will the question of whether the metabolic syndrome should be treated *per se* or its individual components treated separately.

Setting Weight-Loss Goals

Setting realistic goals is important when discussing strategies for weight loss with an individual subject. Prevention of further weight gain is the first priority. Keeping weight within 5% of its current level would be a worthy goal. Most patients have unrealistic goals for their weight loss, and they need the advice of their clinician in setting realistic ones. When patients were asked about the amount of weight they wanted to lose to achieve their "dream weight" it required a loss of more than 30% of their baseline body weight. This is unrealistic. Setting realistic goals are crucial first steps for both physician and participant.

CLINICAL PERSPECTIVE

From a medical perspective, a successful patient will achieve a weight loss of more than 5% below their initial weight (Goldstein, 1992), which is sufficient to reduce significantly the risk of developing diabetes in individuals with impaired glucose tolerance (Knowler et al., 2002). A weight loss of 5 to 15% will reduce most of the risks factors associated with overweight, such as dyslipidemia (except total cholesterol), hypertension, and diabetes mellitus (Sjostrom et al., 1997). In the Diabetes Prevention Program, a multi-center trial in participants with impaired glucose tolerance, weight loss of 7% reduced the rate of progression from impaired glucose tolerance to diabetes by 58% (Knowler et al., 2002). Similar results have been reported with other programs

Table 1
Use of the Body Mass Index to Select Appropriate Treatments

Treatment	Body mass index category (kg/m²)				
	25–29.9	27–29.9	30–34.9	35–39.9	>40
Diet, exercise, lifestyle	+	+	+	+	+
Pharmacotherapy		With co-morbidities	+	+	+
Surgery				With co-morbidities	+

Table 2
Patient Expectations for Weight Loss at the Beginning of a Weight-Loss Study

Outcome	Weight (lb.)	Reduction (%)
Initial	218	0
Dream	135	38
Happy	150	31
Acceptable	163	25
Disappointed	180	17

Source: Foster et al., 1997.

to prevent progression from impaired glucose tolerance to diabetes using diet and exercise (Pan et al., 1997; Tuomilehto et al., 2001) or maintaining lower blood pressure (Stevens et al., 2001).

PATIENT'S PERSPECTIVE

Patients often have a different perspective on their weight-loss goals than their clinician. This point was made elegantly in a survey of participants in a weight-loss program who were asked how much they would like to lose in five different categories (Foster et al., 1997). These categories were their "dream weight loss," "happy weight loss," "acceptable weight loss," and "disappointed weight loss." The results are shown in Table 2. A dream weight translated into a 31 to 38% weight loss, a happy weight into a 25 to 31% weight loss, and an acceptable weight into 17 to 25% weight loss. A disappointed weight would be a weight loss that was less than 17% below where they started. In the study that was then conducted with these women, only 9% achieved enough weight loss to avoid being disappointed, and none achieved their dream weight. If expectations are higher than the realistic goals, disappointment, frustration, and rejection of the program are likely outcomes. One key goal for the clinician is to provide realistic counsel about achievable goals.

One feature of modest weight loss is that body weight may remain lower over months to years. This can be emphasized to the patient during the discussion of goals for the program. In a study of weight change in young and middle-aged women who were participating in the Nurses Health Study, Field et al. (2001) found two important things. First, they noted that women who lost 5% or more of their weight over a 2-year period (1989–1991) gained less weight than their peers between 1989 and 1995. Second, the ones who engaged in vigorous physical activity gained approximately 0.5 kg less than their inactive peers. Thus, encouraging weight loss to help slow later gain and encouraging physical activity are two important lessons.

Clinical Evaluation of the Overweight Patient

The basic components involved in the evaluation of the overweight patient are a medical examination and a laboratory assessment. This should include a record of the historical events associated with the weight gain problem, a physical examination for pertinent information, and appropriate laboratory evaluation. The criteria recommended by the US Preventive Services Task Force (1989) are used, and the reports from the National Heart, Lung, and Blood Institute (1998) and the World Health Organization (N. A., 2000) are also taken into account. The importance of evaluating overweight individuals has increased as the epidemic of overweight has worsened and the number of potential patients needing treatment has increased.

CLINICAL HISTORY

Among the important features to identify are whether there are specific events that are associated with the increase in body weight. Has there been a sudden increase in weight or has body weight been rising steadily over a long period of time? Weight gain is associated with an increased risk to health. Three categories of weight gain can be identified: less than 5 kg (<11 lb.), 5 to 10 kg (11–22 lb.), and more than 10 kg (>22 lb). In addition to total weight gain, the rate of weight gain after age 20 needs to be considered when deciding the degree of risk for a given patient. The more rapidly they are gaining weight, the more concerned a physician should be.

Etiological factors that cause of overweight should be identified, if possible (Bray, 1997; Bray and Gray, 1988). If there are clear-cut factors, such as drugs that produce weight gain or cessation of smoking, they should be noted on the clinical evaluation form (Table 3).

Successful and unsuccessful weight-loss programs should also be identified. A sedentary lifestyle increases the risk of early death. Individuals with no regular physical activity are at higher risk than individuals with modest levels of physical activity.

FAMILY HISTORY

It is important to determine whether the individual comes from a family where overweight is common—the usual setting—or whether they have become overweight in a family in which few people are overweight. This latter setting suggests a search for environmental factors that may be contributing to weight gain. Recent studies have shown that in children and adolescents with a BMI higher than 30 kg/m^2, alterations in the melanocortin-4 receptor occurs in between 2.5 and 5.5% of these individuals. This genetic defect is among the most common associated with any chronic disease, and evaluation of whether this defect is present may become important in the treatment of overweight people.

PHYSICAL EXAMINATION

Determining BMI: A Vital Sign Associated With Overweight

The first step in clinical examination of the overweight patient (Bray, 1997; Bray et al., 1997) is to determine their vital signs, which include BMI, waist circumference, pulse,

Table 3

Measure	Recorded value
Height (in)	
Weight (lb)	
BMI*	
Weight gain since age 18	
Waist circumference (cm)	
Blood pressure SBP/DBP (mmHg)	
HDL-cholesterol (mg/dL)	
Triglycerides (mg/dL)	
Fasting glucose (mg/dL)	
Sleep apnea (present/absent)	

*Calculated as Weight (kg) divided by Height (m) squared (Wt/Ht^2). Can be obtained from tables or on-line.

and blood pressure. Accurate measurement of height and weight is the initial step in the clinical assessment (American Academy of Pediatrics and US Public Health Service, 1994) because they are needed to determine the BMI. The BMI is calculated as the body weight (kg) divided by the stature (height [m]) squared (wt/ht^2). BMI has a reasonable correlation with body fat, and is relatively unaffected by height. Table 3 provides a form to record the height, weight, BMI, and other relevant clinical and laboratory data during this evaluation. This helps categorize the patient as pre-overweight or overweight, with or without clinical complications.

BMI has a curvilinear relationship to risk, as discussed in Chapter 3. Several levels of risk can be identified. These cut points are derived from data collected on Caucasians. It is now clear, however, that different ethnic groups have different percentages of body fat for the same BMI (*see* Chapter 1). Thus, the same BMI presumably carries a different level of risk in each of these populations. These differences need to be taken into consideration when making clinical judgments about the degree of risk for individual patients. During treatment for weight loss, body weight is more useful than the BMI, because the height is not changing and the inclusion of the squared function of height makes it more difficult for physician and patient to evaluate.

Determining Waist Circumference: A Second Vital Sign Associated With Overweight

Waist circumference is the second vital sign in the evaluation of the overweight individual. The waist circumference is the most appropriate measurement for determining central adiposity. It is determined using a metal or non-distensible plastic tape. Measurements at the level of the umbilicus or at the level of the supra iliac crest are the two most common locations. Although visceral fat can be measured more precisely with computed tomography or magnetic resonance imaging, these are expensive and clinical studies show that the waist circumference is a good and much less difficult measure to obtain (Bray et al., 2006; Wang et al., 2005).

Measuring the change in waist circumference is a good strategy for following the clinical progress of weight loss. It is particularly valuable when patients become more physically active. Physical activity may slow loss of muscle mass and thus slow weight loss while fat continues to be mobilized. Waist circumference can help in making this

Table 4
Recommendations for Waist Circumference Values by Three Expert Groups

Recommendation	Value for males (cm)	Value for females (cm)
National Heart, Lung and Blood Institute	<102 (<40 in.)	<88 (<35 in.)
International Diabetes Federation	<94	<80
Asian Obesity Task Force	<90	<80

Table 5
Criteria for Classification of Blood Pressure According to the Joint National Commission VII Recommendations

Categories of blood pressure	
Normal	<120/80
Prehypertension	120–139/80–89
Hypertension	>140/90
Stage 1	140–159/90–99
Stage 2	>160/100

distinction. The relationship of central fat to risk factors for health varies among populations as well as within them (Table 4). Japanese Americans and Indians from South Asia have relatively more visceral fat and are thus at higher risk for a given BMI or total body fat than are Caucasians. Although the BMI is lower than 25 kg/m^2, central fat may be increased and, thus, adjustment of BMI for central adiposity is important, particularly with BMI between 22 and 29 kg/m^2.

Blood Pressure

Careful measurement of blood pressure is important. Hypertension is amenable to improvement with diet (Appel et al., 1997), and is an important criterion for the metabolic syndrome. Having the patient sit quietly for 5 minutes before measuring the blood pressure with a calibrated instrument will help stabilize it. The blood pressure criteria from the Joint National Commission VI recommendations are shown in Table 5.

Other Items for the Physical Examination

Acanthosis nigricans deserves a comment. This is a clinical condition with increased pigmentation in the folds of the neck, along the exterior surface of the distal extremities, and over the knuckles. It may signify increased insulin resistance or malignancy, and should be evaluated.

Laboratory Evaluation

One strategy for refining the meaning of the BMI and the waist circumference is with laboratory measurements of lipids, glucose and C-reactive protein (CRP). An increased fasting glucose, low levels of high-density lipoprotein cholesterol and high triacylglycerol values are atherogenic components of the metabolic syndrome that have been defined earlier. Along with elevated blood pressure, it is possible to categorize the patient as having metabolic syndrome by one of several sets of criteria, two of which are shown in

Table 6
Criteria for Metabolic Syndrome

Criterion	Revised ATP III criteria		International diabetes federation	
Waist circumference				
Female	>35 in.	(>88 cm)	>31 in.	>90 cm
Male	>40 in.	(>102 cm)	>37 in.	>94 cm
High-density lipoprotein-cholesterol				
Female	<50 mg/dL	<1.29 mmol/L	<50 mg/dL	<1.29 mmol/L
Male	<40 mg/dL	<1.03 mmol/L	<40 mg/dL	<1.03 mmol/L
Glucose	100–125[a] mg/dL	(5.5–7.1 mmol/L)	100–125 mg/dL	(5.5–7.1 mmol/L)
Blood pressure	130/85	130/85	130/85	130/85

[a]ATP III revised criteria have lowered glucose to 100 mg/dL or 5.5 mmol/L.
ATP, Adult Treatment Panel.

Table 6. (*see* Chapters 1 and 10 for more details.) In the International Diabetes Federation criteria, presence of increased central adiposity is required with abnormalities in two of the other four criteria. This is the preferred criterion because it helps focus on the importance of the central adiposity. In addition to lipids, which are determined as part of the assessment of the metabolic syndrome, a patient should have a measurement of their low-density lipoprotein cholesterol, which is a key risk factor. Also important is a measurement of high sensitivity CRP. It is now clear that risk for heart disease can be predicted from both the low-density lipoprotein cholesterol and high sensitivity CRP.

PREVENTION

The approaches to preventing overweight have been the subject of several reviews (Daniels et al., 2005; James and Gill, 2004; Jeffery and French, 1999; Koplan et al., 2005; Kuller et al., 2001; Kumanyika and Daniels, 2006; Seidell et al., 2005; Simkin-Silverman et al., 2003; Summerbell et al., 2005; Swinburn et al., 2004).

The epidemic of overweight occurs on a genetic background that has not changed significantly in the last 100 years and certainly not since the epidemic began 20 years ago. Nonetheless, it is clear that genetic factors play a critical role in the susceptibility to becoming obese in a toxic environment. One analogy is that "genes load the gun and a permissive or toxic environment pulls the trigger." Modification of environmental factors acting on genes must be the strategy to prevent the disease. The belief that this can be done by the individual alone is to miss the argument of how environmental factors have acted on these genes to produce the current epidemic, with major emphasis on the imprinting of the plastic brain of the growing child and adolescent and the low cost of tasty energy-dense foods.

The first law of thermodynamics argues that individuals, through "will-power," increased food choices, or more places to exercise, can overcome the current epidemic of overweight. "Cognitive" approaches relying on individual commitment and resolve have so far been unsuccessful in stemming the epidemic and nothing suggests that they will be more successful in the future.

It is what the first law of thermodynamics does not tell us about overweight that is important. In this context, it is the unconscious host systems on which environmental factors operate that produces the disease. If the vending machines that now provide kickbacks to schools contained beverages with no added sugar or high-frustose corn syrup, available calories would be reduced. The exposure of young children to high-frustose corn syrup may produce detrimental imprinting of the brain, making overweight more likely and more difficult to control (Chapter 2).

At least three preventive strategies are available to deal with the epidemic: education, regulation, and modification of the food supply. Education in the school curriculum about good nutrition and healthy weight would be beneficial in helping all children learn how to select appropriate foods and should be included in schools. Foods used in school breakfast and lunch programs should match these educational messages.

However, it is unwise to rely on educational strategies alone, because they have not prevented the epidemic of overweight so far. Regulation is a second strategy. Regulating an improved food label would be one good idea. Regulations on appropriate serving sizes might be part of the information provided by restaurants when requested.

Modification in some components of the food system is a third and most important strategy. Because energy comes from food, individuals need to modify this system to provide smaller portions and less energy density to succeed in combating the epidemic of overweight. One approach is to use differentiated food taxes to promote healthy diets. This strategy has been argued both at the academic level (N. A., 2000; Smed and Denver, 2005; Smed et al., 2005) and at the policy level (Joint WHO/FAO Expert Consultation, 2003). It may be that economic tools that will shift food choices; cost is the "fluoride" for treating the epidemic of overweight.

Strategies Aimed at the Entire Population

Population-based messages and approaches aimed at the public concerning food and exercise could be of a cognitive nature, that is, with no teeth (Kumanyika and Daniels, 2006), or they could be like the "fluoride" described previously—activities that do not require active intervention. Examples of the former are messages assuming that the "individual" has the responsibility for their action and therefore good public health messages should be sufficient. The low-fat message of the 1990s would be one example. The recent report shows that the low-fat message may not have produced weight loss, but it also is not associated with weight gain (Howard et al., 2006). Another would be the America on the Move program in which individuals enrolled individually to increase their activity using step counters.

The alternative approach might involve re-engineering the environment to make it both easier to walk and more likely that individuals would make this choice rather than getting into their cars (Sallis and Glanz 2006). The current model—a cluster of houses off a main street where the automobile is essential for mobility—makes this a long-term strategy whose effectiveness is doubtful.

FOOD

The food industry favors providing healthy alternatives in food stores as a strategy to help overcome the growing problem of overweight. However, because healthy food items are likely to be more expensive than the ones already present, and because newer technologies and marketing are needed, it is unclear whether a price-sensitive public can be moved in this direction, even if it is appropriate. These population approaches cannot be linked to benefit for any given individual (28), and this makes them easy targets for opposition from those who argue that policy or environmental changes threaten personal freedoms (James and Gill, 2004; Kumanyika and Daniels, 2006).

Strategies for improving access to healthful foods often focus on fruits and vegetables. Regular farmers' markets, subsidizing the availability of free fresh fruits and vegetables to school children, lowering the cost of fruits and vegetables while increasing the price of high-fat or high-sugar foods in school or worksite cafeterias, or changing marketing strategies in other ways that increase fruit and vegetable consumption could be helpful (Buzby et al., 2003; French and Wechsler, 2004; Glanz and Hoelscher, 2004; Glanz and Yaroch, 2004; Kennedy et al., 2006). Because we are all price-sensitive, these might move choices of food from the lower cost, less healthy ones to more healthy choices. However, as Drewnowski has pointed out, the high-fat, high-sugar alternatives provide much more energy for the money than the so-called healthier options (Drewnowski and Darmon, 2005).

Another strategy toward this end is to "limit" availability of higher energy foods by making them more expensive. A review of the use of price by Smed et al. has shown that in Europe increasing the tax on "unhealthy" items and reducing the tax on "healthy" items through the value-added tax system could shift consumption toward healthier foods (Smed et al., 2005). The federally funded programs, such as food stamps, school lunches, and meals on wheels, could be used toward this end. Pending the willingness of the public and politicians to tackle some of the political implications of tax policy to combat the epidemic of obesity, this strategy is likely to remain in the background.

PHYSICAL ACTIVITY

Increasing energy expenditure through exercise is highly desirable, and altering the "built environment," such as sidewalks and shopping centers, is one way to do this (Sallis and Glanz, 2006). Because there is a 30- to 40-year lag between initiation of changing architectural land use and real changes in configuration of sidewalks, this is unlikely to impact this problem in the foreseeable future.

Work places are another place where activity occurs. Becuase the days of manual work are fading for many people who now work at home, this becomes an even less tenable strategy. Also, workplaces in the United States have ceased being places where much physical activity occurs. The idea of making stairways more visible has been attractive, but current fire safety laws put significant problems in the way. When the option is available of walking up stairs or taking an escalator, few people chose the escalator.

Schools have also changed. They were once a place where children could be very active. With security issues and concerns about safety with children walking home from school there is less opportunity for physical exercise. Providing safe pedestrian walkways to school could increase physical activity for children more easily than changing the built environment for adults.

The nutrition transition in China is an interesting example of how the modern way of life makes preservation of physical activity so difficult. As recently as 10 years ago, the bicycle was a major mode of transport for Chinese individuals, but now the automobile and public transportation systems are relegating the bicycle to the museums. Whether understanding the need for people to move can provide a rescue for bicycle paths and so on is doubtful.

One element in trying to combat the epidemic of overweight is to focus on the needs of selective groups—so-called social marketing. Such a strategy was one of the approaches the Swedish Department of Health considered more than 20 years ago. The idea is to provide focused messages targeted at selected groups. They eventually decided to focus on increasing consumption of bread and ran a major campaign to that end. The program by the National Cancer Institute to increase fruit and vegetable consumption through the 5 a Day for Better Health program is a modern-day American example of this approach.

Although we would all agree that this is a desirable approach, its effectiveness in changing average fruit and vegetable intake has not been overwhelming (Stables et al., 2002). The VERB™—It's What you Do! program developed by the US Centers for Disease Control and Prevention is another example of a social marketing strategy. It is designed to increase physical activity among ethnically diverse 9- to 13-year-olds (Wong et al., 2004). The question of whether it is really possible to get long-term behavioral change in a society in which the advertising industry and other societal policies favor labor-saving devices remains to be seen. The most recent program for getting Americans more physically active is America on the Move (www.americaon-themove.org). It encourages state involvement in public–private partnerships to improve eating and activity patterns of the public.

CHILDREN

Children of overweight parents are a high-risk group for development of overweight. For this reason, a number of studies have been aimed at this group. The basic message would appear to be that we can change behaviors related to food choices, but that the ability to shift the long-term trajectory for weight seems limited with current approaches.

The recent Cochrane Collaboration review of preventive strategies for children divided studies in this field into long- and short-term studies. Short-term studies were those with data between 12 and 52 weeks. Long-term studies were those with data beyond 52 weeks. This section deals with the long-term studies.

One study by Epstein et al. (2001) was a randomized controlled trial conducted in the United States. Twenty-six children and their families were randomized to two conditions: increasing fruits and vegetables and decreasing fat and sugar. There were 13 children in each arm. The children were 6 to 11 years old and at least one parent accompanied them. They received a comprehensive behavioral program. At the end of 12 months, the decrease in percentage of overweight was −1.10% in the fruit and vegetable group and −2.40% in the decreased fat and sugar group, which were not statistically significant, but nonetheless tantalizing.

A second study judged to be of good quality was conducted by James et al. (2004) in which 644 children were randomized by school class into 15 intervention and 14 control classes in 6 schools. The prevalence of overweight was comparable. The intervention focused on decreasing consumption of carbonated beverages. The intervention was delivered in three 1-hour sessions by trained personnel with the assistance of teachers. At 12 months, the change in BMI Z-score was not significantly different between intervention and control classes (mean Z-score 0.7, standard deviation 0.2). There was, however, a reduction in the self-reported consumption of soft drinks.

A third trial was conducted in Thailand and randomized subjects by class (Mo-suwan et al., 1998). Kindergarten children were randomized by class into an exercise group and a control group with five classes in each arm. The reduction in the prevalence of obesity tended toward significance ($p = 0.07$).

In a US trial, Sallis et al. included 549 children from 6 schools who were stratified by percentage ethnicity. The intervention, called Sports, Play and Active Recreation for Kids (SPARK) was a physical education program with a self-management component. The results for boys showed that the control group had significantly lower BMIs at 6 and 12 months, but not at 18 months. In contrast, the girls in the control group had lower BMI at each time point that reached significance at 18 months.

The Pathways Study (Caballero et al., 2003) is one of the largest studies in children. The participants included 1704 children aged 8 to 11 from 41 American Indian schools. Pathways was a school-based multi-component, multi-center intervention for reducing percentage body fat. There were four components: changing dietary intake, increasing physical activity, a classroom curriculum focused on healthy eating and lifestyle, and a family-involvement program. At the end of the 3-year study, no significant differences were found in BMI, skinfolds, or percentage body fat. Knowledge improved and fat intake at lunch decreased, but there were no changes in either body composition or activity level measured by motion sensor.

Planet Health is a high-quality randomized controlled trial (Gortmaker et al., 1999) conducted among 1295 ethnically diverse children in 10 US schools in New England who were randomized by school. The children were 11 to 12 years old and in grades 6 to 8. The program was a behavioral choice intervention and concentrated on the promotion of physical activity, modification of dietary intake, and reduction of sedentary behavior with an emphasis or reducing time watching television. At follow-up, the percentage of obese girls in the intervention schools was reduced compared with controls (odds ratio [OR] 0.47 [95% confidence interval CI 0.24–0.93]). Each hour of reduction in television time predicted a 15% reduction in obesity (OR 0.85 [95% CI 0.75–0.97]; Fig. 1). Among the boys there was a decline in BMI in both groups, but no significant difference between them. Time spent viewing television was reduced among both boys and girls and fruit and vegetable consumption increased significantly. Gortmaker concluded that the decline in television watching was a major factor.

In another randomized clinical trial from Germany by Mueller et al. (2001), an initial group of 414 children were recruited from 6 schools and randomized into the control or intervention groups (Kiel Obesity Prevention Study [KOPS]). The key messages in the intervention group were to eat more fruits and vegetables each day, reduce high-fat foods, to keep active for at least 1 hour a day, and to decrease television viewing to less than 1 hour a day. At the end of 1 year there was no significant difference in change of BMI between the intervention and control groups.

In a program called Active Program Promoting Lifestyle in School (APPLES), 634 children in 10 schools were randomized to intervention or control groups. The intervention group included teacher training and resources, modification of school meals, support for physical education, and playgroup activities. At 1 year, there was no difference in change in BMI between the children in the two groups, nor was there any difference in dieting behavior. However, children reported a higher consumption of vegetables.

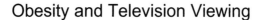

Obesity and Television Viewing

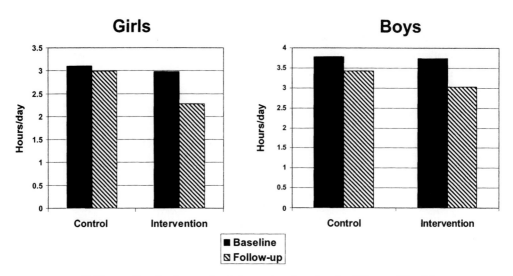

Effect of reducing television viewing in the Planet Health
Study Arch

Fig. 1. Effect of intervention on the hours of television viewed by boys and girls in the Planet Health study comparing baseline and end of intervention. (Drawn from data of Gortmaker et al., 1999.)

Although APPLES was successful in changing the ethos in the schools and the attitudes of the children, the trial was ineffective in changing weight status.

In a final long-term randomized clinical trial, Warren et al. (2003) included 218 children randomized to four conditions: a nutrition group, a physical activity group, a combination nutrition and physical activity group, and a control group. The intervention included raising the value of desired behaviors with reinforcement messages, healthy food tastings, non-competitive activities, and the development of related skills. At the end of 1 year, however, there was no significant difference in the rate of overweight in any of the three intervention groups, although the study may have been underpowered to provide clear-cut answers.

The basic conclusion from the studies of prevention of overweight in children is that behavioral programs aimed at children can change behaviors toward food and activity, but that this only occasionally translates into any impact on the rate at which overweight develops. Thus, in the current climate, preventive behavioral strategies have not been very effective in preventing the current epidemic. It would seem time to explore other ideas, such as those proposed by the fluoride hypothesis identified earlier.

A similar and somewhat pessimistic conclusion is reached by reviewing the literature on prevention in adults. A number of trials have been reviewed in detail by Kumanyika and Daniels in a review published in *Endocrine Update* (2006). Among the studies in adults, The Pound of Prevention study (*see* Table 1; Jeffery and French, 1999; Sherwood et al., 2000) is probably the largest and most general study for prevention of overweight reported to date. This study demonstrated the feasibility of reaching a large number of people and producing some positive behavioral changes. However, as with the children's studies described earlier, the interventions were not successful in preventing weight gain relative to the control condition. The decrease of fat intake and increased physical activity were the strongest predictors of weight maintenance (Sherwood et al., 2000). Again, behavioral changes were positive and perhaps a higher intensity might have produced different results, but at the present time there is a reasonable argument to be made that money spent on behavioral efforts at changing behavior is wasted. The results of the 5-year trial from the Healthy Women's Study are also worth noting (Kuller et al., 2001; Simkin-Silverman et al., 2003). Behavioral counseling at 6 months was effective in preventing a weight gain during the transition to menopause. The intervention program appears to have been well received, judging from retention rates, but it seems to be labor- and cost-intensive to deliver.

INTRODUCTION TO TREATMENT

Risk–Benefit Assessment

Once the work-up for etiological and complicating factors is complete, the risk associated with elevated BMI and increased waist circumference can be evaluated. Several algorithms can be used for this purpose (Bray and Gray, 1988; N. A., 2000; National Heart, Lung and Blood Institute et al., 1998).

The algorithm in Fig. 2, taken from the National Heart, Lung and Blood Institute monograph (1998), will be used. The BMI provides the first assessment of risk. Individuals with a BMI lower than 25 kg/m^2 are at very low risk but, nonetheless, nearly half of those in this category at ages 20 to 25 will become overweight by ages 60 to 69. Thus, a large group of pre-overweight individuals need preventive strategies. Risk rises with a BMI higher than 25 kg/m^2. The presence of complicating factors further increases this risk. Thus, an attempt at a quantitative estimate of these complicating factors is important.

Treatments of overweight can be risky. This is shown in Table 7, which summarizes a number of the untoward events that have happened after the introduction of new treatments for overweight. As can be seen, many treatments have been associated with a therapeutic disaster. The use of thyroid hormone was associated with symptoms of hyperthyroidism. Dinitrophenol produced neuropathies and cataracts. Amphetamine was addictive. Fenfluramine produced aortic value regurgitation. These unwanted side effects must temper enthusiasm for new treatments unless the risk of the new medication is very low. Because overweight is stigmatized, any treatment approved by the Food and Drug Administration will be used to achieve improved self-image (cosmetically desired weight loss) by people who suffer the stigma of being overweight. Thus, drugs to treat overweight must have very high safety profiles.

COSMETICALLY SIGNIFICANT VERSUS CLINICALLY SIGNIFICANT WEIGHT LOSS

As noted earlier, there can be both medical and cosmetic (self-image) benefits to weight loss. However, they do not necessarily occur together. For example, a 10% weight loss, which would be clinically significant for a 300-pound (145-kg) person would only reduce body weight by 30 pounds to 270—a weight change that many people might not notice. At the other extreme, a 10% weight loss for an individual weighing 150 pounds would lower their weight to 135 pounds, which would have a very positive impact on self-image. We also know that cosmetically significant weight losses may not

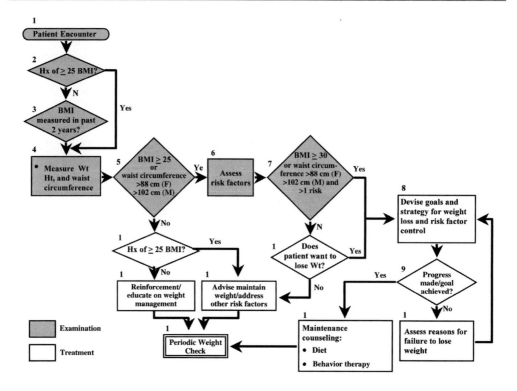

Fig. 2. Algorithm for evaluating risk from overweight and approaches to treatment. (From National Heart, Lung and Blood Institute monograph.)

Table 7
Unintended Consequences Associated With Use of a Number of Treatments for Overweight

Year	Drug	Consequence
1892	Thyroid	Hyperthyroidism
1932	Dintrophenol	Cataracts/neuropathy
1937	Amphetamine	Addiction
1968	Rainbow pulls	Deaths/arrhythmias
1985	Gelatin diets	Cardiovascular deaths
1997	Phen/Fen	Valvulopathy
1998	Phenylpropanolamine (PPA)	Strokes
2003	Ma Huang	Heart attacks/strokes

© 2005 George A. Bray.

produce clinically significant effects. After liposuction that removed about 6% of body weight, there were no improvements in the health-related risk factors (Chapter 11). These distinctions are summarized in Table 8.

Patient Readiness

Before initiating any treatment, the patient must be ready to make behavioral changes that facilitate weight loss. A series of questions developed by Brownell (1990) in the

Table 8
Evaluation of Treatment Outcomes From the Self-Image of the Patient (Cosmetic)
and the Clinical Outcome for the Health Care Giver

Type of procedure	Weight loss	Clinically significant	Cosmetically significant
Diet/exercise	10% from 300 to 270 lb.	Yes	No
	10% from 200 to 180 lb.	Yes	Probably No
	10% from 150 to 135 lb.	Yes	Yes
Liposuction	7% from 220 to 200 lb.	No	Probably No
	7% from 160 to 149 lb.	No	Yes
Surgery (gastric bypass)	40% loss from 264 to 165	Yes	Yes

Dieting Readiness Test can make this assessment. When counseling patients who are ready to lose weight, accommodation of their individual needs as well as ethnic factors, age, and other differences is essential. The approach outlined is not rigid and must be used to help guide clinical decision making, and not serve as an alternative to considering individual factors and clinical judgment in developing a treatment plan. Because of increasing complications of overweight, more aggressive efforts at therapy should be directed at people in each of the successively higher risk classifications.

Doctor–Patient Expectations

The doctor or assistant who identified an elevated BMI or waist circumference in an overweight patient should take a moment to make sure the patient knows how to interpret the BMI or waist circumference. If the patient knows their BMI, it means that the physician or assistant also knows the BMI. However, a recent survey showed that only 42% of overweight patients seen for a routine medical check-up were told they needed to lose weight (Galuska et al., 1999). We need to do better for our patients. The realities of treatment for overweight often conflict with patients' expectations. Patients were asked to give the weights they wanted to achieve in several categories, from their dream weight to a weight loss that would leave them disappointed. These are listed in column two of Table 2 (Foster et al., 1997). Patients then participated in a weight-loss program. The percentage achieving each goal is listed in the right-hand column. None of the patients achieved their dream weight, which was an average 38% below baseline. Nearly half failed to achieve even a weight-loss outcome that at baseline they would consider a disappointment. The patient's desired weight loss from the standpoint of their self-image almost always conflicts with realistically achievable goals for weight loss. This mismatch between patient expectations and the realities of weight loss provides clinicians and their patients with an important challenge as they begin treatment. A weight-loss goal of 5 to 15% can be achieved by most patients and is clinically reasonable.

SLOWING AND CESSATION OF WEIGHT LOSS DURING TREATMENT: WEIGHT PLATEAU

One complaint about treatments for overweight is that they frequently fail; that is, they do not produce continuing weight loss and thus are "no good." A plateau in response to treatment occurs with every treatment, thus an alternative interpretation may be better for why a plateau occurs during weight loss (Fig. 3). Overweight is not curable, but can be treated in many ways. When treatment is stopped, weight is regained. This is similar to what happens to patients with hypertension who are treated with drugs and who stop taking their antihypertensive drugs or patients with high cholesterol who stop taking their hypocholesterolemic drugs. In each case, blood pressure or cholesterol rises. Like the problem of excess body fat, these chronic diseases have not been cured, but rather palliated. When treatment is stopped, the risk factor recurs and so does body fat.

A decrease in body weight of 5 to 15% from baseline improves most comorbidities associated with overweight (Thomas et al., 1995). Patients who are ready to lose weight and have a reasonable expectation for their weight loss are ready to begin a weight-loss program. An ideal outcome is a return of body weight to a BMI below 25 kg/m^2, with no weight gain thereafter (Rossner, 1992). This is rarely achieved and is unrealistic for most patients; thus, they need guidance in accepting a realistic goal, usually a weight loss of 5 to 15% (Thomas et al., 1995). A satisfactory outcome is maintenance of body weight over the ensuing years. A good outcome would be a loss of 5 to 15% of initial body weight and regain no faster than the increase in body weight of the population (0.5 kg/year; Rossner, 1992). Patients who achieve this goal should be applauded. An excellent outcome would be weight loss of more than 15% of body weight. An unsatisfactory outcome is a loss of less than 5% with regain above the population weight.

Criteria for Successful Weight Loss

CRITERIA FOR WEIGHT LOSS

Figure 4 is a model of the natural history of weight change and potential criteria for success (Rossner, 1992). Weight rises slowly but inexorably in most of the population. The principal preventive strategy is to stop further weight gain. This alone would dramatically reduce the ravages of weight gain and prevent progression of the epidemic of overweight. A weight loss of less than 5% is unsatisfactory for any active treatment program for overweight. Several levels of efficacy are shown, ranging from adequate to ideal. Before initiating treatment, a review of likely outcomes is appropriate. An ideal outcome is a return of body weight to the normal range with no weight gain thereafter.

QUALITY OF LIFE

As the comparison of clinically significant and cosmetically significant weight loss makes clear, quality of life is important for all overweight patients. This has effects in many areas. From the health care perspective, a reduction in comorbidities is a significant improvement. Remission of type 2 diabetes or hypertension can reduce costs of treating these conditions, as well as delay or prevent the development of disease. Weight loss can reduce wear and tear on joints, slow the development of osteoarthritis, and usually resolve sleep apnea.

Psychosocial improvement is greatly important to patients. Studies of patients who achieved long-term weight loss from surgical intervention comment on the improved social and economic function of previously disabled overweight patients.

Loss of 5% or more of initial weight almost always translates into improved mobility, improvement in sleep disturbances, increased exercise tolerance, and heightened self-esteem. A focus on these, rather than cosmetic outcomes, is essential.

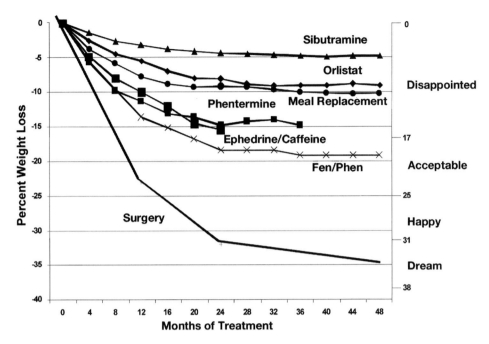

Fig. 3. Slowing of weight loss over the first 6 months of treatment is often called the weight-loss plateau.

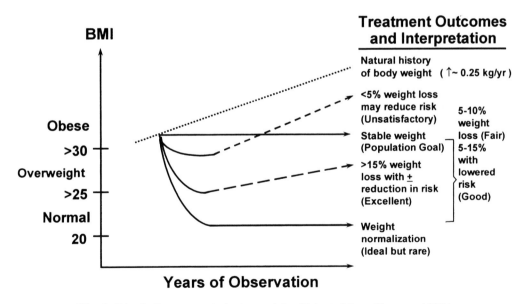

Fig. 4. Criteria for success in losing weight. (Adapted from Rossner, 1992.)

A weight loss of more than 5% from initial body weight is clinically significant and patients maintaining this loss can be called "conditionally successful." At this level, one would expect improvement in the associated risk factors. If this does not occur with the 5% weight loss, then the treatment plan should be reconsidered. A weight loss of 5 to 10% is the outcome seen with most dietary, behavioral, and pharmacological treatments. Provided there are improvements in associated risk factors, this loss would be successful.

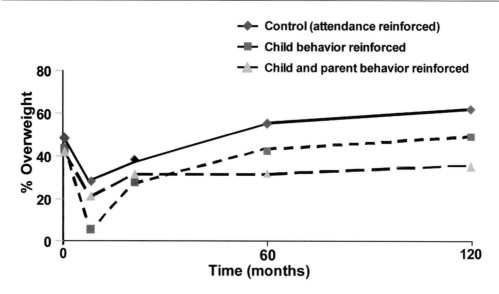

Fig. 5. Long-term weight loss with behavioral therapy. (Redrawn Epstein et al., 1990.)

A weight loss of more than 15% of initial body weight and maintenance of this weight loss is an extremely good result, even if the subject does not reach his or her dream weight.

TREATMENT STRATEGIES BY AGE GROUP

Dividing treatment strategies by age group allows the physician, patient, and family, when appropriate, to focus on the most important components related to their stage in life. After evaluating a patient and deciding that he or she is ready to lose weight, the patient can be placed in one of the categories based on the risk-adjusted BMI and waist circumference. The basic approaches to prevention and treatment are based on this characterization and the patient's age.

Strategies for the Age Group 1–15

Table 9 shows the strategies available for children who are overweight or at risk for overweight. A variety of genetic factors can enhance body weight in this age group, which also contains a high percentage of pre-overweight individuals. Identifying individuals at highest risk for becoming overweight in adult life allows for a focus on preventive strategies. Among these strategies are the need to develop patterns of physical activity and good eating habits, including a lower fat intake and a lower-energy-dense diet. Table 10 lists some predictors for developing overweight. Some of these are evident in children; others are not evident until adult life. For growing children, medications should be used to treat comorbidities directly. Drugs for weight loss are generally inappropriate until the patient reaches adult height, and surgical intervention should only be considered after consultation with medical and surgical experts.

Strategies for Age Group 16–60

Table 11 outlines the available strategies for overweight adults. Because nearly two-thirds of pre-overweight individuals move into the overweight categories in this age

Table 9
Treatment Strategies for the Age Group 1–15 Years

Age	Predictors of overweight	Therapeutic strategies		
		Pre-overweight at risk	Preclinical overweight	Clinical overweight
1–15 years	Positive family history of genetic defects (dysmorphic Prader-Willi syndrome, Bardet-Biedl, Cohen), hypothalamic injury, low metabolic rate, mother with diabetes	Family counseling, reduce inactivity	Family behavioral therapy, exercise, low-fat, low-engery-dense diet	Treat comobidities, exercise, low-fat, low-engery-dense diet

Table 10
Early Life Risk Factors for Obesity in Childhood:
The Avon Cohort Study

Factors	Odds ratio	(95% confidence interval)
High parental body mass index	10.44	(5.11, 23.12)
Birth weight (per 100 g)	1.05	(1.03, 10.7)
Weight gain in first year	10.6	(1.02, 1.1)
Catch-up growth	2.6	(1.09, 6.16)
Standard deviation (SD) for weight at 8 months	3.13	(1.43, 6.85)
SD for weight at 18 months	2.65	(1.25, 5.59)
Adiposity rebound	15	(5.32, 42.3)
More than 8 hours watching television (3 years old)	1.55	(1.13, 2.12)
Short sleep at 30 months (<10.5 hours)	1.45	(1.10, 1.89)

Source: Reilly et al., 2005.
Obesity is defined as body mass index more than 95th percentile.
$N = 8234$ children at age 7.

range, this age is quantitatively the most important. Preventive strategies should be used for patients with predictors of weight gain. These should include advice on lifestyle changes, including increased physical activity, which would benefit almost all adults, and good dietary practices, including a diet lower in saturated fat.

For patients in the overweight category, behavioral strategies should be added to these lifestyle strategies. This is particularly important for overweight adolescents, because 10-year data show that intervention for this group can reduce the degree of overweight in adult life (Epstein et al., 1990). Data on the efficacy of behavior programs carried out in controlled settings show that weight losses average nearly 10% in trials lasting more than 16 weeks. The limitation is the likelihood of regaining weight once the behavior treatment ends, although as shown in Fig. 5, the long-term behavioral therapy in an early adolescent group did provide long-term weight loss (Epstein et al., 1990).

Table 11
Treatment Strategies for Individuals Ages 16–60

Age	Predictors of overweight	Therapeutic strategies		
		Pre-overweight at risk	Preclinical overweight	Clinical overweight
16–60 years	Positive family history of diabetes or obesity, endocrine disorders (polycystic ovarian syndrome), multiple pregnancies, marriage, smoking cessation, medication	Reduce sedentary lifestyle, low-fat, low-engery-dense diet, portion control	Behavioral therapy, low-fat, low-engery-dense diet, reduce sedentary lifestyle	Treat comobidities, drug treatment for over weight, reduce sedentary lifestyle, low-fat, low-engery-dense diet, behavioral therapy, surgery

Medication should be seriously considered for clinically overweight individuals in this group. Two strategies can be used. The first is to use drugs to treat each comorbidity (i.e., individually treating diabetes, hypertension, dyslipidemia, and sleep apnea [*see* Chapter 10]). Alternatively, or in addition, patients with an adjusted BMI higher than 30 kg/m^2 could be treated with a weight-loss drug (Chapter 9). Current drugs include appetite suppressants (sibutramine, phentermine, diethylpropion, benzphetamine, and phendimetrazine) that act on the central nervous system, an endocannabinoid receptor antagonist (rimonabant, not yet approved), and a pancreatic lipase inhibitor (orlistat). The availability of these agents differs from country to country, and any physician planning to use them should be familiar with the local regulations. Most of the drugs on the market were reviewed and approved more than 20 years ago, and are approved for short-term use only. The basis for the short-term use is twofold. First, almost all the studies of these agents are short term. Second, the regulatory agencies are concerned about the potential for abuse, and thus have restricted most of them to prescription use with limitations. The recent withdrawal of fenfluramine and dexfenfluramine because of concerns about their role in the development of valvular heart disease further compounds the concern of health authorities about the safety of these drugs. Because of the regulatory limitations and the lack of longer-term data on safety and efficacy, the use of the drugs approved for short-term treatment must be carefully justified. They may be useful in initiating treatment and in helping a patient who is relapsing (*see* Chapter 9).

Strategies for the Age Group Over 61

Table 12 shows the proposed treatments for this age group. By age 61, almost all of the people who become overweight have done so. Thus, preventive strategies are no longer important, and the focus is on treatment for those who are overweight. The basic treatments and treatment considerations are similar to those of the younger group. However, in the older age group, the argument may be stronger for directly treating comorbidities and paying less attention to treating the clinically overweight by weight loss. For patients in this group who wish to lose weight, however, the considerations for patients between ages 16 and 60 still apply. Surgery should only be considered for

Table 12
Therapeutic Strategies for Individuals Over 61 Years

Age	Predictors of overweight	Therapeutic strategies		
		Pre-overweight at risk	*Preclinical overweight*	*Clinical overweight*
61–75 years	Menopause, declining growth hormone, declining testosterone, smoking cessation, medication	Few individuals remain in this subgroup	Behavioral therapy, low-fat, low-energy-dense diet, reduce sedentary lifestyle	Treat comobidities, drug treatment for overweight, reduce sedentary lifestyle, low-fat, low-engery-dense diet, behavioral therapy, surgery

individuals who are severely overweight. This form of treatment requires skilled surgical intervention, and should only be carried out in a few places.

CONCLUSION

In this chapter, the stage has been set for therapy. The best strategy is to prevent overweight from developing, but even with the best efforts there will always be people who become overweight. For them, treatment may be appropriate, and the remaining chapters of this book look at the therapeutic options.

REFERENCES

American Academy of Pediatrics and US Public Health Service. (1994). Body measurements. In: Clinician's Handbook of Preventive Services: Put Prevention into Family Practice. Elk Grove Village, IL: American Academy of Pediatrics; pp. 141–146.

Appel, L. J., et al. (1997). A clinical trial of the effects of dietary patterns on blood pressure. DASH Collaborative Research Group. N Engl J Med 336(16):1117–1124.

Bish, C. L., et al. (2005). Diet and physical activity behaviors among Americans trying to lose weight: 2000 Behavioral Risk Factor Surveillance System. Obes Res 13(3):596–607.

Bray, G. A. (1997). Classification and evaluation of the overweight patient. In: Handbook of Obesity, edited by Bray, G. A., Bouchard, C., and James, W. P. New York: Marcel Dekker; pp. 831–854.

Bray, G. A., et al. (2007). Computed tomography versus waist circumference as a measure of visceral fat: its uses in the Diabetes Prevention Program (in press).

Bray, G. A., et al. (1997). Definitions and proposed current classification of obesity. In: Handbook of Obesity, edited by Bray, G. A., Bouchard, C., and James, W. P. New York: Marcel Dekker; pp. 31–40.

Bray, G. A. and Gray, D. S. (1988). Obesity. Part II—treatment. West J Med 149:555–571.

Brownell, K. (1990). Dieting readiness. Weight Control Digest 1:1–9.

Buzby, J. C., et al. (2003). Evaluation of the USDA Fruit and Vegetable Pilot Program: Report to Congress. US Department of Agriculture, Economic Research Service.

Caballero, B., et al. (2003). Pathways: a school-based, randomized controlled trial for the prevention of obesity in American Indian schoolchildren. Am J Clin Nutr 78(5):1030–1038.

Daniels, S. R., et al. (2005). Overweight in children and adolescents: pathophysiology, consequences, prevention, and treatment. Circulation 111(15):1999–2012.

Drewnowski, A. and Darmon, N. (2005). The economics of obesity: dietary energy density and energy cost. Am J Clin Nutr 82(1 Suppl):265S–273S.

Epstein, L. H., et al. (2001). Increasing fruit and vegetable intake and decreasing fat and sugar intake in families at risk for childhood obesity. Obes Res 9(3):171–178.

Epstein, L. H., et al. (1990). Ten-year follow-up of behavioral, family-based treatment for obese children. JAMA 264(19):2519–2523.

Field, A. E., et al. (2001). Relationship of a large weight loss to long-term weight change among young and middle-aged US women. Int J Obes Relat Metab Disord 25(8):1113–1121.

Foster, G. D., et al. (1997). What is a reasonable weight loss? Patients' expectations and evaluations of obesity treatment outcomes. J Consult Clin Psychol 65(1):79–85.

French, S. A. and Wechsler, H. (2004). School-based research and initiatives: fruit and vegetable environment, policy, and pricing workshop. Prev Med 39(Suppl 2):S101–S107.

Galuska, D. A., et al. (1999). Are health care professionals advising obese patients to lose weight? JAMA 282(16):1576–1578.

Glanz, K. and Hoelscher, D. (2004). Increasing fruit and vegetable intake by changing environments, policy and pricing: restaurant-based research, strategies, and recommendations. Prev Med 39(Suppl 2): S88–S93.

Glanz, K. and Yaroch, A. L. (2004). Strategies for increasing fruit and vegetable intake in grocery stores and communities: policy, pricing, and environmental change. Prev Med 39(Suppl 2): S75–S80.

Goldstein, D. J. (1992). Beneficial health effects of modest weight loss. Int J Obes Relat Metab Disord 16(6):397–415.

Gortmaker, S. L., et al. (1999). Reducing obesity via a school-based interdisciplinary intervention among youth: Planet Health. Arch Pediatr Adolesc Med 153(4):409–418.

Howard, B. V., et al. (2006). Low-fat dietary pattern and weight change over 7 years: the Women's Health Initiative Dietary Modification Trial. JAMA 295(1):39–49.

James, J., et al. (2004). Preventing childhood obesity by reducing consumption of carbonated drinks: cluster randomised controlled trial. BMJ 328(7450):1237.

James, W. P. T. and Gill, T. P. (2004). Prevention of Obesity. In: Handbook of Obesity: Clinical Applications, edited by Bray, G. and Bouchard, C. New York: Marcel Dekker; pp. 75–96.

Jeffery, R. W. and French, S. A. (1999). Preventing weight gain in adults: the pound of prevention study. Am J Public Health 89(5):747–751.

Joint WHO/FAO Expert Consultation on Diet, Nutrition and the Prevention of Chronic Diseases. (2003). Diet, Nutrition and the Prevention of Chronic Diseases. Geneva, Switzerland: World Health Organization.

Kennedy, B. M., et al. (2006). Socioeconomic status and health disparity in the United States. J Hum Behav Soc Environ (in press).

Knowler, W. C., et al. (2002). Reduction in the incidence of type 2 diabetes with lifestyle intervention or metformin. N Engl J Med 346(6):393–403.

Koplan, J. P., et al. (2005). Preventing Childhood Obesity. Health in the Balance. Washington, D. C.: National Academies Press.

Kuller, L. H., et al. (2001). Women's Healthy Lifestyle Project: A randomized clinical trial: results at 54 months. Circulation 103(1):32–37.

Kumanyika, S. and Daniels, S. R. (2006). Obesity prevention. In: Overweight and the Metabolic Syndrome: From Bench to Bedside, (Bray, G.A., Ryan, D., eds). Boston: Springer; pp. 233–253.

Mo-suwan, L., et al. (1998). Effects of a controlled trial of a school-based exercise program on the obesity indexes of preschool children. Am J Clin Nutr 68(5):1006–1011.

Muller, M. J., et al. (2001). Prevention of obesity—more than an intention. Concept and first results of the Kiel Obesity Prevention Study (KOPS). Int J Obes Relat Metab Disord 25(Suppl 1): S66–S74.

N. A. (2000). Obesity: preventing and managing the global epidemic. Report of a WHO consultation. World Health Organ Tech Rep Ser 894:i–xii, 1–253.

National Heart, Lung and Blood Institute in cooperation with The National Institute of Diabetes and Digestive and Kidney Diseases Appendices. (1998). Clinical Guidelines on the Identification, Evaluation, and Treatment of Overweight and Obesity in Adults—The Evidence Report. Obes Res 6(Suppl 2):51S–209S.

Pan, X. R., et al. (1997). Effects of diet and exercise in preventing NIDDM in people with impaired glucose tolerance. The Da Qing IGT and Diabetes Study. Diabetes Care 20(4):537–544.

Reilly, J. J., et al. (2005). Early life risk factors for obesity in childhood: cohort study. BMJ 330(7504):1357–1367.

Rossner, S. (1992). Factors determining the long-term outcome of obesity treatment. In: Obesity, edited by Bjorntorp, P. and Brodoff, B. N. Philadelphia: J. B. Lippincott; pp. 712–719.

Sallis, J. F. and Glanz, K. (2006). The role of built environments in physical activity, eating, and obesity in childhood. Future Child 16(1):89–108.

Seidell, J. C., et al. (2005). Cost-effective measures to prevent obesity: epidemiological basis and appropriate target groups. Proc Nutr Soc 64(1):1–5.

Sherwood, N. E., et al. (2000). Predictors of weight gain in the Pound of Prevention study. Int J Obes Relat Metab Disord 24(4):395–403.

Simkin-Silverman, L. R., et al. (2003). Lifestyle intervention can prevent weight gain during menopause: results from a 5-year randomized clinical trial. Ann Behav Med 26(3):212–220.

Sjostrom, C. D., et al. (1997). Relationships between changes in body composition and changes in cardiovascular risk factors: the SOS Intervention Study. Swedish Obese Subjects. Obes Res 5(6):519–530.

Smed, S. and Denver, S. (2005). Taxing as Economic Tools in Health Policy. 97th EAAE Seminar, University of Reading.

Smed, S., et al. (2005). Differentiated food taxes as a tool in health and nutrition policy. Copenhagen, Denmark: Eleventh Congress of the European Association of Agricultural Economists.

Stables, G. J., et al. (2002). Changes in vegetable and fruit consumption and awareness among US adults: results of the 1991 and 1997 5 A Day for Better Health Program surveys. J Am Diet Assoc 102(6):809–817.

Stevens, V. J., et al. (2001). Long-term weight loss and changes in blood pressure: results of the Trials of Hypertension Prevention, phase II. Ann Intern Med 134(1):1–11.

Stookey, J. O., et al. (2007). The altered fluid distribution in obesity may reflect plasma hypertonicity. Eur J Clin Nutr 61(2):190–199.

Summerbell, C. D., et al. (2005). Interventions for preventing obesity in children. Cochrane Database Syst Rev (3):CD001871.

Swinburn, B. A., et al. (2004). Diet, nutrition and the prevention of excess weight gain and obesity. Public Health Nutr 7(1A):123–146.

Thomas, P. R., et al. (1995). Weighing the Options: Criteria for Evaluating Weight-Management Programs. Washington, D.C.: The National Academies Press.

Tuomilehto, J., et al. (2001). Prevention of type 2 diabetes mellitus by changes in lifestyle among subjects with impaired glucose tolerance. N Engl J Med 344(18):1343–1350.

US Preventive Services Task Force. (1989). Guide to Clinical Preventive Services: Screening for Obesity. US Department of Health and Human Services; p. 219–229.

Wang, Y., et al. (2005). Comparison of abdominal adiposity and overall obesity in predicting risk of type 2 diabetes among men. Am J Clin Nutr 81(3):555–563.

Warren, J. M., et al. (2003). Evaluation of a pilot school programme aimed at the prevention of obesity in children. Health Promot Int 18(4):287–296.

Wong, F., et al. (2004). VERB—a social marketing campaign to increase physical activity among youth. Prev Chronic Dis 1(3):A10.

6 Diet

CONTENTS

KEY POINTS

- Current diets can be divided into those that reduce fat or carbohydrate selectively or that reduce overall intake of energy.
- The dietary approaches to stop hypertension (DASH) diet is one of two diets recommended by the Dietary Guidelines.
- Drink adequate amounts of water, tea, coffee, and non-calorically sweetened beverages.
- Reduce intake of calorie-sweetened soft drinks and fruit drinks.
- Eat a variety of foods.
- Eat all foods in moderation.
- Low-calorie diets produce significantly more weight loss than control diets.
- Low-carbohydrate diets can produce ketosis.
- Low-fat diets in one meta-analysis are more effective than control diets, but not in another.
- Head-to-head comparison of four popular diets found no difference in weight loss in a group of men and women of all ages, but low-carbohydrate diets appeared better in a group of women. There is considerable individual variation in response in both studies.
- Controlling calorie intake with foods that measure the energy for the client (portion-controlled diets) have been useful.
- Commercial weight-loss programs can be helpful. Look for a program in which the diet has been tested.

INTRODUCTION TO DIET

The dictionary defines "diet" as the "customary allowance of food and drink taken by any person from day to day, particularly one especially planned to meet specific requirements of the individual, and including or excluding certain items of food" (Dorland, 2003). The foods and drink that comprise our diet must contain the nutrients our bodies need to grow and function properly. One can be well nourished and either normal weight or overweight. Conversely, one can be poorly nourished and normal

From: *The Metabolic Syndrome and Obesity*
By: G. A. Bray © Humana Press Inc., Totowa, NJ

weight or overweight. That is, good nutrition and weight status are not directly related. This chapter deals with the elements of good nutrition as well as the use of nutritional techniques for reducing body weight.

Obtaining a diet of food and beverage that provides good nutrition for the population is a subject reviewed regularly by the Dietary Guidelines Committee, whose findings are published by the US Department of Agriculture (USDA) and the Department of Health and Human Services. Table 1 provides information about the major nutrients from the most recent edition of the dietary guidelines (HHS and USDA, 2005), modified to reflect the actual numbers in the studies. The Institute of Medicine recommendations are for women ages 19 to 30 are expressed either as adult minimum daily requirement or as a range of adequate intake. The data in Table 1 show the nutrient requirements for men and women. These include adequate intakes, recommended dietary allowances, and recommended dietary intakes. They can be used to compare the quality of diets and when examining the nutrient content of vitamins and minerals in dietary supplements.

The two dietary patterns recommended in this report were the Dietary Approaches to Stop Hypertension (DASH) eating plan and the USDA food guide plan. The DASH diet is derived from studies on dietary patterns that lower blood pressure (Appel et al., 1997; Moore et al., 2003; Sacks et al., 2001) and the USDA food guide from the MyPyramid Guide. The numbers listed in Table 1 have been slightly modified to reflect more accurately the studies on which they are based (Craddick et al., 2003). For both diets, the protein as a percent of calories is similar. However, there is a small difference in the percentages of fat and carbohydrates, but the distribution of fat between saturated, monounsaturated, and polyunsaturated fatty acids is only slightly different. Calcium, magnesium, and potassium are higher in the DASH diet, as planned by the investigators.

Two words, variety and moderation, are good general concepts to employ in selecting foods and beverages. Because each food has a different complement of nutrients, selecting a variety of foods from all food groups is a good idea. Moderation, that is, controlling the amount of food eaten, is necessary throughout life. When moderation is not practiced, overweight or malnutrition may be the result.

Guidelines have also recently appeared for beverages (Popkin et al., 2006). Water is needed as part of a daily diet, and all beverage needs can be met with water. However, in addition to water, beverages also contain many other nutrients, including vitamins and minerals found in fruit juices. However, many beverages provide only water and calories. Reducing the intake of calorie-containing beverages would be good for everyone, and is particularly important when trying to lose or control weight. Beverage consumption is obviously important when diet is considered for weight loss. Table 2 provides guidance for the consumption of beverages from various categories. Water and non-calorie-containing tea and coffee are preferred. Beverages prepared from whole fruit rather than concentrate and skim or low-fat milk are also good beverages. The beverages made from concentrate, another word for added sugar, and soft drinks that have only water, caloric sweetener, and flavoring are the least valuable for nutritional purposes. The relationship of drinking water to the quantity of food and beverage eaten has been examined by Stookey et al., (2007). They find that there is a linear decrease in energy intake across the quartiles of increasing water consumption, suggesting that drinking more water would be a useful strategy in the battle of the bulge (*see* Chapter 2). The number of servings from each of the food groups and subgroups for the DASH and USDA food guide are shown in Table 3.

Diet is also used to describe the nutritional programs designed to help people lose weight. Many weight-loss diets have been published and some of them will be discussed

Table 1
IOM Recommendations Comparing Two Eating Plans Recommended by the Dietary Guidelines 2005

Nutrient	IOM recommendations for women 19–30	DASH eating plan	USDA food guide plan
Protein (%)	AMDR: 18–35%	18%	18%
Fat (%)	AMDR: 20–35%	27%	29%
Carbohydrate (%)	AMDR: 45–55%	55%	53%
Saturated fat (%)	—	6.2%	7.8%
Monounsaturated fat (%)	—	11.2%	11%
Polyunsaturated fat (%)	—	7.8%	9.0%
Cholesterol (mg)		136	230
Total dietary fiber (g)	AI: 28	30	31
Potassium (mg)	AI: 4700	4706	4044
Sodium (mg)	AI: 1500	2329	1779
Calcium (mg)	AI: 1000	1619	1316
Magnesium (mg)	RDA: 310	500	380

Adapted from the Dietary Guidelines. The DASH diet has been adapted to correct the errors in the published guidelines. Other minerals and vitamins have not been included.

IOM, Institute of Medicine; USDA, US Department of Agriculture; DASH, Dietary Approaches to Stop Hypertension; AMDR, adult minimum daily requirement; AI, adequate intake; RDA, recommended dietary allowance.

Table 2
Guidance for Beverage Intake

Category	Maximum number of servings per day[a]	
	Men	Women
Total daily intake	13	9
Water	13	9
Coffee (unsweetened = 0 cal)	4	4
Tea (unsweetened = 0 cal)	8	8
Skim/low-fat milk	2	2
Diet soft drinks or tea and coffee with artificial sweetener	4	4
100% fruit juice/whole milk or sports drinks	1	1
Soft drinks/juice drinks	1	1

[a]A serving is considered 8 ounces (240 mL).

in detail later. Because overweight develops when energy intake exceeds energy expenditure, for whatever reason, all diets must reduce energy intake relative to energy expenditure. This means restricting some foods or beverages in the diet. Beverages with added sugar or high-fructose corn syrup (HFCS) are obvious candidates because they usually contain nothing but sweet taste, energy (calories), and water. Substituting water or non-calorically sweetened beverages would be a good strategy to reduce energy.

The modern diet has taken many centuries to develop (Cordain et al., 2005). Much of the development depended on technical innovation, such as development of slavery in the

Table 3
Comparison of the USDA Food Guide and DASH Diet Eating Plans

Food groups and subgroups	USDA food guide amount	DASH diet amount	Equivalent amounts
Fruit group	2 cups = 4 servings	2–2.5 cups = 4–5 servings	½ cup = ½ cup fresh, frozen, or canned fruit; 1 medium fruit, ¼ cup dried fruit, USDA: ½ cup fruit juice, DASH: ¼ cup fruit juice
Vegetable group	2.5 cups – 5 servings	2–2.5 cups	½ cup is equivalent to ½ cup of cut-up raw or cooked vegetables, 1 cup raw leafy vegetables; USDA: ½ cup vegetable juice, DASH: ¾ cup vegetable juice
Dark green vegetables	3 cups/week		
Orange vegetables	2 cups/week		
Legumes (dry beans)	3 cups/week		
Starchy vegetables	3 cups/week		
Other vegetables	6.5 cups/week		
Grain group	6-oz. equivalents	7 to 8-oz. equivalents (7–8 servings)	1-oz. equivalent = 1 slice of bread, 1 cup dry cereal, ½ cup cooked rice, pasta or cereal; DASH: 1 oz. dry cereal (½ –1¼ cup depending on cereal type [check label])
Whole grains	3-oz. equivalents		
Other grains	3-oz. equivalents		
Meat and beans group	5.5-oz. equivalents	6 oz. or less of meat, poultry, or fish; 4–5 servings per week of nuts, seeds, and dry beans	1-oz. equivalent = 1 oz. cooked lean meat, poultry, or fish, 1 egg; USDA: ¼ cup cooked dry beans or tofu, 1 Tbsp. peanut butter, ½ oz. nuts or seeds, DASH: 1½ oz. nuts, ½ oz. seeds, ½ cup cooked dry beans
Milk group (low fat)	3 cups	2 to 3 cups	1-cup equivalent = 1 cup low-fat/fat-free milk or yogurt, 1½ oz. low-fat or fat-free natural cheese, 2 oz. low-fat or fat-free processed cheese
Oils	23 g (6 tsp.)	8–12 g (2–3 tsp.)	1-tsp equivalent = DASH: 1 tsp soft margarine, 1 Tbsp. low-fat mayo, 2 Tbsp. light salad dressing, 1 tsp. vegetable oil
Discretionary calorie	267 calories		1-Tbsp. equivalent = DASH: 1 Tbsp. jelly or

(Continued)

Table 3 (*Continued*)

Food groups and subgroups	USDA food guide amount	DASH diet amount	Equivalent amounts
allowance			jam, ½ oz jelly beans, 8 oz. lemonade
Example of distribution			
Solid fat	18 g		
Added sugars	8 tsp.	About 1 tsp. (5 Tbsp. per week)	

USDA, US Department of Agriculture; DASH, Dietary Approaches to Stop Hypertension.

West Indies and United States, which was essential for mass production of sugar; the processing of whole grains into refined wheat, corn, and rice; the hydrogenation of liquid oils to produce saturated (solid) fats, which often contain trans fats and which in turn increase the risk of cardiovascular disease; and the isomerization of glucose to produce HFCS. With these industrial advances and federal subsidies to keep prices low, consumption of a high-fat, high-sugar diet was an obvious outcome, with overweight to follow.

In this setting, it is important to remember that good nutrition and adequate energy intake do not necessarily go together. A person can be well nourished at both normal and high body weights. Equally, an individual can be poorly nourished at normal and high body weights. In the remainder of this chapter, the dietary approaches and behavioral strategies that have been used to redress the energy imbalance that resulted in excess body fatness are examined.

RATE OF WEIGHT LOSS

Total Energy Requirement

The energy stored in fat cells can be viewed as a kind of bank account. A pound of fat tissue has approximately 3500 kcal of energy (7000 kcal/kg fat tissue), so that if an individual weighs 100 kg (220 lb.) and has 40% body fat, the fat tissue represents 40 kg of weight and has 280,000 kcal of stored energy. If an individual eats 1600 kcal per day, 30% of which is fat, nearly 500 kcal of fat energy is received each day, or less than 0.5% of what is stored in fat. If an individual eats 500 kcal less each day than the body needs to maintain its functions, the body will withdraw 500 kcal from body fat. Over 7 days, this will be 3500 kcal, or 1 lb. (0.45 kg) of weight loss, which is why it takes so long to lose 50 lb. of fat tissue and why techniques for "rapid" weight loss are so popular.

As part of the planning process for a new diet, physicians need some estimate of the energy expenditure for their patients. Although there are several methods of estimating caloric expenditure, the Food and Agriculture Organization/World Health Organization criteria are suggested (Table 4). This method allows a calculation of resting metabolic rate (RMR), from which daily energy needs can be obtained by multiplying by an activity factor for individual patients. The low activity level for sedentary individuals is about 1.3 times the estimated RMR. A high activity level has an activity factor of 1.7, which is multiplied by the calculated RMR to give an

Table 4
Estimated Energy Needs Revised WHO Equations
for Estimating Basal Metabolic Rate (RMR)

Men	
18–30 years	$(0.0630 \times \text{actual weight in kg} + 2.8957) \times 240 \text{ kcal/d}$
31–60 years	$(0.0484 \times \text{actual weight in kg} + 3.6534) \times 240 \text{ kcal/d}$
Women	
18–30 years	$(0.0621 \times \text{actual weight in kg} + 2.0357) \times 240 \text{ kcal/d}$
31–60 years	$(0.0342 \times \text{actual weight in kg} + 3.5377) \times 240 \text{ kcal/d}$
Estimated total energy expenditure	BMR × ativity factor

Activity Level	Activity Factor
Low (sedentary)	1.3
Intermediate (some regular excercise)	1.5
High (regular activity or demanding job)	1.7

estimate of total energy expenditure. People with an activity factor of 1.7 are those in jobs requiring manual labor or with regular daily vigorous physical exercise programs (Lin et al., 2003).

The fundamental truth is that if a patient eats more food energy than is burned over a prolonged period of time, they will gain weight. This is referred to as positive energy balance and has been gospel in this field since the early 20th century, when Wilbur Olin Atwater showed that the energy balance concept applied to human beings by using people who lived in calorimeters.

Translating this concept into every day use is challenging. In studies in calorimeters similar to those of Atwater, how close an individual can come to zero energy balance has been explored; that is, how small a difference can be achieved between energy intake over 24 hours and energy expenditure for an individual during the same time interval. Figure 14 in Chapter 2 shows the data from one subject in the chambers at the Pennington Center. Food intake was intermittent while energy expenditure went up and down in relation to exercise and meals and then declined at night during sleep. Over 4 consecutive days, the subject never got closer than 25 kcal to energy balance and was usually 50 to 100 kcal in positive or negative energy balance. From these studies, we concluded that human beings are never in energy balance within a single day, and that it is adjustments over several days or weeks that are important in becoming overweight or not. This day-to-day variability is shown for a group of dietitians in Fig. 1. Ten women who were trained as dietitians were asked to record what they ate as accurately as possible for 1 week, during which time their energy expenditure was measured.

For the patient who wants to lose weight, the essential message is that if they are eating fewer calories than their body needs it will withdraw the extra calories from the fat stores and they will lose weight. Many years ago, Dr. Kinsell and his colleagues hospitalized a number of overweight patients in a metabolic ward and gave them a predetermined amount of energy and varied the sources of food that made up the energy supply. Thus, they had high-protein, high-fat, or high-carbohydrate diets. The rate of weight loss was determined by the caloric content of the diet, not by the dietary

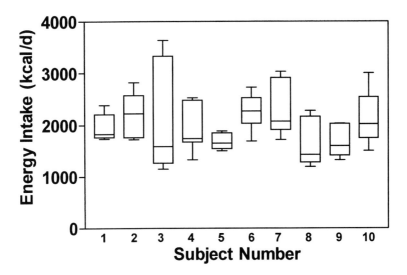

Fig. 1. Variability of food intake during 1 week in 10 healthy women.

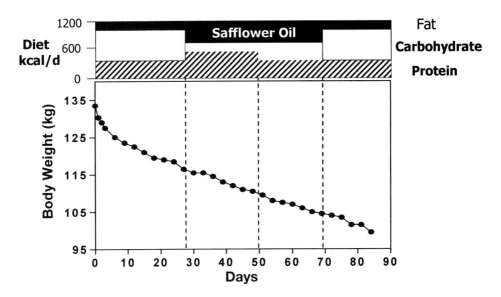

Fig. 2. Weight loss while in the hospital eating a 1200-kcal/d diet with differing composition. (Redrawn from Kinsell et al., 1965.)

composition. This is shown in Fig. 2 (Kinsell et al., 1964). The important message is that to lose weight a patient must be in negative energy balance; that is, energy intake must be lower than energy expenditure for an extended period of time.

Because we know that people under-report the amount of food they eat and that overweight people are even more inaccurate, it is necessary to interpret patient records of food intake cautiously. Even dietitians who are used to recording food intake report slightly less, about 10%, than what is determined using the doubly labeled water method to measure energy expenditure (Champagne et al., 2002) (Chapter 2).

One of the key messages for patients and physicians alike is that when caloric intake is reduced below that needed for daily energy expenditure, there is a predictable rate of weight loss. It is thus essential to adhere to the diet and the amount of food energy actually ingested (Keys et al., 1950; Kinsell et al., 1964; National Heart, Lung and Blood Institute, 2000).

Prediction of weight loss for an individual patient can be difficult because of marked intersubject variability in energy expenditure and adherence. When weight loss was evaluated in subjects on a metabolic ward, the degree of weight loss in a group of overweight women who ate 800 kcal per day (3.4 MJ/day) for 3 weeks while hospitalized on a metabolic ward varied from 1 kg to more than 10 kg (Garrow, 1981). The rate of weight loss could be predicted from the woman's metabolic expenditure. Body weight was the major predictor of metabolic expenditure: heavier women lose weight more rapidly.

Another important fact to keep in mind is that men generally lose weight faster than women of similar height and weight on any given diet because men have more lean body mass and therefore higher energy expenditure. Similarly, older patients have a lower metabolic expenditure and as a rule lose weight more slowly than younger subjects because metabolic rate declines by approximately 2% (or about 100 kcal) per decade (Lin et al., 2003).

When food intake is recorded with food records, actual energy expenditure is usually underestimated. Using doubly labeled water provides a way to estimate energy expenditure over an interval of 10 to 14 days that includes energy expended on resting metabolism and exercise. With this method, most normal-weight people are found to under-report what they eat by 10 to 30%. Overweight people are even less accurate and tend to under-report their intake by 30 to 50% or more (Champagne et al., 2002).

The important message is that adherence to dietary programs is the essential component of success. In a small study in which foods were labeled with non-radioactive carbon so that the amount eaten could be quantified (Lyon et al., 1995), the level of success was directly related to how well the subject adhered to the diet.

The rate of weight loss on any diet is directly related to the difference between the subject's energy intake and energy requirements. An average deficit of 500 kcal per day should result in weight loss of 0.45 kg per week (1 lb./week). When individuals are asked to record their intake, there is considerable variation from day to day, even when the subjects know that their energy expenditure is being measured with doubly labeled water. This is shown in Fig. 1, which shows data on 10 dietitians who recorded what they ate each day for 7 days. As a group, they reported food intake that was within 10% of that measured with doubly labeled water. However, there was wide variability between subjects, often varying by twofold (Edholm et al., 1955; Champagne et al., 2002).

Breakdown of some protein is to be expected during weight loss. When weight increases as a result of overeating, approximately 75% of the extra energy is stored as fat and the remaining 25% as lean tissue. If the lean tissue contains 20% protein, then 5% of the extra weight gain would be protein. Thus, it should be anticipated that during weight loss at least 5% of weight loss will be protein. A desirable feature of any calorie-restricted diet, however, is that it results in the lowest possible loss of protein, recognizing that this will not be less than 5% of the weight that is lost.

Genetic factors are important in determining both weight gain and weight loss. Bouchard et al. (1990) reported a study in which 12 identical male twins ate an extra 1000 kcal per day 6 days a week for 84 days to induce weight gain (*see* Chapter 4). The weight gain varied from 4.3 to 13.3 kg, but most of this difference resulted from genetic factors, not environmental ones.

DIETS REDUCED IN ENERGY OR SPECIFIC MACRONUTRIENTS

Overview

The number of diets is enormous and grows each year as entrepreneurs and health care providers bring forth their latest "ideas" about how to reduce excess fat in the body. As noted earlier, reducing energy intake below expenditure is essential for weight loss to occur. A focus on reducing energy intake is one strategy used by some diets. A second strategy is to change the intake of one or more major nutrients, carbohydrates or fat, or to increase the intake of protein. We will discuss each of these in turn. The overall effect on energy and nutrients from each of these approaches has been analyzed by Freedman et al. (2001) and the Consumers Union, whose data is shown in Table 5.

Diets can be defined by whether they are reduced in energy with a balanced reduction of foods, or whether they focus on reduction of either macronutrients or specific foods.

Types of Reduced Energy Diets

1. Very low-calorie diets (VLCDs) have an energy level at or below 800 kcal per day. (These diets are also called protein-sparing modified fasts because they provide sufficient protein but reduce other macronutrients to very low levels.)
2. Balanced energy deficit diets in which all dietary components are reduced but the total calorie intake is above 800 kcal per day, and usually above 1200 kcal per day for women and 1500 kcal per day for men.
3. Portion-controlled diets using prepared meals (frozen or otherwise low-calorie level), food bars, or portion-sized liquid beverages.
4. Macronutrient-reduced diets
   a. Low-carbohydrate diets.
   b. Low-fat diets.
   c. Fad diets (diets involving unusual combinations of foods or eating sequences).

VERY LOW-CALORIE DIETS

Diets with energy levels between 200 and 800 kcal per day are called very low-calorie diets (VLCDs) or very low-energy diets. If the calorie intake is below 200 kcal per day, the diet is no longer a VLCD, but rather a starvation diet. Complete starvation is the ultimate result of this concept and produces the most rapid weight loss. However, starvation produces problems like hair loss, postural hypotension, uric acid renal stones, and an increased risk of gallstones. Fasting is rarely used for treatment of overweight any more.

The theory behind the VLCD or protein-sparing modified fasting diet is that the lower the energy intake, the more energy would be withdrawn from fat stores and thus accelerate weight and fat loss. Contrary to this theory, weight loss when using a 400 kcal per day VLCD compared with an 800 kcal per day diet was not different, probably because the subjects adapted to the difference by modifying their energy expenditure during activity or during sleep. A systematic review of 29 studies on VLCD that were conducted in the United States has been published. Participants were in a structured weight-loss program that lasted more than 2 years. Anderson et al. (2001) found that

Table 5
Nutritional Content of Several Popular Diets

Diet	Protein (%)	Fat (%)	Saturated fat (%)	Carbohydrate (%)	Fiber g/1000 kcal	Fruit and vegetable daily servings
Atkins	29	60	20	11	12	6
e-Diets	24	23	5	53	19	12
Jenny Craig	20	18	7	62	16	6
Ornish	16	6	1	77	31	17
Slim-Fast	21	22	6	57	21	12
South Beach	22	39	9	38	19	3
Volumetrics	22	23	7	55	20	14
Weight Waters	20	24	7	56	20	11

Adapted from *Consumer Reports*, May 2005, p. 21.

participants on the VLCD lost significantly more than those on hypoenergetic balanced diets (Fig. 3). In the studies that provided data at 5 years, those who had been on the VLCD programs and were available for follow-up body weights maintained a 7.1 kg loss compared with a 2.0 kg loss for those on the hypoenergetic diet groups.

Table 6 shows the commercial programs that are based on use of VLCDs as adapted from the review by Tsai and Wadden (2005).

Protein loss is rapid during the early phases of a VLCD as the body's amino acids are used to produce glucose. With time, protein loss slows to about 3 to 4 g per day. Other benefits include reduction in blood pressure and improvement in hyperglycemia in patients with diabetes. A fall in blood pressure is characteristic during the first week of fasting, and may result in postural hypotension. Antihypertensive drugs, especially calcium channel blockers and diuretics, should usually be discontinued when a VLCD is begun. Most people with diabetes eating VLCDs have marked improvement in hyperglycemia. Blood glucose concentrations fall within the first 1 to 2 weeks, and remain low as long as the diet is continued. Those patients taking less than 50 U insulin or an oral hypoglycemic drug will usually be able to discontinue therapy (Blackburn et al., 1985). In my view, VLCDs should be reserved for subjects who require rapid weight loss for a specific purpose, such as surgery. The weight regain when the diet is stopped is often rapid, and it is better to take a more sustainable approach than to use a method that cannot be sustained. For short periods and under appropriate supervision, these diets have produced significant weight loss. However, after accounting for secondary regain, the average weight loss is no different from that achieved with a balanced energy reduction of lesser magnitude (Wadden et al., 1992; Walsh and Flynn, 1995).

BALANCED ENERGY DEFICIT DIETS

A number of dietary studies have been done using lower calorie (600 kcal per day deficit) diets to treat the complications of overweight, such as hypertension and asthma. A meta-analysis of these studies Avenell et al. (2004) identified 12 studies that evaluated diet versus a control that lasted more than 12 months. Five of these studies examined hypertensives (Treatment of Hypertension Prevention I and II, Hypertension Prevention Trial, Hypertension Optimal Treatment, Trial of Anti-Hypertension

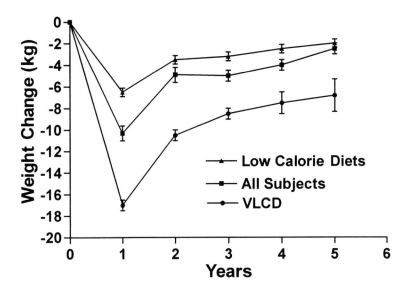

Fig. 3. Weight loss on very low-calorie diets ([VLCDs]; as Redrawn from Anderson VLCD).

Intervention Management, Trial of Non-Pharmacological in the Elderly, and Dietary Intervention Study of Hypertension). One trial examined those with borderline hypertension, one study recruited participants with diabetes, one study recruited participants with asthma, and one studied individuals with a myocardial infarction. At the end of 12 months, the difference between control and treated groups in these 12 studies was –5.31 kg (95% confidence interval [CI] –5.86 to – 4.77 kg). When the group was divided into those with cardiovascular components and those without, there was a clear difference. Those with cardiovascular risk had a 12-month weight loss of – 4.19 kg (95% CI –4.90 to –3.48 kg), compared with those who did not have any risk factors who had a weight loss of –6.98 kg (95% CI –7.83 to – 6.12 kg; Avenell et al., 2004). In another systematic review of studies having more than 100 subjects and a duration of more than 1 year, without pharmacological intervention, Douketis et al. (2005) found 16 studies that met their criteria. After 2 to 3 years, weight loss was usually less than 5 kg below baseline (–3.5 ± 2.4 kg; range 0.9–10.0 kg) and after 4 to 7 years (where there was data) it was –3.6 ± 2.6 kg (Douketis et al., 2005).

The food guide pyramid was developed by the USDA to provide dietary guidance for Americans. The new pyramid depicts an individual walking up stairs to highlight the importance of exercise in a healthy lifestyle. Colors for each of the food groups run up the side of the pyramid. Six different categories are identified in Table 7. The grains group is at one side followed by vegetables, fruits, meat and beans, dairy products, and oils. Several points are emphasized. Whole-grain products are preferred to "highly refined" grain products, such as white bread, white pasta, and white rice. For fruits and vegetables, variety is the word with plenty of blue and red fruits. Bananas tend to be higher in energy and should be eaten in moderation. One hundred percent fruit juices, preferably not from concentrate, are preferred. In the meat and beans group, emphasis should be on fish, poultry (skinless), beans, and nuts with moderated consumption of

Table 6
Commercial VLCD Programs

Name	Group or individual	Diet	Physical activity	Staff
HMR (Health Management Resources)	Group sessions and weekly classes	Low-calorie or VLCD provided by meal replacement products	Walking and calorie charts	Physician and other health care providers
Medifast	Group classes included in Take Shape for Life	Low-calorie or VLCD provided by meal replacement products	May be included in Take Shape for Life	?
Optifast	Group classes and telephone support	Low-calorie diet provided through meal replacement products	Physical activity modules in lifestyle classes	Physician and other health care providers

Adapted from Tsai and Wadden, 2005.
VLCD: very low-calorie diet.

red meat, appropriately trimmed of fat. For the dairy products group, emphasis should be on skim milk and low-fat dairy products and yogurt. In the oils group, liquid vegetable oils that are free of trans fats should be selected. Labels on foods should be examined to select those that have no trans fats.

Planning a low-calorie diet requires the selection of a caloric intake and then selection of foods to meet this intake. It is desirable to eat foods with adequate amounts of protein, carbohydrate, and essential fatty acids. Thus, weight-reducing diets should eliminate alcohol, sugar-containing beverages, and most highly concentrated sweets, because they rarely contain adequate amounts of other nutrients besides energy. One concept is to buy and consume foods that are naturally nutrient-rich. This would mean eating more fruits, vegetables, whole grains (this leaves more of the vitamins from the grain), lower fat meats, fish, poultry, beans, 100% fruit juices (not from concentrate), and yogurt, and eating less of the processed foods in which the nutrients that are naturally present have not been altered, removed, diluted, or otherwise changed (Drewnowski, 2005).

PORTION-CONTROLLED DIETS

Portion-controlled diets (Fig. 4) are another way of achieving a balanced caloric deficit. This can be done most simply by use of individually packaged foods. Formula diet drinks using powdered or liquid formula diets, nutrition bars, and frozen food are alternatives. Frozen low-calorie meals containing 250 to 350 kcal per package can be convenient and nutritious. The use of formula diets or breakfast bars for breakfast, formula diets or a frozen entree for lunch, and a frozen calorie-controlled entree with additional vegetables for dinner has often been recommended. In this way, it is easily possible to obtain a calorie-controlled diet with 1000 to 1500 kcal per day. In one 4-year study, this approach resulted in early initial weight loss, which then was maintained (Flechtner-Mors et al., 2000). The use of formula diets alone is not recommended.

Table 7
New Food Pyramid (MyPyramid)

Food group	Servings	Comments
Grains	7 oz. (men) 6 oz. (women)	Emphasize whole-grain bread, pasta, and brown rice. Be careful with white bread, white pasta, and white rice because refined grains are linked to higher risk of type 2 diabetes.
Vegetables	3 cups	Emphasize variety. Be careful about fried potatoes because these are the leading vegetable with more fat.
Fruits	2 cups	Emphasize variety with plenty of blue and red fruits. Moderation with bananas. Emphasize 100% fruit juices. Limit juices and punches made from concentrate, which is another name for sugar.
Meat and beans	6 oz.	Emphasize fish, poultry (skinless), beans and nuts. Fish can be a good source of omega-3 fatty acids. Trim meats of fat and eat less red meat to reduce saturated fat intake.
Dairy products	3 cups	Emphasize skim milk and low-fat yogurt. If you do not drink milk, take calcium and vitamin D supplements. Be careful with ice cream, butter, and cream.
Oils	6 tsp.	Liquid vegetable oils without trans fats are preferred. Avoid products with trans fats because they are linked to high rates of heart disease.

Adapted with comments from www.MyPyramid.gov.

Low-Carbohydrate Diets

DIETARY CARBOHYDRATE, DIETARY FIBER, AND GLYCEMIC INDEX

Dietary carbohydrate comes from the starch in plant foods and from the small molecules that contain glucose, fructose, galactose, maltose, lactose, or sucrose found in many fruits and milk. Dietary fiber represents the plant carbohydrates that are difficult or impossible for the normal enzymes in the human body to digest. Fibers are usually divided into water-soluble and -insoluble kinds, depending on whether they can be dissolved in water or not. Within the human body, the major source of carbohydrate is glycogen stored in the liver or muscles, along with glucose that is formed by breakdown of the glycogen.

Sugars are often added to food and provide an additional source of carbohydrates. Of the foods that provide more than 5% of added sugar to the diet, the following items are major contributors: regular soft drinks contribute 33%; sugars and candies, 16.1%; cakes, cookies, and pies, 12.9%; fruit drinks (including fruit punch), 9.7%; dairy desserts and milk products, 8.6%; and other items 5.8% (2005b). (So that the buyer can beware, added sugars can be listed as "brown sugar, corn sweetener, corn syrup, dextrose, fructose, fruit juice concentrate, glucose, HFCS, honey, invert sugar, lactose, maltose, malt syrup, molasses, raw sugar, sucrose, sugar, and syrup"). When shopping, try to avoid any juice that is made from concentrate, if possible.

LOW-GLYCEMIC-INDEX DIETS

The glycemic index is one way of expressing the ease with which glucose can be made available from plant foods. It is based on measurement of the rise in blood glucose

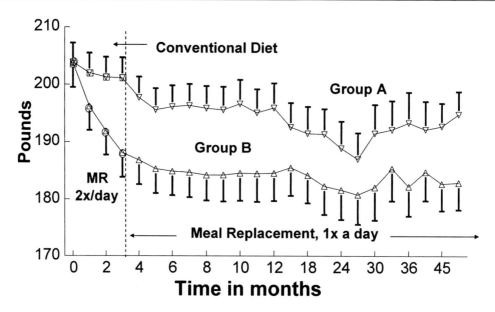

Fig. 4. Portion-controlled diet and body weight over 4 years.

Table 8
Table of Glycemic Index Values for Various Foods

Food	Glycemic index	Glycemic load
Instant rice	91	24.8
Baked potato	85	20.3
Corn flakes	84	21.0
White bread	70	21.0
Rye bread	65	19.5
Banana	53	13.3
Spaghetti	41	16.4
Apple	36	8.1
Lentil beans	29	5.7

Source: Adapted from Ludwig, 2002.

in the test food compared with the rise after a 50-g portion of white bread (Ludwig, 2002). Foods with a high glycemic index are those that have a rapid digestion and rapid rise in blood glucose. Low-glycemic-index foods usually come with fiber and are more slowly digested and thus produce a slower rise in blood glucose. Table 8 is a list of the glycemic index of some foods. The glycemic load refers to the quantity of carbohydrate in a food multiplied by the glycemic index of that food. Carrots, for example, have a high glycemic index because the carbohydrate they have is rapidly digested. However, they have a low glycemic load because there is not much carbohydrate in carrots. In a review of six studies, investigators documented that the consumption of foods with a high glycemic index was associated with higher energy intake than when the foods had a low glycemic index (Ludwig, 2002). In his review, Ludwig (2002) notes that lower satiety, increased hunger, and/or increased voluntary food intake was noted in 15 of 16 single-day studies comparing high- and low-glycemic-index test meals. Among 13 studies, 10 showed that subjects eating a low-glycemic-index diet had lower triglycerides and lower total/high-density lipoprotein (HDL)-cholesterol ratios.

Thus, higher-fiber foods with a low glycemic index, which release carbohydrates more slowly, stimulate less food intake than foods with a high glycemic index in which glucose is rapidly released. In addition to the role of the glycemic index, data have shown that high-fiber diets are associated with decreased weight. However, a randomized clinical trial of a low-glycemic-load diet and a conventional diet failed to show any difference in weight loss between the two diets. However, those on the lower glycemic load diet had a higher resting energy expenditure, lower triglycerides, and less insulin resistance (Pereira et al., 2004). Thus, to eating foods with more fiber can have benefits over and above any effect on body weight and make good nutritional sense.

LOW-CARBOHYDRATE HIGH-PROTEIN DIETS

Low-carbohydrate high-protein diets have been popular for nearly 150 years when a layman named William Banting published a small pamphlet describing how he had lost weight. His weight loss of more than 50 pounds during the year he used his diet is shown in Fig. 5. His diet became an immediate hit, and for much of the last half of the 19th century, weight-loss programs were referred to as Bantingism. The low-fat high-protein theme he introduced has been revived over and over again for more than 150 years, with the Atkins diet being one of the most profitable renditions.

In spite of the popularity of low-carbohydrate high-protein diets, they have been widely criticized by health care providers because these diets are often high in saturated fat with unproven benefits. The safety of low-carbohydrate high-protein diets have been criticized because they are high in protein and fat, and because they are ketogenic and may induce calcium loss. These concerns have been tested in several clinical trials that have shown little effect on lipids but have left the concern about bone health. In a clinical trial in which 32 subjects aged 50 years were randomly assigned to a high- or low-protein diet (meat supplements of approximately 55 g per day or 3 g per day exchanged isocalorically for carbohydrates), urinary calcium excretion was the same in both groups, but the high-protein diet was associated with an increase in serum insulin-like growth factor-1 concentrations and a decrease in urinary N-telopeptides (Dawson-Hughes et al., 2004), which suggests that high-protein diets can cause calcium loss (Reddy et al., 2002).

The concern about detrimental effects on serum lipids has been largely eliminated (Hays et al., 2003; Willett, 2004). In three clinical trials (Brehm et al., 2003; Foster et al., 2003; Samaha et al., 2003), a very low-carbohydrate, high-protein diet designed after that of Dr. Atkins was compared with a control diet. All three of these studies agreed in finding no significant effects on lipids. In a meta-analysis of low-carbohydrate versus low-fat diets including these three studies plus two others, Nordmann et al. (2006) found significantly more weight loss at 6 months favoring the low-carbohydrate diet (–3.3 kg, 95% CI –5.3 to –1.4 kg) but that this benefit had been lost by 12 months (–1.0 kg 95% CI –3.5 to 1.5 kg) (Fig. 6). Changes in lipids varied between diets. The low-carbohydrate diet produced a more favorable change in triglycerides and HDL-cholesterol, whereas the low-fat diets were more favorable for changes in total cholesterol and low-density lipoprotein (LDL)-cholesterol.

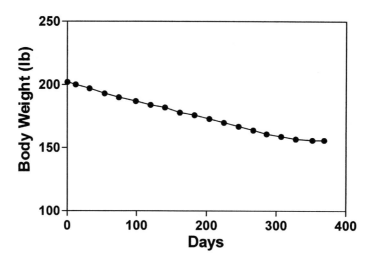

Fig. 5. Weight loss curve for Mr. Banting during the first year on this diet during 1861–1862.

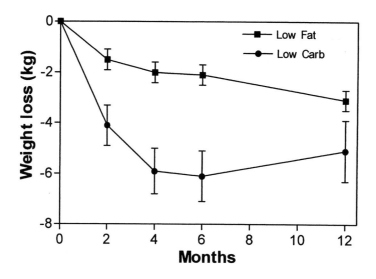

Fig. 6. Weight loss on a very low-carbohydrate diet compared with a control diet over 1 year. (Redrawn from Stern et al., 2004.)

From the patient's perspective, the advantage of the very low-carbohydrate high-protein diet is that it produces rapid weight loss because of the acute reduction in glycogen stores, with loss of the associated water. A systematic review of 107 studies using low-carbohydrate diets concluded that there was insufficient evidence to recommend for or against them (Bravata et al., 2003). However, data from four randomized clinical trials of at least 6 months duration that have compared low-carbohydrate diets (with no restrictions on amount or type of fat) with low-fat diets show greater increases in serum HDL-cholesterol in two of the studies (Foster et al., 2003; Yancy et al., 2004) and greater decreases in serum triglyceride concentrations were observed in three of the trials (Foster et al., 2003; Stern et al., 2004; Yancy et al., 2004). There were no significant differences in serum LDL-cholesterol or glucose. Unfortunately, the dropout rates were high in these trials, ranging from 21 to 39% with both types of diet. In addition, some of the additional early weight loss observed with the low-carbohydrate diets could be a result of fluid loss (although information on this was not provided) (*see* below for head-to-head comparison of diets).

High-Protein Diets

Dietary protein is essential for all aspects of growth and development, and it may play a role in modulating food intake and body weight regain after weight loss (Westerterp-Plantenga, 2003). The quantity of protein in the diet has been nearly constant for the past century since Atwater first estimated it to be about 15% of energy intake. Protein comes from both plant and animal sources. The percentage distribution of individual amino acids in animal proteins is closer to those of humans than it is to plant proteins, which are often low in one or another amino acid. It is thus desirable to get protein from a variety of sources, including meat, fish, poultry, beans, and nuts.

Effects of varying protein have been tested in weight-loss diets. One study compared 15 and 25% protein diets. Each diet had the same fat content and thus differed in carbohydrate content. Weight loss over 6 months was greater with the higher-protein diet (Skov et al., 1999). In follow-up at 12 and 24 months, Due et al. (2004) found that the higher-protein diet group had regained weight, but were still less heavy than the medium protein group and still 6 kg below their baseline weight, which was similar to the 5.5-kg weight loss in the control group. At the 2 year follow-up, there were only 5 of the original 23 in the medium protein group and 11 of the 23 in the high protein group (Fig. 7). The body weights were the same and about 8 to 10 kg below their initial baseline. This is indeed a very impressive 2-year result for a lower-fat diet, but does not suggest that one protein level is superior to the other (Hu, 2005).

The interaction of dietary protein with exercise on body composition and weight loss was examined in a 4-month trial by Layman et al. (2005). A total of 48 women with a BMI lower than 26 kg/m^2 and a body weight less than 160 kg were randomized to four groups. Two groups received 15% protein diets and the other two received 30% protein with energy levels of 7.1 MJ per day (1500 kcal per day). The two diet groups were divided into either a lifestyle activity group or a supervised exercise group that did supervised walking 5 days a week plus resistance training 2 days per week. At the end of 4 months, the high-protein group with or without exercise lost more body weight and body fat than the low-protein group. Exercise preserved lean body mass and enhanced fat loss. In another pair of 3-month studies, however, there was no difference in weight loss with high-protein compared with moderate-protein diets, but there was no exercise program included, which may have been an important oversight (Luscombe-Marsh et al., 2005; Noakes et al., 2005).

High-protein diets have also been shown to enhance weight maintenance (Westerterp-Plantenga et al., 2004). Following weight loss with a VLCD for 4 weeks, 148 male and female subjects with a baseline BMI of 29.5 kg/m^2 were stratified by age, BMI, body weight, restrained eating, and resting energy expenditure and randomized to a control condition or a supplement of 48.2 g per day of additional protein. Both groups received regular visits and counseling by the dietitian at the university clinic. At the end of 3 months, the group receiving the protein supplement (which brought protein intake to 18%) had a 50% lower body weight regain, which consisted only of protein, than the unsupplemented group (whose protein intake was about 15%). The protein-supplemented

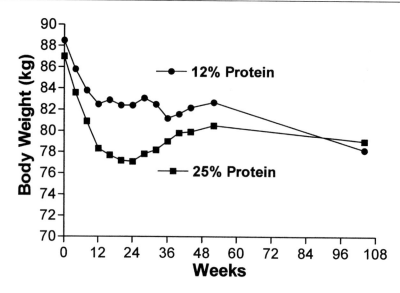

Fig. 7. Effect of high- and low-protein diets on weight loss. (Redrawn from Due & Astrup 2004.)

group had increased satiety and lower increases in triglycerides and leptin. Resting energy expenditure, Respiratory Quotient (RQ), and total energy expenditure were similar between the two groups.

Dietary Fat, Energy Density, and Low-Fat Diets

Dietary fat includes the fats and oils used in cooking, those hidden in foods, as well as sterols, of which cholesterol is the most widely recognized. Whether the fats and oils in one's diet are solid or liquid depends on the kind of fatty acids of which they are made. From the nutritional perspective, saturated fats and trans fats pose the greatest health risk. There is no health value in eating foods with trans fats in them, but these fats, which are the result of commercial hydorgenization, are cheap to make and are often found in processed foods. Eliminating trans fats from the diet and reducing saturated fats to less than 10% is a worthwhile nutritional goal. Table 9 shows the way in which reducing fats in the diet can also reduce energy intake. A number of food items have a considerable amount of fat and might easily be reduced in the diet of normal weight and overweight people. For example, cheese can contain up to 13% saturated fat; beef, 11.7%; oils, 4.9%; ice cream, 4.7%; butter, 4.6%; salad dressing, 4.4%; poultry, 3.6%; and sausage, 3.2% (2005a). In commercial foods, trans fats have been found in up to 40% of the fat in cakes, cookies, crackers, pies, and bread. In animal products, trans fats can be up to 20% or more of the fat. In some margarines, they are up to 17%. Fried potatoes can have 8%; potato chips, corn chips, and popcorn, 5%; and household shortening, 4% (2005a). Buyers should look for foods that say they contain no trans fats.

Low-fat diets range in fat from 10% in the Ornish diet to diets with 25 to 30% fat as recommended by the American Heart Association (AHA). Diets with fat levels less than 30% of total intake are consistent with the recommendations of the AHA. Low-fat diets decrease total cholesterol and LDL-cholesterol levels. In the short term, they may also decrease HDL-cholesterol levels, but with continued dieting and weight loss, HDL-cholesterol levels usually increase over 3 to 6 months (Kris-Etherton et al., 1999).

Table 9
Comparison of Normal and Lower-Fat Options

Food item	Full-fat option		Lower fat option	
	Saturated fat (g)	Energy (kcal)	Saturated fat (g)	Energy (kcal)
Cheese (1 oz.)	6.0	114	1.2	49
Ground beef (3 oz. cooked)	6.1	236	2.6	148
Milk (1 cup or 8 oz.)	4.6	146	1.5	102
Breads (medium croissant versus medium bagel)	6.6	231	0.2	227
Frozen dessert (regular ice cream versus low-fat frozen yogurt [½ cup])	4.9	145	2.0	110
Table Spreads (butter versus soft margarine with zero trans fat)	2.4	34	0.7	25
Chicken (fried chicken leg with skin versus roasted chicken breast no skin [3 oz.])	3.3	212	0.9	140
Fish (fresh fish versus baked fish [3 oz.])	2.8	195	1.5	129

Adapted from the Dietary Guidelines 2005.

The amount of weight lost with low-fat diets is related to the degree of fat reduction. A 10% decrease in dietary fat will reduce body fat by approximately 6 g per day, or more than 4 kg in 6 months (Astrup, 2001; Bray and Popkin, 1998). The rate weight is regained is slower in patients eating a low-fat diet than in patients eating a calorie-restricted diet (Toubro, 1997). However, the use of low-fat diets is not associated with long-term maintenance of reduced body weight, implying that older eating habits with higher calorie intake return.

LOW-FAT DIETS

Low-fat diets are one of the standard strategies to help patients lose weight. A key reason is that high-fat diets, especially diets high in saturated and trans fatty acids, have been associated with the development of overweight, heart disease, and certain forms of cancer, among other adverse effects (Bray and Popkin, 1998). Almost all dietary guidelines recommend a daily intake of fat of 20 to 35% of energy intake or less (HHS and USDA, 2005). In addition, one report noted that people who successfully keep their weight reduced adopt three strategies, one of which is eating a lower-fat diet (Forcyt and Goodrick, 1991). The effect of low-fat diets has been examined in a meta-analysis. One concern about the recommendation of low-fat diets is that the population has continued to gain weight and some have suggested that the low-fat recommendation may have played a detrimental role. A recent large randomized clinical trial of low-fat versus control diets that included 48,835 women made this interpretation of the obesity epidemic unlikely. Howard et al. (2006) randomly assigned women from the Women's Health Initiative to low-fat or control diets and followed them. The food records showed that the group assigned to the low-fat diet did reduce fat intake from 38.8% to an average of 29.8% compared with 38.8% in the control group, which remained almost constant (38.1% at end of study). Weight loss was 2.2 kg at 1 year and 0.6 kg at an average of 7.5 years of follow-up. The reduction was similar across BMI groups, but there was a clear relationship between the decrease in percent fat and weight loss ($p < 0.001$ for trend). Weight loss was also associated with greater consumption of fruits and vegetables. Thus low-fat diets can produce modest and prolonged benefit.

In contrast with the value of low-fat diets for prevention of weight gain as discussed earlier, is the issue of their role in weight loss. In the analysis by Bray and Popkin (1998), the reduction of dietary fat intake of 10% predicted an early fat loss of about 6 g per day or about 4 kg in 6 months. In a meta-analysis of weight-loss studies, Astrup et al. (2000) found that over the first 6 months low-fat diets produced weight loss and that heavier individuals lost more weight. A few randomized clinical trials of low-fat diets have been conducted, and Pirozzo et al. (2003) conducted a meta-analysis of them. The five randomized controlled trials that were included in the analysis compared low-fat diets with a control diet. The authors concluded that low-fat diets produced significant weight loss, but no more so than the control diets against which they were compared (Fig. 8). Weight regain occurs when treatments for overweight are discontinued, whether they be low-fat or low-carbohydrate diets.

A low-fat diet can be implemented in two ways. First, the dietitian can provide the subject with specific menu plans that emphasize the use of reduced fat foods. As a guideline, remember that if a food "melts" in your mouth, it probably has fat in it.

Second, subjects can be instructed in counting fat grams. Fat has 9.4 kcal/g. It is thus very easy to calculate the number of grams of fat a subject can eat for any given level of energy intake. Counting fat grams is an alternative to counting calories. Many experts recommend keeping calories from fat to below 30% of total calories. In practical terms, this means eating about 33 g of fat for each 1000 calories in the diet. For simplicity, I use 30 g of fat or less for each 1000 kcal. For a 1500 calorie diet, this would mean about 45 g/d or less of fat, which can be counted using the nutrition information labels on food packages.

MODERATE-FAT MEDITERRANEAN-TYPE DIETS

A clinical trial of a Mediterranean-style diet, similar to the Mediterranean step-1 diet of the AHA, provided instruction in nutrition to reduce body weight by 10% by eating a diet consisting of 1300 kcal per day with 50 to 60% carbohydrates, 15 to 20% protein, less than 30% fat (<10% saturated fat) with 10 to 15% from monounsaturated fats and 5 to 8% from polyunsaturated fat. Fiber was prescribed at 18 g per 1000 calories. Women were also given behavioral weight-loss instruction on setting personal weight-loss goals and self-monitoring with food diaries with regular behaviorally oriented sessions (Esposito et al., 2003). After 2 years in the trial, body weight had decreased 14 kg in the intervention group of 60 women but only 3 kg in the control group. Blood pressure, glucose, and insulin also improved more in the group with the Mediterranean diet, as did adiponectin, interleukin 6 and 18, and C-reactive protein. This moderate weight-loss diet is clearly one of the most impressive longer-term follow-up studies.

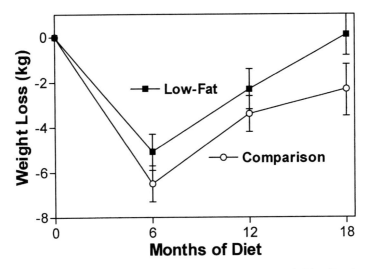

Fig. 8. Meta-analysis of five low-fat diets. (Pirozzo et al. Obes Rev.)

POPULAR DIETS

Overview

Many popular diets are on the bookshelf, and a new crop appears each year promising success where the others failed (Dansinger et al., 2005; Freedman et al., 2001; Gardner et al., 2007). Among the current crop are The Sonoma Diet, which touts small portion sizes of sun-drenched California cuisine with red or white wine; How the Rich Get Thin, which stresses daily exercise, avoidance of processed foods, a high intake of calcium and high-quality protein; The Flavor Point Diet, which has monotony as its buzz-word—that is, limiting your choices; The Rice Diet Solution whose title tells the story; The Supermarket Diet, which steers you toward produce and away from processed foods; and The QOD (every other day) Diet, which touts alternating 400 kcal on one day with a larger intake on the next. The major differences are the gimmicks, which are designed to lower the intake of calories, fat and/or carbohydrates, or to increase energy expenditure or both.

Ignoring the gimmicks, most popular diets can be grouped into very low-fat, moderate-fat, or high-fat categories. A recent analysis of these diets by Consumers Union has been adapted in Table 5. Included in this analysis are low-carbohydrate diets (Atkins), low-fat diets (Ornish), low-glycemic-index diet (South Beach), computer diets (e-Diets), energy density diets (Volumetrics), portion-controlled diets (Slim-Fast), and commercial groups (Jenny Craig and Weight Watchers). The Ornish diet (Ornish, 1993) and the Pritikin diet (Pritikin, 1991,which is not included in the table) are two examples of very low-fat diets. Nutritional analysis has shown that the Ornish diet provides only 13 g of fat (6%; Freedman et al., 2001) Carbohydrate intake in this dietary program is the highest of all the popular diets. Maintaining a very low-fat diet can be difficult in this society with its abundance of high-fat foods, but for those who do adhere to the diet, weight loss can be substantial. An additional benefit from this very low level of fat is the slowing or reversal of coronary artery disease. The Atkins diet is clearly the highest in fat, with the South Beach second highest. The Ornish diet and the Volumetrics diet have the highest amount of fruits and vegetables (Table 5).

Two examples of the moderate-fat low-calorie diet are the Sugar Busters! diet (Steward et al., 2002) and the Weight Watchers diet. Fat intakes with these diets are nearly the same, at 44 and 42 g per day, respectively (Freedman et al., 2001). Carbohydrate intakes also are similar, but the type of carbohydrate differs. The Sugar Busters! diet emphasizes the use low-glycemic-index foods (that is, foods that have higher fiber content and thus absorb glucose more slowly). The Glucose Revolution (Brand-Miller et al., 2003) is another popular diet that uses foods with a low glycemic index as the basis for a higher-fiber, lower-calorie diet.

The third group of diets is the very low-carbohydrate, high-fat, high-protein diets. The most popular example in this category is the Atkins diet (Atkins, 2002). Nutritional analysis of the Atkins diet has shown 75 g of fat in the induction diet, which increased to 114 g of fat during the maintenance diet (Freedman et al., 2001). Carbohydrate intake on the Atkins diet is 13 g per day during induction, and this level increases to 95 g per day during maintenance. The Carbohydrate Addict's diet (Heller, 1993) has a similarly high level of fat but a somewhat less restrictive level of carbohydrates, at 87 g per day (Freedman et al., 2001). When carbohydrate intake is less than 50 g per day, ketosis uniformly develops. One concern with ketosis is the source of the cations needed to excrete the ketones. If the cations consist of calcium from the bone, this process may enhance the risk of bone loss.

Comparison of Popular Diets

Any diet that results in a decrease in calorie intake will achieve weight loss. This was nicely demonstrated in a head-to-head comparison of four popular diets, including the Atkins diet, the Ornish diet, Weight Watchers, and the Zone diet (Dansinger et al., 2005) (Fig. 9). In this randomized 12-month trial, each diet produced weight loss of about 5 kg, but there was no difference between diets. In a second head-to-head comparison of four diets, the subjects were young women. Here, the Atkins diet was modestly but significantly better than the Ornish, LEARN, or Protein Power approaches (Gardner et al., 2007). With each diet some patients lost significant amounts of weight. Adherence to the diet was the most important single criterion of success in the first trial. With most diets, however, these losses were not maintained, and patients tended to regain weight as their previous eating habits returned. Thus, the physician should encourage patients to try different diets because the placebo effect is an important component of each of them.

COMMERCIAL WEIGHT-LOSS PROGRAMS

A number of commercial and self-help programs, including Overeaters Anonymous, Take Off Pounds Sensibly, Weight Watchers, Jenny Craig, Herbalife, OPTIFAST, LA Health, and e-Diets are available to help the consumer. Tsai and Wadden (2005) examined the effectiveness of a number of these programs (Table 10). Balanced-deficit diets, such as the Weight Watchers diet (derived from the Prudent Diet of Jolliffe), are the other way of reducing calories by using a balanced decrease in macronutrients. They included randomized trials that lasted at least 12 weeks and enrolled only adults as well as case series that met their criteria and stated the number of enrollees with an evaluation of 1 year or longer. Ten studies met their selection criteria.

There are three commercial weight-loss programs shown in Table 10. The effects of the Weight Watchers program was evaluated in three randomized controlled trials. In one trial lasting 2 years and including 423 subjects, the participants in the intervention group attended the Weight Watchers meetings and experienced a mean

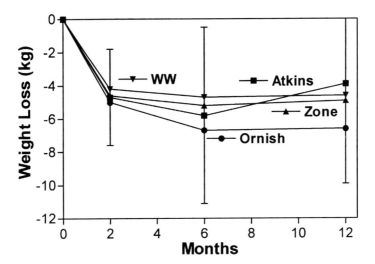

Fig. 9. Comparison of four popular diets. (Dansiger JAMA 2005.)

Table 10
Components of Commercial Weight-Loss Programs

Name	Group or individual	Diet	Physical activity	Staff
Weight Watchers	Group	Low-calorie exchange	Yes	Successful lifetime member
Jenny Craig	Individual	Pre-packaged foods	Yes	Company-trained counselor
LA Weight Loss	Individual	Low-calorie	Yes	Licensed physician and other health care providers

Adapted from Tsai and Wadden, 2005.

weight loss of 5.3% at 1 year and 3.2% at 2 years compared with 1.5% at 1 year and 0% weight loss for the control group that received the self-help intervention with two visits to a dietitian (Heshka et al., 2003). The Weight Watchers diet does not focus on the glycemic index, but rather uses a balanced nutrient reduction to lower calories (Fig. 10). The Volumetrics diet (Rolls and Barnett, 2000) emphasizes the need to eat less energy-dense foods. The theory is that filling the stomach with low-fat, high-fiber foods that have low energy density will reduce hunger and produce satiety.

In two other smaller studies, there was evidence favoring those who attended the Weight Watchers program (Tsai and Wadden, 2005). In their review, they presented two case series with the Weight Watchers program, one case series with the Jenny Craig program, but no published evaluation of LA Weight Loss.

CONCLUSION

This chapter focused on dietary strategies as a way to reduce energy intake. From the perspective of an overweight patient, the reduction in energy intake is the most

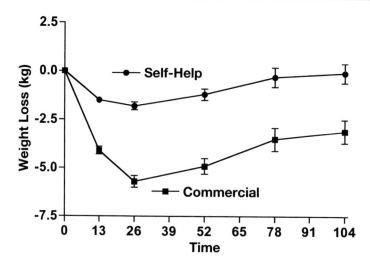

Fig. 10. Commercial versus self-help plans for weight loss.

effective way of acutely redressing the energy imbalance that has over months to years produced the extra body fat. The next two chapters consider the important techniques flowing from behavior modification and exercise that can be used to augment any dietary program and turn to the use of physical activity as a way to bolster efforts to maintain lower body weight.

REFERENCES

(2005a). Dietary Fats. Retrieved April 10, 2006. Available from: http://www.nhlbisupport.com/chd1/ Tipsheets/tipsheet.satfat.htm.

(2005b). Dietary Guidelines for Americans 2005. Retrieved April 7, 2006. Available from: http://www. healthierus.gov/dietaryguidelines/.

Department of Health and Human Services (HHS) and the Department of Agriculture (USDA). (2005). Dietary Guidelines for Americans 2005. Retrieved April 7, 2006. Available from: http://www.healthierus.gov/ dietaryguidelines/.

Anderson, J. W., et al. (2001). Long-term weight-loss maintenance: a meta-analysis of US studies. Am J Clin Nutr 74(5):579–584.

Appel, L. J., et al. (1997). A clinical trial of the effects of dietary patterns on blood pressure. DASH Collaborative Research Group. N Engl J Med 336(16):1117–1124.

Astrup, A. (2001). The role of dietary fat in the prevention and treatment of obesity. Efficacy and safety of low-fat diets. Int J Obes Relat Metab Disord 25(Suppl 1):S46–S50.

Astrup, A., et al. (2000). The role of low-fat diets in body weight control: a meta-analysis of ad libitum dietary intervention studies. Int J Obes Relat Metab Disord 24(12):1545–1552.

Atkins, R. C. (2002). Dr. Atkins's New Diet Revolution. New York: Avon.

Avenell, A., et al. (2004). Systematic review of the long-term effects and economic consequences of treatments for obesity and implications for health improvement. Health Technol Assess 8(21):iii–iv, 1–182.

Blackburn, G. L., et al. (1985). Management of obesity by severe caloric restriction. Littleton, MA: PSG Publishing.

Bouchard, C., et al. (1990). The response to long-term overfeeding in identical twins. N Engl J Med 322(21):1477–1482.

Brand-Miller, J., et al. (2003). The New Glucose Revolution: The Glycemic Index Solution for a Healthier Future. New York: Avalon Publishing Group.

Bravata, D. M., et al. (2003). Efficacy and safety of low-carbohydrate diets: a systematic review. JAMA 289(14):1837–1850.

Bray, G. A. and Popkin, B. M. (1998). Dietary fat intake does affect obesity! Am J Clin Nutr 68(6): 1157–1173.

Brehm, B. J., et al. (2003). A randomized trial comparing a very low carbohydrate diet and a calorie-restricted low fat diet on body weight and cardiovascular risk factors in healthy women. J Clin Endocrinol Metab 88(4):1617–1623.

Brehm, B. J., et al. (2005). The role of energy expenditure in the differential weight loss in obese women on low-fat and low-carbohydrate diets. J Clin Endocrinol Metab 90(3):1475–1482.

Champagne, C. M., et al. (2002). Energy intake and energy expenditure: a controlled study comparing dietitians and non-dietitians. J Am Diet Assoc 102(10):1428–1432.

Cordain, L., et al. (2005). Origins and evolution of the Western diet: health implications for the 21st century. Am J Clin Nutr 81(2):341–354.

Craddick, S. R., et al. (2003). The DASH diet and blood pressure. Curr Atheroscler Rep 5(6):484–491.

Dansinger, M. L., et al. (2005). Comparison of the Atkins, Ornish, Weight Watchers, and Zone diets for weight loss and heart disease risk reduction: a randomized trial. JAMA 293(1):43–53.

Dawson-Hughes, B., et al. (2004). Effect of dietary protein supplements on calcium excretion in healthy older men and women. J Clin Endocrinol Metab 89(3):1169–1173.

Dorland, W. A. N. (2003). Dorland's Illustrated Medical Dictionary. Philadelphia: W.B. Saunders Company.

Douketis, J. D., et al. (2005). Systematic review of long-term weight loss studies in obese adults: clinical significance and applicability to clinical practice. Int J Obes (Lond) 29(10):1153–1167.

Drewnowski, A. (2005). Concept of a nutritious food: toward a nutrient density score. Am J Clin Nutr 82(4):721–732.

Due, A., et al. (2004). Effect of normal-fat diets, either medium or high in protein, on body weight in overweight subjects: a randomised 1-year trial. Int J Obes Relat Metab Disord 28(10):1283–1290.

Edholm, O. G., et al. (1955). The energy expenditure and food intake of individual men. Br J Nutr 9(3): 286–300.

Esposito, K., et al. (2003). Effect of weight loss and lifestyle changes on vascular inflammatory markers in obese women: a randomized trial. JAMA 289(14):1799–1804.

Flechtner-Mors, M., et al. (2000). Metabolic and weight loss effects of long-term dietary intervention in obese patients: four-year results. Obes Res 8(5):399–402.

Foreyt, J. P. and Goodrick, G. K. (1991). Factors common to successful therapy for the obese patient. Med Sci Sports Exerc 23(3):292–297.

Foster, G. D., et al. (2003). A randomized trial of a low-carbohydrate diet for obesity. N Engl J Med 348(21):2082–2090.

Freedman, M. R., et al. (2001). Popular diets: a scientific review. Obes Res 9(Suppl 1):1S–40S.

Gardner, C. D., Kiazand, A., Alhassan, S., et al. (2007). Comparison of the Atkins, Zone, Ornish, and LEARN diets for change in weight and related risk factors among overweight, premenopausal women. JAMA 297:969–977.

Garrow, J. S. (1981). Treat Obesity Seriously: A Clinical Manual. New York: Churchill Livingston.

Hays, J. H., et al. (2003). Effect of a high saturated fat and no-starch diet on serum lipid subfractions in patients with documented atherosclerotic cardiovascular disease. Mayo Clin Proc 78(11):1331–1336.

Heller, R. F. (1993). The Carbohydrate Addict's Diet: the Lifelong Solution to Yo-Yo Dieting. New York: Signet.

Heshka, S., et al. (2003). Weight loss with self-help compared with a structured commercial program: a randomized trial. JAMA 289(14):1792–1798.

Howard, B. V., et al. (2006). Low-fat dietary pattern and weight change over 7 years: the Women's Health Initiative Dietary Modification Trial. JAMA 295(1):39–49.

Hu, F. B. (2005). Protein, body weight, and cardiovascular health. Am J Clin Nutr 82(1 Suppl):242S–247S.

Keys, A., et al. (1950). The Biology of Human Starvation, vols. 1 and 2. Minneapolis: University of Minnesota Press.

Kinsell, L. W., et al. (1964). Calories do count. Metabolism 13:195–204.

Kris-Etherton, P. M., et al. (1999). High-monounsaturated fatty acid diets lower both plasma cholesterol and triacylglycerol concentrations. Am J Clin Nutr 70(6):1009–1015.

Layman, D. K., et al. (2005). Dietary protein and exercise have additive effects on body composition during weight loss in adult women. J Nutr 135(8):1903–1910.

Lin, P. H., et al. (2003). Estimation of energy requirements in a controlled feeding trial. Am J Clin Nutr 77(3):639–645.

Ludwig, D. S. (2002). The glycemic index: physiological mechanisms relating to obesity, diabetes, and cardiovascular disease. JAMA 287(18):2414–2423.

Luscombe-Marsh, N. D., et al. (2005). Carbohydrate-restricted diets high in either monounsaturated fat or protein are equally effective at promoting fat loss and improving blood lipids. Am J Clin Nutr 81(4):762–772.

Lyon, X. H., et al. (1995). Compliance to dietary advice directed towards increasing the carbohydrate to fat ratio of the everyday diet. Int J Obes Relat Metab Disord 19(4):260–269.

Metcalf, N. (2005). Rating the diets from Atkins to Dr. Sears Zonc. Consumer Reports, May 7, 2005.

Moore, T., et al. (2003). The DASH Diet for Hypertension. New York: Simon & Schuster.

National Institute of Health, National Heart, Lung and Blood Institute, et al. (2000). Practical guide in identification, evaluation and treatment of overweight and obesity in adults. Bethesda, MD: National Institutes of Health.

Noakes, M., et al. (2005). Effect of an energy-restricted, high-protein, low-fat diet relative to a conventional high-carbohydrate, low-fat diet on weight loss, body composition, nutritional status, and markers of cardiovascular health in obese women. Am J Clin Nutr 81(6):1298–1306.

Nordmann, A. J., et al. (2006). Effects of low-carbohydrate vs low-fat diets on weight loss and cardiovascular risk factors: a meta-analysis of randomized controlled trials. Arch Intern Med 166(3):285–293.

Ornish, D. (1993). Eat More, Weigh Less: Dr. Dean Ornish's Life Choice Program for Losing Weight Safely While Eating Abundantly. New York: HarperCollins.

Pereira, M. A., et al. (2004). Effects of a low-glycemic load diet on resting energy expenditure and heart disease risk factors during weight loss. JAMA 292(20):2482–2490.

Pirozzo, S., et al. (2003). Should we recommend low-fat diets for obesity? Obes Rev 4(2):83–90.

Popkin, B. M., et al. (2006). A new proposed guidance system for beverage consumption in the United States. Am J Clin Nutr 83(3):529–542.

Pritikin, R. (1991). The New Pritikin Program: The Easy and Delicious Way to Shed Fat, Lower Your Cholesterol, and Stay Fit. New York: Pocket Books.

Reddy, S. T., et al. (2002). Effect of low-carbohydrate high-protein diets on acid-base balance, stone-forming propensity, and calcium metabolism. Am J Kidney Dis 40(2):265–274.

Rolls, B. J. and Barnett, R. A. (2000). Volumetrics: Feel Full on Fewer Calories. New York: HarperCollins.

Sacks, F. M., et al. (2001). Effects on blood pressure of reduced dietary sodium and the Dietary Approaches to Stop Hypertension (DASH) diet. DASH-Sodium Collaborative Research Group. N Engl J Med 344(1):3–10.

Samaha, F. F., et al. (2003). A low-carbohydrate as compared with a low-fat diet in severe obesity. N Engl J Med 348(21):2074–2081.

Skov, A. R., et al. (1999). Randomized trial on protein vs carbohydrate in ad libitum fat reduced diet for the treatment of obesity. Int J Obes Relat Metab Disord 23(5):528–536.

Stern, L., et al. (2004). The effects of low-carbohydrate versus conventional weight loss diets in severely obese adults: one-year follow-up of a randomized trial. Ann Intern Med 140(10):778–785.

Steward, H. L., et al. (2002). The New Sugar Busters! Cut Sugar to Trim Fat. New York: Ballantine.

Stookey, J. D., et al. (2007). The altered fluid distribution in obesity may reflect plasma hypertonicity. Eur J Clin Nutr 61(2):190–199.

Toubro, S., et al. (1997). Randomized comparison of diets for maintaining obese subjects weight after major weight loss: ad lib, low fat, high carbohydrate diet V fixed energy intake. BMJ 314(7073):29–34.

Tsai, A. G. and Wadden, T. A. (2005). Systematic review: an evaluation of major commercial weight loss programs in the United States. Ann Intern Med 142(1):56–66.

Wadden, T. A., et al. (1992). A multicenter evaluation of a proprietary weight reduction program for the treatment of marked obesity. Arch Intern Med 152(5):961–966.

Walsh, M. F. and Flynn, T. J. (1995). A 54-month evaluation of a popular very low calorie diet program. J Fam Pract 41(3):231–236.

Westerterp-Plantenga, M. S. (2003). The significance of protein in food intake and body weight regulation. Curr Opin Clin Nutr Metab Care 6(6):635–638.

Westerterp-Plantenga, M. S., et al. (2004). High protein intake sustains weight maintenance after body weight loss in humans. Int J Obes Relat Metab Disord 28(1):57–64.

Willett, W. C. (2004). Reduced-carbohydrate diets: no roll in weight management? Ann Intern Med 140(10):836–837.

Yancy, W. S., et al. (2004). A low-carbohydrate, ketogenic diet versus a low-fat diet to treat obesity and hyperlipidemia: a randomized, controlled trial. Ann Intern Med 140(10):769–777.

7 Behavior Modification

KEY POINTS

- Behavioral strategies are a cornerstone for treatment of overweight.
- Behavioral strategies are based on the theory that obesity results from maladaptive behavior that can be improved by behavioral strategies.
- The extent of self-monitoring of behavior is related to weight loss.
- Reducing environmental stimuli that increase food intake is a good idea.
- Eating more slowly may allow satiety signals to be activated.
- It is important to set realistic goals and to take small steps toward them.
- Behavioral contracting with rewards is a valuable strategy.
- Nutrition education and use of portion-controlled meals helps.
- Increasing physical activity is associated with maintaining lower weight.
- A supporting family environment is helpful, whereas a destructive one is unhelpful.
- Learning positive thinking and assertiveness training is part of the plan.
- Behavioral weight-loss programs can produce weight losses of 10% over 6 months.
- The Internet may be useful for delivering behavioral program and for helping with weight maintenance.
- Some of the best results with behavioral strategies are in children.

INTRODUCTION TO THE USE OF BEHAVIORAL STRATEGIES TO TREAT OVERWEIGHT

Behavioral treatment of obesity has become a standard part of most treatment programs in the last 35 years. The goal of this approach is to help patients modify their eating habits, increase their physical activity, and become more conscious of both of these activities, thereby helping them make healthier choices.

Behavior, as the visible or outward evidence of often unknown internal processes, can be modified by two broad but different approaches. The first of these, known as

From: *The Metabolic Syndrome and Obesity*
By: G. A. Bray © Humana Press Inc., Totowa, NJ

Pavlovian or conditioned behavior, uses the ability of people to change their behavior in response to the association of external stimuli with unconditioned behavior patterns (Pavlov, 1927). The classic example is the salivation response to food, an unconditioned response when it is connected to the sound of a bell or a flashing light. Animals and humans learn to respond to the flashing light or sound of a bell with salivation before presentation of the food. This conditioned salivary response will last for many trials when food is not presented, but will eventually be extinguished. Thus, changing association patterns is one approach to behavioral change.

The second approach is usually referred to as operant conditioning (Skinner, 1988). It makes use of the behaviors animals and humans perform spontaneously, and increases the likelihood of performing the desired ones by providing an appropriate reward system. It is this latter approach that has been most widely used for changing behavior in relation to food intake.

The first report of successful application of these behavioral principles to treatment of overweight patients was by Stuart (1967). This was a landmark study of 11 patients, 8 of whom completed the trial. Using a variety of techniques based on learning theory, Stuart reported among the largest weight losses that have been published using behavior modification. In the three decades since his report, there have been many significant contributions to this field. The length and aggressiveness of treatment techniques has been extended and intensified. Weight losses with the current programs range from 7 to 10% of initial body weight (Knowler et al., 2002; Williamson et al., 2006; Wing, 2004; Espeland, 2007). Weight losses are maximal within the first 6 months after the initiation of treatment. Regrettably, maintenance of these initial weight losses has been difficult.

There are two basic assumptions underlying behavior therapy for overweight patients. The first is that obese individuals have learned maladaptive eating and exercise patterns that are contributing to weight gain and/or maintenance of their overweight state. The second is that these behaviors can be modified and that weight loss will result. With this theory, principles of learning from schools of classical and operant conditioning are applied in training new behaviors. Thus, behavioral treatment for the overweight patient seeks to alter the environment and environmental reinforcement contingencies and shape eating behavior and physical activity.

One of the key elements of human nature is that "if at first you don't succeed try, try again." This concept applies admirably to the search for new ways to lose weight that happens on an almost annual basis. Polivy and Herman (2002) have labeled this cycle of failure and renewed effort as a "false hope syndrome." They posit a number of reasons why self-change attempts fail. First, expectations often exceed what is feasible. Second, people often predict that they will change more quickly and more easily than is possible. Third, people overestimate their abilities in many domains and are unaware that they are inaccurate. Finally, people often believe that making a change will improve their lives more than can reasonably be expected. Dieters go through a number of explanations for their failure. The failure was because something outside of them caused a relapse, and if they only tried harder to control their environment they could succeed. The plateau that occurs with all weight-loss efforts can be viewed by the dieter as the result of not trying hard enough—maybe next time they could try harder and succeed. If a particular diet did not work, it is the diet's fault. For the counselor, the option is to try another diet, which is why there is a ready market for new diets. Polivy and Herman see disadvantages to cycling through the false hope syndrome. The weight regain produces negative feelings and frustrations for the dieter. Obsessions with food may also be a consequence of this cycling through failure. At present, some people overcome these barriers and succeed, as the national Weight Loss Registry attests. The goal of behavioralists is to increase these numbers.

ELEMENTS OF BEHAVIORAL STRATEGIES

The behavioral package that is currently used in most programs contains a number of components that will be discussed individually, although they are usually used together. These include keeping food diaries and activity records, so-called self-monitoring, control of the stimuli that activate eating, slowing down eating, goal setting, behavioral contracting and reinforcement, nutrition education, meal planning, modification of physical activity, social support, cognitive restructuring, and problem solving. The leading manual to help patients learn behavioral strategies is *The LEARN Program for Weight Management,* 10th Edition by Brownell (2004).

Behavioral programs can be successful when administered individually as was done with the Diabetes Prevention Program (DPP) in which weight loss averaged 7% below baseline by 6 months with only a slow gradual regain over the ensuing 3 years (Knowler et al., 2002; Wing et al., 2004). It can also be done using groups, which provides a more economical setting, because a single therapist can handle 15 or more participants (Espeland, 2007) In a meta-analysis of four trials comparing group and individual therapy, Avenell et al. (2004) found no difference in the weight loss between the two approaches after 12 months (1.59 kg [95% confidence interval {CI} −1.81 to 5.00 kg]).

Self-Monitoring or Keeping Food Diaries and Activity Records

Self-monitoring is one of the key elements in a successful behavioral weight-loss program. The participants are instructed in how to record everything they eat and the calories in the food as well as the situation in which they are eating. It is predictive of success during a weight-loss program and is used daily during the first 4 to 6 months and then continued as needed (Guare et al., 1989). The National Weight Control Registry, which is following a group of individuals who lost weight and have maintained that weight loss, finds that self-monitoring is one of the techniques that is most frequently used among this successful group (Wing and Phelan, 2005). In a recent study comparing placebo and drug therapy for overweight children, those who self-monitored their behavior lost more or gained less in either placebo or drug-treated groups than those adolescents who did not adhere well to self-monitoring (Berkowitz et al., 2003). In this trial, the adolescents who were "high" at self-monitoring and took sibutramine lost 11.5% in body mass index (BMI) units compared with 6.3% for the "low" self-monitoring group who took sibutramine. A similar result was seen in the placebo-treated group. Here, the high self-monitoring group lost 6.3% BMI units compared with only 1.2% for the low self-monitoring group. The value of self-monitoring has also been shown in a study using sibutramine in adults. Those participants who recorded their food intake more frequently lost more than twice as much weight as those who did not (18.1 ± 9.8 versus 7.7 ± 7.5 kg; Wadden et al., 2005). The graded effect of self-monitoring and weight loss is shown in Fig. 1.

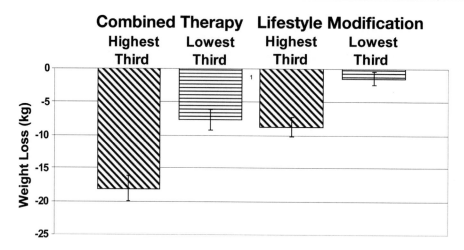

Fig. 1. Comparison of those in the highest versus the lowest third of self-monitoring on weight loss in individuals treated with sibutramine or the combination of sibutramine and lifestyle. (Adapted from Wadden et al. 2005.)

Gaining Control Over the Environmental Factors That Activate Eating (Also Called Stimulus Control)

Stimulus control is considered a key element in a behavioral program (Stuart, 1967; Wing, 2004). Because food is a key issue in weight gain, participants are taught to buy more fresh fruits and vegetables, to prepare easy-to-eat lower calorie foods, and to place these foods prominently in the refrigerator or on the counter. The proximity of food and the kinds of containers that are used to serve it can influence how much is eaten. The elegant studies of Wansink and associates showed that when foods are close at hand, more is eaten, and that people pour out more fluid when they pour it into a short squat container than when they pour it into a tall, thin container. Stimulus control focuses on eliminating or modifying the environmental factors that facilitate overeating. Part of this process is also to make the act of eating a focus of its own. Thus turning off the television set and putting down reading materials can allow the individual to concentrate on eating.

Slowing Down the Rate of Eating

Because eating is central to ingesting food, slowing down the process may give "physiological" signals for fullness time to come into play. A couple of ways of slowing down eating can be to concentrate on the "tastes" of the food—to savor what is being eaten. Other techniques might involve leaving the table during a meal to do something else if you are eating alone, or going to the bathroom, if eating out. Drinking water between bites can be another strategy to slow down eating.

Setting Realistic Goals

New ways of eating will not be learned overnight. It is important for the patient and their therapist to set realistic goals. Small steps are better than trying to conquer the entire weight-loss problem at once. It is also important to set concrete, achievable goals that the participant and the therapist agree on (Bandura and Simon, 1977). A weight loss of 0.5 to 1 kg per week is a realistic goal. To achieve this goal, participants are encouraged to reduce energy intake by 1000 kcal per day, which can be done with diet instruction, provision of food, or the use of portion-controlled foods.

Behavioral Contracting and Reinforcement

Reinforcing successful outcomes is important. Providing small tokens for success, such as gasoline purchase cards when gasoline prices are high or a small amount of money on a card for purchases at a local store can be beneficial. Rewarding women with a new hair-do or a manicure can be a way to motivate them to achieve the goals that they set. We all respond to positive encouragement, and this is particularly important when trying to lose weight.

Nutritional Education and Meal Planning

Providing a defined meal structure including portion control has helped individuals lose more weight than in the absence of such structure (Wing, 2004). Use of portion-controlled diets is one of the strategies for providing this structured environment for eating. A lower-fat diet is another approach that has been used. This was one of the strategies, along with lower-calorie goals that were used in the successful intensive lifestyle arm of the DPP (Wing et al., 2004). In a meta-analysis, Avenell et al. (2004) found in four trials that adding behavioral therapy to diet increased the weight loss after 12 months by –7.67 kg (95% CI –11.97 to –3.36 kg).

Increasing Physical Activity

Increasing physical activity is another part of the successful behavioral program. As with the using of self-monitoring, increasing physical activity was a key element in success for members of the National Weight Control Registry (Wing and Phelan, 2005). In this group of more than 4000 individuals who had lost a least 13.6 kg (30 pounds) and kept it off for at least 1 year, increasing physical activity was an important element in success. These individuals had lost an average of 33 kg and maintained it for an average of 5.7 years. Women in the registry reported expending 2545 kcal per week and men 3293 kcal per week. This would be equivalent to about 1 hour a day of moderate-intensity activity, such as brisk walking (Klem et al., 1997).

Social Support

Enhancing social support may also be a means for improving long-term weight loss (McLean et al., 2003). Inclusion of family members or spouses is one of the best ways to accomplish this support. There are both short- and long-term benefits to programs that include strong family support. In a meta-analysis of four behavioral programs that included family members, Avenell et al. (2004) found that after 12 months, a family-based intervention had a weight loss of –2.96 kg (95% CI –5.31 to –0.60 kg) more than the control behavioral programs.

Cognitive Restructuring, Problem Solving, Assertiveness Training, and Stress Reduction

All of these behavioral tools have been used to help increase the success of behavioral programs. We have internal conversations going all of the time. These can be negative or positive. For example, if you eat a piece of cake, you can either blame yourself or you can decide to do some additional exercise to make up for the extra cake. Self-blame is negative self-talk. Cognitive restructuring is intended to increase positive self-talk, like exercising more to overcome the caloric excess from the unintended cake. Problems dealing with food arise all the time. Learning how to handle restaurant situations, cocktail parties, and so on is essential for success. Part of this is learning to control portion sizes of food and part is learning to say no and continuing to say no, even when food is being pushed on you. This is the task of assertiveness training. Finally, stress should be reduced because, for some people, stress is a "stimulus" to eat. One approach is to think of a relaxing beach where you can take a deep breath and just relax. Whatever technique is used, stress reduction in this busy world is an important goal for a successful behavioral program.

EFFECTIVENESS: DURATION AND INTENSITY OF PROGRAMS

One of the major lessons of the past 30 years is that programs of greater length are more effective than shorter ones. An average of 8 weeks was in vogue in 1974 and has increased to an average of 21 weeks by the 1990s as treatment duration lengthened (Williamson et al., 2006). In 1974, the average weight loss was 3.8 kg after 8 weeks. As treatment lengthened in the 1990s, the average weight loss increased to 8.5 kg after 21 weeks of treatment. In 2000, Jeffery et al. (2000) estimated that average weight losses in behavioral treatment for overweight had increased by approximately 75% between 1974 and 1994. In a 40-week program, Perri et al. (1992) reported that after 40 weeks, weight loss was significantly greater than after treatment for 20 weeks. In a review of this research in 1998, Perri (1998) concluded that extended contact with participants yielded better weight loss.

Behavioral programs have also been effective in producing weight loss and improving the status of individuals with diabetes (Wing et al., 1985) and those at risk for diabetes (Knowler et al., 2002). The weight loss with the behavioral program from the DPP is shown in Fig. 2. A review of long-term effectiveness of lifestyle and behavioral weight-loss interventions by Norris et al. (2004) found 22 studies that examined weight loss in this group of patients, with some studies lasting up to 5 years. Compared with weight loss among more than 500 people with diabetes receiving usual care, behavioral strategies produced an added –1.7 kg of weight loss (95% CI 0.3 to 3.2 kg). If physical activity and behavioral strategies were combined with a very low-calorie diet ($N = 117$ people with diabetes) weight loss was –3.0 kg more than in the very low-calorie diet comparison groups. With more intense physical activity added on top of behavioral and dietary advice, added weight loss was –3.9 kg. The authors conclude that weight-loss strategies involving behavior change, diet, and physical activity were associated with small between-group improvements in weight loss for people with diabetes.

INTERNET-BASED PROGRAMS

The Internet is all around us, and it would be surprising if were not used as a strategy to deliver behavioral therapy to overweight individuals. The first use of computer-assisted therapy for weight-loss programs was reported in 1985 (Burnett et al., 1985). Since 2000, there have been several studies on its effectiveness (Harvey-Berino et al.,

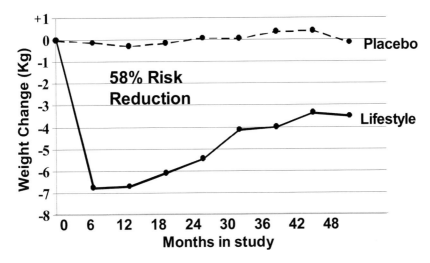

Fig. 2. Weight loss in the lifestyle and placebo-treated groups from the Diabetes Prevention Trial. (Adapted from Knowler et al. 2002.)

2002a; Harvey-Berino et al., 2002b; Harvey-Berino et al., 2004; Napolitano et al., 2003; Tate et al., 2001; Tate et al., 2003; Winett et al., 2005; Womble et al., 2004) and the introduction of commercial weight-loss programs involving the Internet (www.e-Diets.com). The Internet provides one means of increasing therapist contact to improve long-term weight maintenance.

Several studies have examined the use of the Internet to deliver weight management programs to adults. Encouraging preliminary results were reported by Tate et al. (2001). A total of 91 participants were randomly assigned to either an Internet education program ($N = 32$ completers) or an Internet behavioral program. All participants had one face-to-face weight-loss session. The Internet behavioral group received 24 weekly behavioral lessons via e-mail and individualized responses to weekly online submission of their self-monitoring diaries. Attrition rate was 15% at 3 months and 22% at 6 months. The Internet behavioral group lost –4.0 kg in 3 months and –4.4 kg in 6 months compared with –1.7 and –1.6 kg for the Internet educational group. Using a 5% weight-loss criterion, 45% of those in the Internet behavioral intervention achieved this goal, compared with 22% for the Internet education group. They also noted that login frequency predicted the degree of success. A second single-site randomized clinical trial from the same group compared the efficacy of interactive Internet-based counseling program with an Internet health education website (Tate et al., 2003). Using an intent-to-treat analysis, the weight loss at 12 months was –4.4 kg in the behavioral e-counseling group compared with –2.0 in the basic Internet group.

Two studies by Harvey-Berino et al. (2002a, 2002b) examined the value of the Internet in maintaining weight loss produced by direct patient contact. In the first study, 122 participants were treated with an intensive behavioral program for 6 months and then joined the group to which they had been randomly assigned (2002a). One of groups was an Internet support group, the second was an in-person support group, and the third was a minimal in-person support program. The randomized part of the trial began at the end of the 6 months of in-person treatment and continued for the ensuing 12 months.

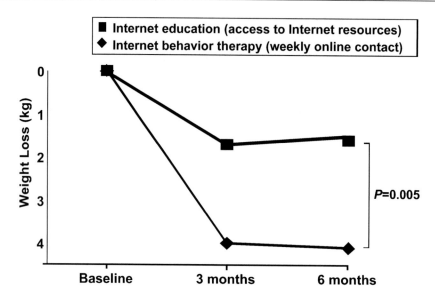

Fig. 3. A comparison of Internet delivery of a weight-loss program versus an educational program.

Attrition was 18% at 6 months and 24% over the entire 18 months. In this study, Internet support did not appear to be as effective (–5.7 kg at 18 months) as either the frequent in-person support or minimal in-person support (–10.4 kg at 18 months for both groups) In a subsequent study, the group assigned to the Internet support group did just as well as those with continued face-to-face contact (Harvey-Berino et al., 2004). In a second trial from this group, the initial 6-month treatment for which 255 individuals enrolled was conducted over interactive television. The mean weight loss for those completing 6 months was –7.8 kg or about 8.9%. The subjects were then randomized to an Internet support group, minimal in-person support, or frequent in-person support. At the end of 18 months, there was no significant difference between maintenance of weight loss between the three conditions (–8.2% for the Internet support, –5.6% for the frequent in-person support, and –6.0% for the minimal in-person group), suggesting that Internet strategies, when appropriately used, can be as helpful with weight mainte-nance as the more expensive in-person meetings. In this study, attendance at treatment meetings and chat room sessions as well as frequency of self-monitoring was related to successful maintenance.

One study compared the effects of treatment for 62 subjects randomly assigned to the use of the Internet with 61 subjects having treatment through the Internet plus in-person support (Micco et al., 2004). At 6 months, the Internet group lost –9.2 kg compared with –6.9 kg for the Internet plus in-person support ($P = 0.08$) and at 12 months the Internet group lost –8.1 kg compared with –5.6 kg for the Internet plus in-person support ($p = 0.15$). The login rate was correlated with success ($r = 0.55$) as was posting to an Internet journal ($r = 0.33$), use of the Internet bulletin board ($r = 0.31$), use of progress graphs ($r = 0.36$), and use of the BMI calculator ($r = 0.26$).

The response to a commercial Internet website (www.e-Diets.com) has been compared in a randomized trial with a program that provided the LEARN manual in 47 women. The subjects had an initial visit and were then seen at 8, 16, 26, and 52 weeks

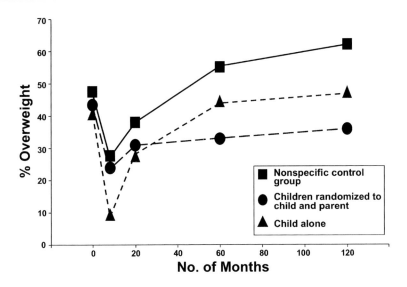

Fig. 4. Comparison of weight over 10 years in overweight children who were treated alone or with one parent. (Redrawn from Epstein et al. 1990.)

to review their progress. At 16 and 52 weeks, the weight loss of women assigned to the commercial program was smaller (–0.9% at 16 weeks and 1.1% at 52 weeks) than for the women using the weight-loss manual (–3.6% at 16 weeks and –4.0% at 52 weeks). The significance of the data depended on the analysis used. The last observation carried forward provided a statistically significant advantage for the women using the weight-loss manual, but the baseline carried forward and completers analyses did not. Thus, the differences were small (Gold et al., 2004; Womble et al., 2004).

Finally, the Internet has been used as a strategy to prevent weight regain. In the Study to Prevent Regain, Wing et al. (2006) have investigated five cohorts enrolled between 2000 and 2005 with the goal of preventing a more than 2.4 kg (5 lb.) regain. A total of 314 adults who had lost more than 10% of their body weight in the previous 2 years were enrolled. They were on average 51 years old, had a BMI of 28.6 kg/m^2, and a weight loss of 20 kg (44 lb.). They were divided into three groups. The control group received only a newsletter, one intervention group received their program via the Internet and chat room with a leader, and the other intervention group had face-to-face group meetings for 4 weeks and then monthly. Lesson content was identical and they were to exercise 60 minutes per day and weigh themselves daily. Weight gains were classified into three categories: less than 3 lb., 3 to 4 lb., and more than 5 lb. The latter group received active intervention with use of pedometers, calorie books, scales, and menu plans. Both intervention groups did better than the control group in maintaining their weight loss, but there was no difference whether the maintenance techniques were delivered via Internet or in person. Weighing frequently was related to success.

BEHAVIORAL TREATMENT FOR CHILDREN AND ADOLESCENTS

Some of the most promising studies of behavior therapy have been conducted in children. Epstein et al. (1990) made two important contributions to this area. First, they showed that when overweight children aged 10 to 12 were treated with members of the

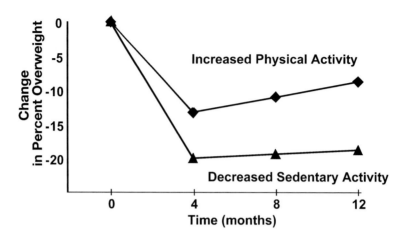

Fig. 5. A comparison of advice to adolescents to be more physically active or to be less physically inactive. (Redrawn from Epstein et al. 1995.)

family, as opposed to individually, there was a weight loss that was largely retained over a 10-year period than when the children were treated without parents or when the parents were treated in separate sessions (Epstein et al., 1990) (Fig. 4).

In a second study, Epstein et al. (1995) showed that motivating adolescents to reduce inactivity (mainly decreasing television time) was more important than focusing on increasing activity (Fig. 5). Not only did the adolescents gain less weight (or lose more), but there was a significant effect on reducing food intake.

The Internet has also been utilized for weight loss and weight maintenance in adolescents and children. Baranowski et al. (2003) found that an 8-week Internet-based intervention for overweight 8-year-old African-American girls did not yield significant weight changes in comparison with a control group. In contrast, a second study by Williamson and colleagues showed that in a program called Health Information Program for Teens weight increased 2.29 kg in the control group, but only 0.70 kg in the Internet-treatment group ($p < 0.05$). The body fat of the adolescent girls decreased −1.12% in the behavioral group compared with a gain of 0.43% in the control group. Their parents also showed a greater decrease in body weight and body fat (Williamson et al., 2005).

As with adults, parent involvement in treatment is recommended (Kumanyika et al., 2006) to promote the enhancement of social support for children and adolescents who are losing weight. Parents need to learn to be supportive of their child's progress and avoid actions sabotaging progress. It is clear that for younger children (not necessarily adolescents) parents have control over the home environment, including types and amounts of foods available, food preparation methods, and opportunities for physical activity.

REFERENCES

Avenell, A., et al. (2004). Systematic review of the long-term effects and economic consequences of treatments for obesity and implications for health improvement. Health Technol Assess 8(21):iii–iv, 1–182.

Bandura, A. and Simon, K. M. (1977). The role of proximal intentions in self-regulation of refractory behavior. Cognitive Therapy Research 1:177–193.

Baranowski, T., et al. (2003). The Fun, Food, and Fitness Project (FFFP): the Baylor GEMS pilot study. Ethn Dis 13(1 Suppl 1):S30–S39.

Berkowitz, R. I., et al. (2003). Behavior therapy and sibutramine for the treatment of adolescent obesity: a randomized controlled trial. JAMA 289(14):1805–1812.

Brownell, K. (2004). The LEARN Program for Weight Control: 10th Edition. Dallas: American Health Pub.

Burnett, K. F., et al. (1985). Ambulatory computer-assisted therapy for obesity: a new frontier for behavior therapy. J Consult Clin Psychol 53(5):698–703.

Epstein, L. H., et al. (1990). Ten-year follow-up of behavioral, family-based treatment for obese children. JAMA 264(19):2519–2523.

Epstein, L. H., et al. (1995). Effects of decreasing sedentary behavior and increasing activity on weight change in obese children. Health Psychol 14:109–115.

Espeland, M. (2007). Reduction in weight and cardiovascular risk factors in individuals with type 2 diabetes: one-year results of the Look AHEAD Trial. Diabetes Care E-pub date: March 15.

Gold, E. C., et al. (2004). Weight loss on the web: A pilot study comparing a commercial website to a structured online behavioral intervention. Obes Res 12:A24.

Guare, J. C., et al. (1989). Analysis of changes in eating behavior and weight loss in type II diabetic patients. Which behaviors to change. Diabetes Care 12(7):500–503.

Harvey-Berino, J., et al. (2002a). Does using the Internet facilitate the maintenance of weight loss? Int J Obes Relat Metab Disord 26(9):1254–1260.

Harvey-Berino, J., et al. (2002b). The feasibility of using Internet support for the maintenance of weight loss. Behav Modif 26(1):103–116.

Harvey-Berino, J., et al. (2004b). Effect of internet support on the long-term maintenance of weight loss. Obes Res 12(2):320–329.

Jeffery, R. W., et al. (2000). Long-term maintenance of weight loss: current status. Health Psychol 19(1 Suppl):5–16.

Klem, M. L., et al. (1997). A descriptive study of individuals successful at long-term maintenance of substantial weight loss. Am J Clin Nutr 66(2):239–246.

Knowler, W. C., et al. (2002). Reduction in the incidence of type 2 diabetes with lifestyle intervention or metformin. N Engl J Med 346(6):393–403.

Kumanyika, S., et al. (2006). Obesity prevention. In: Overweight and the Metabolic Syndrome: From Bench to Bedside (Bray, G. A., Ryan, D., ed.). Boston: Springer; pp. 233–253.

McLean, N., et al. (2003). Family involvement in weight control, weight maintenance and weight-loss interventions: a systematic review of randomised trials. Int J Obes Relat Metab Disord 27(9): 987–1005.

Micco, M., et al. (2004). Internet weight loss: Stand-alone intervention or adjunct to traditional behavioral treatment? Obes Res 12:A24.

Napolitano, M. A., et al. (2003). Evaluation of an internet-based physical activity intervention: a preliminary investigation. Ann Behav Med 25(2):92–99.

Norris, S. L., et al. (2004). Long-term effectiveness of lifestyle and behavioral weight loss interventions in adults with type 2 diabetes: a meta-analysis. Am J Med 117(10):762–774.

Pavlov, I. P. (1927). Conditioned Reflexes: An investigation of the physiological activity of the cerebral cortex. London: Oxford University Press.

Perri, M. G. (1998). The maintenance of treatment effects in the long-term management of obesity. Clin Psychol Sci Pract 5:526–543.

Perri, M. G., et al. (1992). Improving the Long-Term Management of Obesity: Theory, research, and Clinical Guidelines. New York: Wiley.

Polivy, J. and Herman, C. P. (2002). If at first you don't succeed. False hopes of self-change. Am Psychol 57(9):677–689.

Skinner, B. F. (1988). The operant side of behavior therapy. J Behav Ther Exp Psychiatry 19:171.

Stuart, R. B. (1967). Behavioral control of overeating. Behav Res Ther 5:357–365.

Tate, D. F., et al. (2003). Effects of Internet behavioral counseling on weight loss in adults at risk for type 2 diabetes: a randomized trial. JAMA 289(14):1833–1836.

Tate, D. F., et al. (2001). Using Internet technology to deliver a behavioral weight loss program. JAMA 285(9):1172–1177.

Wadden, T. A., et al. (2005). Randomized trial of lifestyle modification and pharmacotherapy for obesity. N Engl J Med 353(20):2111–2120.

Williamson, D. A., et al. (2006). Behavioral strategies for controlling obesity. In: Overweight and the Metabolic Syndrome: From Bench to Bedside (Bray, G. A., Ryan, D., ed.). Boston: Springer; pp. 219–232.

Williamson, D. A., et al. (2005). Efficacy of an internet-based behavioral weight loss program for overweight adolescent African-American girls. Eat Weight Disord 10(3):193–203.

Winett, R. A., et al. (2005). Long-term weight gain prevention: a theoretically based Internet approach. Prev Med 41(2):629–641.

Wing, R. R. (2004). Behavioral Approaches to the Treatment of Obesity. In: Handbook of Obesity: Clinical Applications, edited by Bray, G. and Bouchard, C. New York: Marcel Dekker; pp. 147–167.

Wing, R. R., et al. (1985). Behavior change, weight loss, and physiological improvements in type II diabetic patients. J Consult Clin Psychol 53(1):111–122.

Wing, R. R., et al. (2004). Achieving weight and activity goals among diabetes prevention program lifestyle participants. Obes Res 12(9):1426–1434.

Wing, R. R. and Phelan, S. (2005). Long-term weight loss maintenance. Am J Clin Nutr 82(1 Suppl): 222S–225S.

Wing, R. R., et al. (2006). A self-regulation program for maintenance of weight loss. N Engl J Med 335(15):1563–1571.

Womble, L. G., et al. (2004). A randomized controlled trial of a commercial internet weight loss program. Obes Res 12(6):1011–1018.

8 Physical Activity and Exercise in the Obese

KEY POINTS

- Fitness improves longevity. It is better to be fit than unfit. If overweight, it is better to be fit and overweight than overweight and unfit.
- There is a genetic component to weight loss during exercise. In overweight identical twins who lost weight exercising, there was more resemblance within pairs in the amount of weight lost than between pairs.
- The three main components of energy expenditure are resting metabolic rate, energy consumed after eating a meal, and physical activity. We only have conscious control over physical activity.
- Exercise alone is not very effective for inducing weight loss.
- Exercise is a most important component in maintaining a lower body weight.

INTRODUCTION

Physical activity is a key component of energy expenditure. Changes in physical activity are particularly important in the pathogenesis of overweight and in its treatment. This is especially true for long-term maintenance of weight loss when it involves the use of one or more large muscle groups and raises the heart rate.

The components of energy expenditure are shown in Fig. 1. They include energy needed for heat production, maintenance of body temperature, maintenance of ionic gradients across cells, resting cardiac and respiratory function, thermogenesis, and physical activity (Fig. 1). A dose–response relationship has been demonstrated in overweight adult women between the amount of exercise and long-term weight loss (Jakicic et al., 1999; Schoeller and Fjeld, 1991; Slentz et al., 2004). Jakicic et al. showed that after losing weight, 200 minutes of exercise per week maintained the lost weight over 18 months, but that 150 and 100 minutes of activity per week did not.

From: *The Metabolic Syndrome and Obesity*
By: G. A. Bray © Humana Press Inc., Totowa, NJ

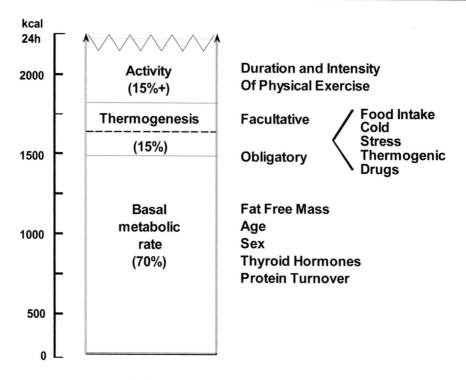

Fig. 1. Components of energy expenditure.

MEASURING ENERGY EXPENDITURE

There are several components of energy expenditure that are shown in Fig. 1. The largest component is involved in "resting" or basal metabolism. The second largest component is physical activity, the theme of this chapter. The smallest component, representing about 10% of the total, is the thermic effect of food (TEF). It is the rise in energy expenditure that follows a meal. This was first measured by Lavoisier more than 200 years ago.

A direct measure of the energy expenditure associated with activity comes from measurements of oxygen consumption determined as the difference between resting oxygen consumption and oxygen consumption for a given activity. Measurement of resting metabolic rate, the oxygen consumed when a subject is resting, is a measure of the energy needed for metabolism other than activity. When resting metabolic rate and TEF are subtracted from the total daily energy expenditure measured by the turnover of doubly labeled water, one has another way to estimate of energy expenditure due to activity. Overall estimated energy requirements for females and males of various ages are shown in Table 1.

Total Energy Expenditure

Total energy expenditure can be measured in two different ways. The first is to house individuals in calorimeters and measure their intake of energy and energy expenditure. The first of these human calorimeters was developed in the mid-19th century, but the widest application came from Atwater and Benedict and those who followed them.

Gender	Age	Activity level		
		Sedentary	Moderately active	Active
Boys and girls	2–3	1,000	1,000–1,400	1,000–1,400
Female	4–8	1,200	1,400–1,600	1,400–1800
	9–13	1,600	1,600–2,000	1,800–2,200
	14–18	1,800	2,000	2,400
	19–30	2,000	2,000–2,200	2,400
	31–50	1,800	2,000	2,200
	>50	1,600	1,800	2,000–2,200
Male	4–8	1,400	1,400–1,600	1,600–2,000
	9–13	1,800	1,800–2,200	2,000–2,600
	14–18	2,200	2,400–2,800	2,800–3,200
	19–30	2,400	2,600–2,800	3,000
	31–50	2,200	2,400–2,600	2,800–3,000
	>51	2,000	2,200–2,400	2,400–2,800

Adapted from the Dietary Guidelines 2005.

They showed that human beings obeyed the laws of conservation of energy, just as other animals did. This important set of studies forms the basis for modern physiological thinking about energy control and its theoretical basis.

Total daily energy expenditure can also be measured with a technique called doubly labeled water. During studies of distribution of oxygen among molecules in the body, Lifson et al. (1949) recognized that oxygen equilibrated with other oxygen molecules in the body. Thus by providing a form of oxygen that was not in the body they could measure the amount of oxygen excreted either as carbon dioxide or water. When deuterium, a second molecule that equilibrated with body hydrogen was given, they could trace its metabolism by measuring hydrogen appearing in the urine as water, because it is the end product of all hydrogen. Because hydrogen can only leave the body as water, whereas oxygen can leave as water or carbon dioxide, they could estimate the energy metabolism by measuring the production of carbon dioxide in the expired air of their animals (Lifson et al., 1949). This technique was soon applied to human beings, and has since been used as a way of measuring total daily energy expenditure in children and adults during 7- to 10-day intervals. The energy expenditure associated with physical activity, as well as the quantity of activity, can be measured in a number of ways. The simplest is to use questionnaires of time spent in activity. Some of the questionnaires used are the Paffenbarger et al. questionnaire, the Modifiable Activity Questionnaire and the Low Level Physical Activity Recall. Somewhat more quantitative methods involve the use of pedometers or wrist actigraphs. Change in heart rate above baseline is another technique. However, it is not effective for low levels of activity and must be calibrated for each individual.

Doubly labeled water is the gold standard for measurement of total daily energy expenditure (Fig. 2). For this method, the subject is given a known dose of water labeled with oxygen-18 and hydrogen-2 (deuterium), both of which are nonradioactive, or

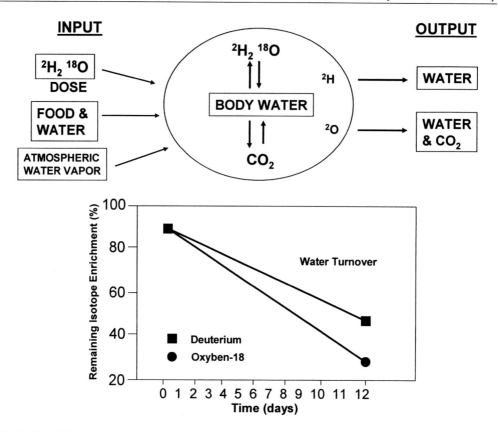

Fig. 2. Model for the measurement of energy expenditure by use of doubly labeled nonradioactive water.

stable, isotopes. The rate of decrease in body ^{18}O and ^2H (deuterium) is a measure of carbon dioxide production and can be converted to energy expenditure if the respiratory quotient is known.

Thermic Effect of Food

The TEF describes the increase in energy expenditure, measured as oxygen consumption that occurs after ingesting food, which Lavoisier was first to note more than 200 years ago. For a given load, protein produces the largest amount of heat, and carbohydrate and fat are similar. When a mixed meal is ingested, the thermic effect accounts for about 10% of the total energy value of the meal. There has been an ongoing argument as to whether overweight people have a reduced TEF. If the thermic response were reduced, this would provide a way to get up to 10% more energy to store after eating a meal. In a review of this subject, it was noted that when similar methods were used, overweight people, particularly those who were more insulin-resistant, had lower thermic responses to meals (de Jonge, 2002).

Energy Expenditure From Physical Activity

Energy expenditure with physical activity is directly related to body weight and thus a reasonable target for weight maintenance and weight-loss strategies. These methods have their limitations, but can nonetheless provide energy expenditure from activity.

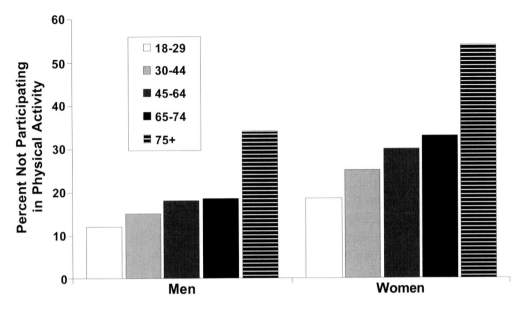

Fig. 3. Energy expenditure among Americans according to the Surgeon General.

Levels of physical activity correlate well with health risks, and suggest that Americans are relatively inactive and become less active as they age. In the Surgeon General's report on physical activity, for example, the percent of time Americans spent in physical activity decreased as their age increased (Fig. 3; CDC, 1996).

PHYSICAL ACTIVITY AND HEALTH

The first National Health and Examination Survey found that low levels of physical activity and recreation were strongly related to weight gain in both men and women (Williamson et al., 1993). Self-reported recreational physical activity was measured and divided into three categories: low, medium, and high. Weight change after 10 years among 3515 men and 5810 women aged 25 to 74 showed that low levels of recreational physical activity were strongly related to major weight gain (>13 kg) during the preceding 10 years. The estimated relative risk of major weight gain for those in the low-activity group at the follow-up survey compared with those in the high-activity group was 3.1 in men and 3.8 in women. The relative risk for subjects whose activity level was low at both the baseline and follow-up surveys was 2.3 in men and 7.1 in women.

The Nurses Health Study found that women who maintain vigorous physical activity have a smaller weight gain over 6 years of follow-up than those who do not (Field et al., 2001).

Exercise levels decrease during adolescence (DeLany et al., 2004; Kimm et al., 2000). In a longitudinal study of adolescents, the level of activity declined each year during adolescence, in both black and white girls. By age 17, there was almost no spontaneous physical activity reported by the black girls and only slightly more by the white girls (Kimm et al., 2002).

There is an important genetic component to the level of physical activity (Stubbe et al., 2005). In a study examining regular exercise among identical and fraternal

Decreasing Television Viewing Leads to Improved Body Mass Index in Children

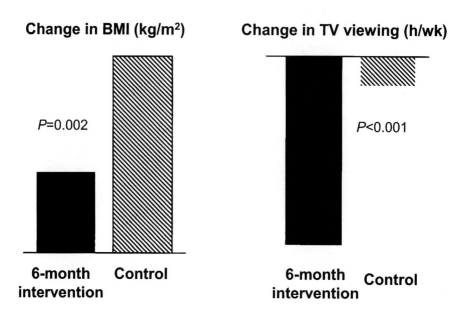

Fig. 4. Effect of BMI after 6 months of an intervention in children aimed at reducing the amount of television. (Adapted from Robinson, 1999.)

twins that included both same and opposite sex pairs, environmental factors shared by children at age 13 accounted for 78 to 84% of sports participation, whereas genetic differences provided almost no contribution. By ages 17 to 18, the genetic influences represented 36% of the variance in the level of participation in sports and by ages 18 to 20 genetic factors accounted for almost all (85%) of the differences in participation in sports (Samaras et al., 1999; Stubbe et al., 2005). In a cross-sectional study of adolescents, a lower percent body fat was associated with high amounts of vigorous physical activity, but not with moderate physical activity.

Improvements in cardiovascular fitness were more strongly associated with vigorous physical activity in black and white adolescents than in those with moderate physical activity (Gutin et al., 2005).

Television appears to be an important factor in the decreasing level of physical activity in children and adolescents (Chapters 2 and 5). There is a graded increase in body mass index (BMI) as the number of hours watching television increases (Crespo et al., 2001). A clinical trial comparing a school-based intervention aimed at reducing TV watching in one school with no intervention in another school found that the increase in BMI could be significantly slowed if TV viewing was reduced (Robinson, 1999) (Fig. 4).

The contribution of physical activity interacts with genetic factors in the pathogenesis of overweight. In a study of 970 healthy female twins, total body and central abdominal fat were 5.6 and 0.6 kg lower, respectively, in women who reported vigorous weight-bearing activity (Samaras et al., 1999). Even in women who had an overweight twin, higher levels of physical activity resulted in significantly lower total body and abdominal fat (4.0 and 0.5 kg, respectively). These findings suggest that physical activity is likely to protect against overweight regardless of an individual's genetic predisposition to it.

However, not everybody benefits from physical training. Improvements in physical conditioning in response to exercise have strong familial and genetic components. The HERITAGE study provided a 20-week program of physical training for 481 family members from two generations, including 95 fathers, 86 mothers, 141 sons, and 159 daughters in which the subjects' level of activity was observed. There were both non-responders and high responders to the exercise training program (Bouchard et al., 1999). Men had more improvement than women, and the children more than their parents. There was a strong intra-family resemblance in their response to physical training, with some families showing considerable improvement in physical fitness after exercise (an increase of 500 mL/minute in max V_{O2}) and others showing much less improvement (less than 300 mL/minute, max V_{O2}).

The amount of time one spends in leisure activity can contribute to a lower body weight. In a comparison of community settings, one of which could be described as "high walkability" versus "low-walkability" environments, Saelens et al. (2003) found that individuals living in the low-walkability neighborhoods had a higher mean BMI than people living in high-walkability neighborhoods. Both leisure time physical activity and regular walking or cycling to work are associated with lower body weight and weight gain over 5 years in middle-aged men (Wagner et al., 2001).

Benefit of Exercise

Exercise and physical activity have several benefits for normal and overweight individuals, including lowering mortality. Physical activity habits over 12 years were analyzed in 10,269 male Harvard alumni in a retrospective study (Paffenbarger et al., 1993). Those men who engaged in moderately vigorous sports had a 23% lower risk of death than those who were less active. The improvement in survival with exercise was equivalent and additive to other lifestyle measures, such as cessation of smoking, control of hypertension, and avoidance of overweight.

The relation of physical activity and adiposity to mortality has also been studied in the Nurses Health Study, which showed that it is better to be thin than fat and better to be active than inactive (Hu et al., 2004). Estimates of moderate (brisk walking) and vigorous activity (strenuous sports and jogging) were done by recall in 1980 and 1982 and then with an eight-item questionnaire from 1988 through 1998. BMI and mortality showed a "j" shaped relationship. Both overweight and physical activity were associated with increased mortality. Women with a BMI lower than 25 kg/m^2 and who had a high level of physical activity (>3.5 hours/week) were the comparison group with an odds ratio (OR) of 1.0 for total mortality. Inactive women (<1.0 hour/week) with a BMI lower than 25 had an OR of 1.55, or a 55% greater mortality. Active obese women with BMI higher than 30 had an OR of 1.91 and the OR was increased even further (OR = 2.42) for inactive obese women.

In the Aerobics Center Longitudinal Study of men with diabetes at various levels of BMI, there was a steep inverse gradient between fitness and mortality that was independent of BMI (Church et al., 2004).

In two cohorts from the Lipid Research Clinics Study, fitness in the American and Russian male cohorts was associated with all-cause and cardiovascular disease mortality, but fatness was not. Compared with the fit, not fat group, the adjusted hazard ratios for the American men were 1.40 (95% confidence interval [CI] 1.07–1.83) among the fit fat group, 1.41 (95% CI 1.12–1.77) among the unfit, but not fat group, and 1.54 (95% CI 1.24–2.06) among the unfit fat group. There were no statistically significant interactions between fitness and fatness in either group of men for all-cause or cardio-vascular disease mortality. The authors concluded that the effects of fitness on mortality may be more robust across populations than fatness (Stevens et al., 2004).

Physical activity can improve glycemic control and insulin sensitivity, and it may prevent the development of type 2 diabetes (Boule et al., 2005). Vigorous exercise and energy restriction were independently and additively able to reduce glucose and insulin concentrations in response to an oral glucose tolerance test (Cox et al., 2003). Although exercise training improves almost all variables obtained by the minimal model of glucose metabolism after an intravenous glucose tolerance test, these improvements disappear within 72 hours after discontinuing exercise. Exercise can also be beneficial in hypertension. Additionally, aerobic exercise training has been shown to improve serum lipoprotein concentrations, body composition, aerobic capacity, and hemostatic factors associated with thrombosis. Finally, several studies also found a strong inverse relationship between habitual exercise and fitness and the risk of coronary disease and death (Blair et al., 1996; Church et al., 2004; Lee et al., 1999; Paffenbarger et al., 1993; Wei et al., 1999). Although most were made in men, some studies have found a similar cardiovascular benefit from fitness in women (Paffenbarger et al., 1993).

Central adiposity with increased abdominal and visceral fat is related to all of the diseases discussed earlier. Exercise programs with or without weight loss can cause a greater decrease in abdominal fat than in total body fat (Despres et al., 1991).

Disadvantages of Exercise

However, exercise is not without its intrinsic risks. It has been associated with an increased risk of musculoskeletal injuries, cardiac arrhythmia, acute myocardial infarction, and bronchospasm.

TREATMENT OF OVERWEIGHT USING EXERCISE

Exercise has been evaluated as a single treatment for overweight and in combination with diet, as well as for maintaining weight loss. Table 2 summarizes studies relating to exercise and weight loss. Ostman et al. (2004) performed a Medline search for studies related to physical exercise and overweight, and identified six randomized control trials among 186 articles that dealt with overweight with physical activity as a treatment, treatment intervals of 12 months (with one exception), and had drop-out rates of less than 40%. Table 2 has been adapted with addition of two newer trials, 16 and 8 months long, respectively.

The two best trials in terms of design and execution are those by Wood et al. (1988; 1991). In men, diet alone produced more weight loss than exercise alone, but when combined, diet and exercise were better than diet alone. In women there were no significant additive effects of exercise to that of diet (–4.2 versus –5.5 kg). In the Pritchard et al. (1997) study, the weight loss was greater with energy restriction than exercise (6.3 versus 2.6 kg), and the loss of fat was essentially the same.

In a 16-week randomized controlled trial in overweight men, Cox et al. (2003) found a significant weight loss with energy restriction, but not with vigorous exercise

Table 2
Clinical Trials of Exercise in Overweight Individuals

Author	Inclusion criteria	Intervention groups	Duration	No. of patients/no. of follow-up	Weight/fat	Comments
Wood 1988	Men 120–160% overweight	1. Diet to give 1 kg/week weight loss; fat reduced by 30%. 2. Individual instruction to lose 1 kg/week; training at 60–80% max physical capacity 40–50 minutes three to four times/week.	1 year	1. 51/42 2. 52/47 3. 52/42	Weight: 1. −7.2 kg; fat: 1. −5.9 kg Weight: 2. −4.0 kg; fat: 2. −4.2 kg Weight: 3. +0.6 kg; fat: 3. −0.3 kg	TG and HDL-cholesterol also improved; diet and physical activity yield same reduction in weight and fat at same negative calorie balance
Wing 1988	Women: 30–60 years with type 2 diabetes; more than 20% above ideal weight	1. Diet (−1000 kcal/day plus 3 mi. three times/week 2. Free diet plus training (+3 mi., four times/week) 3. Diet plus stretching	12 months	1. 12 2. 15 3. 13	1. −7.9 kg 2. −7.9 kg 3. −3.8 kg	Hemoblogin A1C reduced and medications reduced in groups 1 and 2
Wood 1991	Men and women 25–49 years; overweight 120–160%	1. Diet (moderate reduction of energy, fat, cholesterol) 2. Diet (as above) plus physical activity (60–80% of max) 25–45 minutes three times/week	Top of form bottom of form	1. 87/71 2. 90/81 3. 87/79	Men: 1. −5.1 kg; women: 1. −4.2 kg Men: 2. −8.7 kg; women: 2. −5.5 kg Men: 3. +1.7 kg; women: 3. +1.3 kg	Blood pressure decreased in groups 1 and 2; cholesterol decreased in women in both groups 1 and 2; HDL-cholesterol increased in group 2 in both men and women; TG decreased in men in group 2
Svendsen 1994	Women 49–58 years; BMI 25–42 kg/m²	1. Diet (4.2 MJ/day=1000 kcal/day) 2. Diet (as above) plus physical activity (submax aerotics and body building)	12 weeks with 6 months follow-up	1. 51/47 2. 49/47	12 weeks: 1. −6.6 kg; 6 months: 1. −8.0 kg 12 weeks: 2. −10.9 kg; 6 months: 2. −8.0 kg	TG decreased HDL-cholesterol increased; no effect from physical activity

(Continued)

Table 2 (*Continued*)

Author	Inclusion criteria	Intervention groups	Duration	No. of patients/no. of follow-up	Weight/fat	Comments
		3. Controls		3. 21/16	12 months: 3. 0.0 kg; 6 months: 3. 0.0 kg	
Pritchard 1997	Overweight men, mean BMI = 29 kg/m^2	1. Diet: reduction of 500 kcal/d with low fat 2. 65–75% of max physical capacity 45 minutes three to seven times/week 3. Controls	12 months	66/60	1. −6.3 kg 2. −2.6 kg 3. +0.9 kg	Diet "self-controlled"
Irwin 2003	Overweight nonsmoking post-menopausal women ages 50–75 years with a BMI higher than 25 kg/m^2 or BMI 24–25 kg/m^2 and body fat more than 33% by DEXA who were sedentary at baseline <60 minutes/week of moderate to vigorous activity) and maximal oxygen uptake of less than 25 mL/kg/minute	1. Exercise consisted of at least 45 minutes of moderate intensity exercise 5 days/week for 12 months (months 1–3, they attended three sessions/week; months 4–12, they attended one session/week) 2. Weekly stretching sessions of 45 minutes for 12 months	12 months	1. 87/84 2. 86/86	1. Exercise 2. 3 months: B.W. −0.5 kg; 12 months: B.W. −1.3 kg; Fat −1.4 kg; VAT −8.5 cm^2 Top of Form 3 months: B.W. 0.0 kg; 12 months: B.W. 0.1 kg; Fat −0.1 kg; VAT 0.1 cm^2 Bottom of Form	Advised to maintain usual diet; weight loss related to degree of exercise

194

Study	Subjects	Intervention	Duration	N	Results	Conclusion
Donnelly 2003	Overweight men and women age 17 to 36 with a BMI of 25.0 to 34.9 kg/m²	1. Exercise targeted at 400 kcal/d 5 days a week with walking on a treadmill at 55–70% of maximal oxygen uptake	16 months of verified exercise	1. 87/41	16 months: group 1: (men) weight –5.2 kg; fat –4.9 kg; VAT –22.4 cm² (women) weight +0.4 kg; fat –0.2 kg; VAT –3.2 cm²	Exercise produced weight loss in men and prevented weight gain in women
		2. Control group had same testing but no exercise program		2. 44/33	16 months: group 2: (men) weight –0.5 kg; fat –0.7 kg; VAT –6.3 cm² (women) weight +2.9 kg; fat +2.0 kg; VAT +3.1 cm²	
Slentz 2004	Men and women age 40 to 60 years, BMI 25–35 kg/m², and mild to moderate lipid abnormalities	Top of Form Bottom of Form	9 months; exercise was observed; this was not a weight loss study and diet was provided to maintain body weight	1. 44/17	1. High/vigorous intensity: weight –3.5 kg; waist –3.4 cm; fat –4.9 kg;	
				2. 52/24	2. Low/vigorous intensity weight –1.1 kg; fat –2.6 kg; waist –1.4 cm	
				3. 42/14	3. Low/moderate intensity: weight –1.3 kg; fat –2.0 kg; waist –1.1 cm	
				4. 44/7	4. Control: weight –1.1 kg; fat –0.5 kg; waist –0.8 cm	

Source: Ostman et al., 2004.
TG, triglycerides; HDL: high-density lipoprotein; BMI, body mass index; DEXA, dual energy X-ray absorptiometry.

(–10.9 kg with diet and light exercise versus –11.7 kg with diet and vigorous exercise; light exercise with normal diet produced –0.44 kg weight loss compared with –1.55 kg with normal diet and vigorous exercise). In another study, 4 months' supervised exercise or lifestyle were two factors and the protein intake at two levels were the other factors (15% [0.8 g/kg/day] versus 30% [about 1.6 g/kg/day]) protein]. Because the exercise was supervised, both dietary groups lost body fat and preserved lean body mass, and the combined effects of diet and exercise were additive on body composition. Body fat decreased 2 to 3% in the lifestyle groups with either low- or high-protein diet. Differences in the diet produced differential effects on lipids, with the low-protein group having greater decreases in total and low-density lipoprotein-cholesterol, and the higher protein diet having larger decreases in triglycerides and maintaining higher high-density lipoprotein concentrations (Layman et al., 2005).

A meta-analysis of earlier studies of diet and exercise reviewed the period between 1966 and 1994 and found 21 studies that included at least 100 participants. When the 493 participants with a BMI averaging 33 kg/m^2 were compared, those in the diet groups lost about 11 kg compared with 3 kg for those in the exercise groups. In the few studies identified in this meta-analysis that lasted 1 year, the weight loss was 8.7 kg with exercise alone, 9.0 kg with diet alone, and 11.8 kg with exercise plus diet (Miller et al., 1997). In a more recent meta-analysis, Avenell et al. (2004) found that diet and exercise versus control at 12 months produced a weight difference of –4.78 kg (95% CI –5.41 to –4.16 kg) in favor of the diet and exercise group. Even at 24 months, there was a weight difference of –2.70 kg (95% CI –3.60 to –1.80 kg) in favor of exercise.

Exercise as a Single Treatment

Several studies have evaluated the effect of exercise alone in inducing weight loss (Donnelly et al., 2003; Irwin et al. 2003; Pritchard et al., 1997; Slentz et al., 2004; Wood et al., 1988). Weight losses were in general quite small (approximately 0.1 kg/week), except in military recruits (1.8 kg/week; Lee et al., 1994), whose exercise program was more rigorous. Although it may be difficult to lose weight with exercise alone, it may have an effect on body fat. In a 12-week study of diet- versus exercise-induced weight loss on body composition and insulin sensitivity in 52 obese men (Lee et al., 1994), there was a greater reduction in total body fat in the exercise-induced weight-loss group and similar reductions in abdominal adiposity, visceral fat, and insulin resistance in the two treatment groups. In the treatment group assigned to exercise without weight loss who increased caloric intake to match energy expenditure, abdominal and visceral fat was decreased, but to a lesser degree than in the other treatment groups.

Exercise also has beneficial effects on body composition. In a study in postmenopausal women, subjects were randomized to moderate-intensity exercise (most commonly brisk walking, on average 3 hours/week), versus a stretching program (control group) for 12 months. The women in the exercise group lost more weight, and had greater decreases in body, intra-abdominal, and subcutaneous fat (Irwin et al., 2003).

For a given amount of exercise, men appear to lose more weight than women. In a study of 74 sedentary, overweight or moderately obese young men and women randomly assigned to exercise at an energy equivalent of 2000 calories per week, compared with a control group for 16 months, significant decreases in weight, BMI, and fat mass were seen in the men (5.2 ± 4.7 kg, 1.6 ± 1.4 kg/m^2, and 4.9 ± 4.4 kg, respectively;

Donnelly et al., 2003). In contrast, women assigned to exercise maintained their baseline weight, BMI, and fat mass, whereas increases in all three outcomes occurred in women in the control group.

Exercise Plus Diet

Exercise programs added to diets with moderate to severe caloric restriction have little additional effect on weight loss. Whether lean body mass is spared by exercise during caloric restriction is controversial. In one study, 6 of 12 obese families eating a diet of approximately 800 kcal per day were randomly assigned to exercise for 1 hour, 4 days per week at 50 to 60% of their maximum aerobic capacity, or no exercise. Both groups lost 12 to 13 kg, and there was no difference between them in the loss of body weight, body fat, or lean body mass.

Despite these conflicting reports, there is a strong suggestion that exercise reduces the loss of lean body mass during dieting. Such factors as sex, age, quality and type of diet, frequency and intensity of exercise may explain some of the discrepancies among the various studies. If a patient utilizes 100 calories during exercise each day (700 kcal/week) without a change in food intake, it would take 5 weeks to utilize the energy in 1 lb. of fat. It thus takes a considerable amount of time and effort to expend enough extra calories through exercise to produce large weight losses, more than most people realize. However, exercise duration or intensity may be less important than the addition of exercise per se to diet. As an example, in a 12-month study of 184 overweight, sedentary women who were randomly assigned to one of four exercise programs in addition to caloric restriction, weight loss was the same in all groups, regardless of exercise intensity or duration (Jakicic et al., 2003).

EXERCISE AS A STRATEGY TO MAINTAIN WEIGHT LOSS

Exercise is an important factor in maintaining weight loss after any weight reduction (Donnelly et al., 2003; Jakicic et al., 2003; Slentz et al., 2004; Wadden et al., 1997). One example is an 8-week study of diet plus exercise in which the subjects were followed up for 18 months. Weight loss with diet or diet plus exercise was not significantly different. However, during the subsequent follow-up period, the subjects who maintained their activity levels regained less weight than those who became sedentary again. The National Weight Control Registry is another example. The sample in this registry is defined by a 10% weight loss that is maintained and documented for 1 year before entering the registry. This group has on average lost 33 kg and maintained the loss for more than 5 years. The individuals in the registry report high levels of physical activity amounting to an hour or more per day that help them maintain their lower weight (Wing and Phelan, 2005).

Other studies have similarly suggested that inclusion of exercise in a weight control program leads to improved long-term results (Miller et al., 1997; Wadden et al., 1997). Schoeller et al. (1997) showed that the maintenance of weight loss had a graded relation to the amount of exercise that individuals continued after their initial treatment. A meta analysis evaluated 493 studies involving aerobic exercise for short durations (average 15.6 weeks) in moderately overweight subjects (average BMI 33.4 kg/m^2 with an average weight of 92.7 kg; Miller et al., 1997). The subjects who participated in exercise alone lost 2.9 kg, as compared with 10.7 kg for the diet-only group,

Table 3
Energy in Kilocalories Expended in Various Daily Activities

Moderate physical activity	Approximate kcal/hour for a 70 kg (154 lb.) individual
Hiking	370
Light gardening or yard work	330
Dancing	330
Gold (walking and carrying clubs)	330
Bicycling (<10 mph)	290
Waling (3.5 mph)	280
Weight lifting (general light workout)	220
Stretching	180
Vigorous physical activity	
Running or jogging (5 mph)	590
Bicycling (>10 mph)	590
Swimming (flow freestyle laps)	510
Aerobics	480
Waling (4.5 mph)	460
Heavy yard work (chopping wood)	440
Weight lifting (vigorous effort)	440
Basketball (vigorous)	440

Adapted from the Dietary Guidelines.
Includes the "basal" level associate with no effort, which is about 60–100 kcal per hour.

and 11.0 kg for the combination of diet and exercise. However, the diet and exercise group maintained 8.6 kg of weight loss after 1 year compared with 6.6 kg in the diet-only group.

SUGGESTIONS FOR PHYSICAL ACTIVITY

Increasing the level of physical activity would be beneficial to all ages and for all groups. A consensus statement has outlined the types of exercise programs that are recommended (Grundy et al., 1999). Any exercise program should be designed to fit into the health and physical conditions of the subject. Existing medical conditions, age, and preferences for types of exercise should all be considered in the decisions.

Subjects who are about to begin an exercise program, even those whose only exercise will be walking, should be advised of the possibility of musculoskeletal stresses and strains and joint injury. For those who are able, walking 150 to 210 minutes per week (30 minutes/day, 5–7 days/week) would be beneficial.

The role of exercise stress testing before beginning an exercise program has been controversial because of the frequency of false-positive tests. A joint 2002 American College of Cardiology/American Heart Association task force did not recommend routine exercise testing in this setting. However, it did give a class IIa recommendation (weight of evidence supports usefulness) to use exercise testing in asymptomatic persons with diabetes mellitus who plan to start vigorous exercise and a lesser recommendation in patients with multiple risk factors for coronary heart disease (Gibbons et al., 1997; Gibbons et al., 2002).

Physical activity should be performed for 30 to 60 minutes, 5 to 7 days a week. This will increase energy expenditure by 1000 to 2000 calories per week, or slightly more than 100 calories per day. The amount of energy expended depends on the duration and intensity of the exercise, and the subject's initial weight (Table 3). As an example, a 120-pound person walking 3 mph expends slightly less than 2 kcal per minute more than standing still. At 160 pounds, the difference is 2.4 kcal per minute, and at 200 pounds, it is 3 kcal per minute. Thus, a 30-minute walk at 3 mph for a 200-lb. person would dissipate an extra 90 kcal as compared with 60 kcal for a person weighing 120 pounds.

Finding appropriate places to exercise can facilitate any program of exercise. Health clubs may be helpful, but for most people walking is the most appropriate form of exercise. In one study of obese women, the combination of diet plus advice to increase physical activity by incorporating short periods of activity into daily schedules (e.g., walking instead of driving short distances, taking stairs instead of elevators) was as effective for inducing weight loss as diet plus structured aerobic activity (aerobics classes; Andersen et al., 1999).

REFERENCES

Andersen, R. E., et al. (1999). Effects of lifestyle activity vs structured aerobic exercise in obese women: a randomized trial. JAMA 281(4):335–340.

Avenell, A., et al. (2004). Systematic review of the long-term effects and economic consequences of treatments for obesity and implications for health improvement. Health Technol Assess 8(21):iii–iv, 1–182.

Blair, S. N., et al. (1996). Influences of cardiorespiratory fitness and other precursors on cardiovascular disease and all-cause mortality in men and women. JAMA 276(3):205–210.

Bouchard, C., et al. (1999). Familial aggregation of VO(2max) response to exercise training: results from the HERITAGE Family Study. J Appl Physiol 87(3):1003–1008.

Boule, N. G., et al. (2005). Effects of exercise training on glucose homeostasis: the HERITAGE Family Study. Diabetes Care 28(1):108–114.

Centers for Disease Control and Prevention. (1996). Physical activity and health: a report of the Surgeon General. Atlanta: US Department of Health and Human Services.

Church, T. S., et al. (2004). Exercise capacity and body composition as predictors of mortality among men with diabetes. Diabetes Care 27(1):83–88.

Cox, K. L., et al. (2003). The independent and combined effects of 16 weeks of vigorous exercise and energy restriction on body mass and composition in free-living overweight men—a randomized controlled trial. Metabolism 52(1):107–115.

Crespo, C. J., et al. (2001). Television watching, energy intake, and obesity in US children: results from the third National Health and Nutrition Examination Survey, 1988–1994. Arch Pediatr Adolesc Med 155(3):360–365.

DeJonge, L., et al. The thermic effect of food is reduced in obesity. Nutr Rev 60(9):295–297.

DeLany, J. P., et al. (2004). Energy expenditure in African American and white boys and girls in a 2-y follow-up of the Baton Rouge Children's Study. Am J Clin Nutr 79(2):268–273.

Despres, J. P., et al. (1991). Loss of abdominal fat and metabolic response to exercise training in obese women. Am J Physiol 261(2 Pt 1):E159–E167.

Donnelly, J. E., et al. (2003). Effects of a 16-month randomized controlled exercise trial on body weight and composition in young, overweight men and women: the Midwest Exercise Trial. Arch Intern Med 163(11):1343–1350.

Field, A. E., et al. (2001). Relationship of a large weight loss to long-term weight change among young and middle-aged US women. Int J Obes Relat Metab Disord 25(8):1113–1121.

Gibbons, R. J., et al. (1997). ACC/AHA Guidelines for Exercise Testing. A report of the American College of Cardiology/American Heart Association Task Force on Practice Guidelines (Committee on Exercise Testing). J Am Coll Cardiol 30(1):260–311.

Gibbons, R. J., et al. (2002). ACC/AHA 2002 guideline update for exercise testing: summary article: a report of the American College of Cardiology/American Heart Association Task Force on Practice Guidelines (Committee to Update the 1997 Exercise Testing Guidelines). Circulation 106(14): 1883–1892.

Grundy, S. M., et al. (1999). Physical activity in the prevention and treatment of obesity and its comorbidities. Med Sci Sports Exerc 31(11 Suppl):S502–S508.

Gutin, B., et al. (2005). Relations of moderate and vigorous physical activity to fitness and fatness in adolescents. Am J Clin Nutr 81(4):746–750.

Hu, F. B., et al. (2004). Adiposity as compared with physical activity in predicting mortality among women. N Engl J Med 351(26):2694–2703.

Irwin, M. L., et al. (2003). Effect of exercise on total and intra-abdominal body fat in postmenopausal women: a randomized controlled trial. JAMA 289(3):323–330.

Jakicic, J. M., et al. (2003). Effect of exercise duration and intensity on weight loss in overweight, sedentary women: a randomized trial. JAMA 290(10):1323–1330.

Jakicic, J. M., et al. (1999). Effects of intermittent exercise and use of home exercise equipment on adherence, weight loss, and fitness in overweight women: a randomized trial. JAMA 282(16):1554–1560.

Kimm, S. Y., et al. (2002). Decline in physical activity in black girls and white girls during adolescence. N Engl J Med 347(10):709–715.

Kimm, S. Y., et al. (2000). Longitudinal changes in physical activity in a biracial cohort during adolescence. Med Sci Sports Exerc 32(8):1445–1454.

Layman, D. K., et al. (2005). Dietary protein and exercise have additive effects on body composition during weight loss in adult women. J Nutr 135(8):1903–1910.

Lee, C. D., et al. (1999). Cardiorespiratory fitness, body composition, and all-cause and cardiovascular disease mortality in men. Am J Clin Nutr 69(3):373–380.

Lee, L., et al. (1994). The impact of five-month basic military training on the body weight and body fat of 197 moderately to severely obese Singaporean males aged 17 to 19 years. Int J Obes Relat Metab Disord 18(2):105–109.

Lifson, N., et al. (1949). The fate of utilized molecular oxygen and the source of the oxygen of respiratory carbon dioxide studied with the aid of heavy oxygen. J Biol Chem 180:803–811.

Miller, W. C., et al. (1997). A meta-analysis of the past 25 years of weight loss research using diet, exercise or diet plus exercise intervention. Int J Obes Relat Metab Disord 21(10):941–947.

Ostman, M., et al. (2004). Physical exercise. In: Treating and Preventing Obesity, edited by Ostman, M., et al. Weinheim, Germany: Wiley-VCH Verlag GmbH & Co. KgaA.; pp. 142–143.

Paffenbarger, R. S., Jr., et al. (1993). The association of changes in physical-activity level and other lifestyle characteristics with mortality among men. N Engl J Med 328(8):538–545.

Pritchard, J. E., et al. (1997). A worksite program for overweight middle-aged men achieves lesser weight loss with exercise than with dietary change. J Am Diet Assoc 97(1):37–42.

Robinson, T. N. (1999). Reducing children's television viewing to prevent obesity: a randomized controlled trial. JAMA 282(16):1561–1567.

Saelens, B. E., et al. (2003). Neighborhood-based differences in physical activity: an environment scale evaluation. Am J Public Health 93(9):1552–1558.

Samaras, K., et al. (1999). Genetic and environmental influences on total-body and central abdominal fat: the effect of physical activity in female twins. Ann Intern Med 130(11):873–882.

Schoeller, D. A. and Fjeld, C. R. (1991). Human energy metabolism: what have we learned from the doubly labeled water method? Annu Rev Nutr 11:355–373.

Schoeller, D. A., et al. (1997). How much physical activity is needed to minimize weight gain in previously obese women? Am J Clin Nutr 66(3):551–556.

Slentz, C. A., et al. (2004). Effects of the amount of exercise on body weight, body composition, and measures of central obesity: STRRIDE—a randomized controlled study. Arch Intern Med 164(1):31–39.

Stevens, J., et al. (2004). Associations of fitness and fatness with mortality in Russian and American men in the lipids research clinics study. Int J Obes Relat Metab Disord 28(11):1463–1470.

Stubbe, J. H., et al. (2005). Sports participation during adolescence: a shift from environmental to genetic factors. Med Sci Sports Exerc 37(4):563–570.

Wadden, T. A., et al. (1997). Exercise in the treatment of obesity: effects of four interventions on body composition, resting energy expenditure, appetite, and mood. J Consult Clin Psychol 65(2):269–277.

Wagner, A., et al. (2001). Leisure-time physical activity and regular walking or cycling to work are associated with adiposity and 5 y weight gain in middle-aged men: the PRIME Study. Int J Obes Relat Metab Disord 25(7):940–948.

Wei, M., et al. (1999). Relationship between low cardiorespiratory fitness and mortality in normal-weight, overweight, and obese men. JAMA 282(16):1547–1553.

Williamson, D. F., et al. (1993). Recreational physical activity and ten-year weight change in a US national cohort. Int J Obes Relat Metab Disord 17(5):279–286.

Wing, R. R. and Phelan, S. (2005). Long-term weight loss maintenance. Am J Clin Nutr 82(1 Suppl): 222S–225S.

Wood, P. D., et al. (1988). Changes in plasma lipids and lipoproteins in overweight men during weight loss through dieting as compared with exercise. N Engl J Med 319(18):1173–1179.

Wood, P. D., et al. (1991). The effects on plasma lipoproteins of a prudent weight-reducing diet, with or without exercise, in overweight men and women. N Engl J Med 325(7):461–466.

9

Pharmacological Treatment of the Overweight Patient

CONTENTS

KEY POINTS

- Medications significantly increase weight loss compared with placebo in most trials.
- Weight loss from initiation of the diet and exercise program, or without these programs, reaches its nadir between 20 and 36 weeks.
- Patients can expect a weight loss of 8 to 10% from baseline, provided they adhere to the weight-loss program and take medications regularly.
- Clinical trials with sibutramine and orlistat that have been approved by the Food and Drug Administration have lasted for 2 to 4 years with placebo control.
- All medications have side effects that need to be considered.
- For sibutramine, there is a rise in blood pressure and heart rate that may require discontinuation of the drug in a small percent of patients.
- For orlistat, the principal side effects are gastrointestinal resulting from the increased activity of the lower bowel.
- Rimonabant is a cannabinoid receptor antagonist that has completed phase 3 trials and is being reviewed by the Food and Drug Administration.

From: *The Metabolic Syndrome and Obesity*
By: G. A. Bray © Humana Press Inc., Totowa, NJ

- Other medications are in clinical trial and on their way.
- Over-the-counter medications and herbal products are also available, but in the case of the herbal products there is little data on effectiveness or safety.

INTRODUCTION

To use medications properly for treatment of the overweight patient, it is important to start with a framework based on the realities of its treatment. The following is a brief summary:

- Overweight results from an imbalance between energy intake and energy expenditure.
- Drugs can either reduce food intake or increase energy expenditure.
- Drug treatment does not cure the overweight patient.
- The therapeutic armamentarium of physicians is limited to only a few drugs.
- The use of drugs labors under the negative halo of treatment mishaps.
- Drugs do not work when they are not taken.
- Weight-loss plateaus during continued treatment occur when compensatory mechanisms come into play to counterbalance the effect of the drug.
- Monotherapy usually produces weight loss in the range of 10% (5% better than placebo).
- Frustration with the failure to continue to lose weight often leads to discontinuation of therapy and weight regain, with the drug labeled as a failure.

Physicians have several strategies for confronting the problems of the overweight patient. They can counsel the patient that they are concerned about the current level of body weight and, if the patient is interested, they can initiate treatment. Alternatively, if physicians feel uncomfortable with overweight patients, they can ignore the problem and hope that the patient will not raise the issue. Or, finally, they can wait until the complications of excess weight manifest themselves, such as diabetes, dyslipidemia, or hypertension and then institute appropriate therapy for each of these medical problems. With the current high-quality therapies available to treat diabetes mellitus, dyslipidemia, and hypertension, many physicians would prefer this latter strategy. Treatment for the metabolic syndrome often falls in this category and is discussed in Chapter 10.

However, if medical treatment of the overweight patient were more effective, physicians might prefer to treat it and thus delay the onset of the problems related to overweight. This strategy was the basis for the long-term Diabetes Prevention Program (DPP) and the Swedish Obese Subjects study. In the DPP, the onset of new cases of diabetes among individuals with impaired glucose tolerance was reduced 58% in the group that lost weight compared with the control group that did not lose weight. In the Swedish Obese Subjects study, the incidence of new cases of diabetes was reduced to zero over 2 years in patients who lost and maintained a weight loss of 12% or more compared with an incidence of 8.5% for new cases of diabetes in those who did not lose weight (Sjostrom et al., 2004). Thus, effective treatment of the overweight patient can reduce the risk of developing serious diseases in the future.

One reason that most physicians are reluctant to treat overweight patients is that their treatments are limited in number and effectiveness. At this writing, there are only two drugs approved by the US Food and Drug Administration (FDA) for long-term use, but a third one is anticipated in 2007. As monotherapy, these agents can produce an overall weight loss of 8 to 10% among patients who continue to take the medication for more than 6 months. However, to achieve the reduction in the rate of new cases of diabetes noted above, the weight loss needs to exceed 12%, a goal that is not usually achieved with current monotherapy. Thus, there is a great need for new drugs to be used as monotherapy and probably in combinations when prevention fails.

Both physicians and patients know that overweight is a stigmatized disease. One commonly held view is that overweight people are lazy and weak-willed. If fat people just had willpower, they would push themselves away from the table and not be over-weight. This widely held view is shared by the public and health professionals alike. The clamoring of women to be lean and well proportioned supports this view. The declining relative weight of centerfold models in Playboy magazine and of women who are winners of the Miss America contest also supports this view. Many physicians just do not like to see overweight patients come into their offices. Dealing with this problem poses a major challenge to any efforts to improve the lot of people who are overweight.

Three other issues aggravate the problem of treating overweight patient. The first is the "negative halo" that surrounds the use of appetite suppressants because amphetamine is addictive. There was never any evidence that dexfenfluramine was addictive. Nonetheless, the drug was scheduled by the US Drug Enforcement Agency as a schedule IV drug because on paper it had chemical similarities to amphetamine.

The second issue is the concern about the plateau of body weight that is reached when homeostatic mechanisms in the body come into play and stop further weight loss. There is an analogy with treatment of hypertension. When an antihypertensive drug is given, blood pressure drops and then stops falling within a few weeks to reach a "plateau" at a new lower level. The antihypertensive drug has not lost its effect when the plateau occurs, but its effect is being counteracted by physiological mechanisms designed to maintain blood pressure. In the treatment of overweight patients, a similar plateau in body weight is often viewed as a therapeutic failure for the weight-loss drug. This is particularly so when weight is regained when the drug is stopped. These attitudes and biases need to change before any effective new therapy will become widely accepted.

The final issue is the disaster that recently befell many patients who took the combination of fenfluramine and phentermine. Aortic regurgitation occurred in up to 25% of the patients treated with this combination of drugs and led many physicians to say "I told you so," and "I'm certainly glad I didn't use those drugs." Much of this will subside with time, but there will remain a residue of concern among some physicians and regulators about the potential problems that might surface when new treatments for overweight are made available to the public. Although the drug treatment of overweight patients has at least a century long history, progress in drug discovery was given a new impetus by the discovery of leptin in 1994. This peptide demonstrated that overweight can be caused by a hormone deficiency and be reversed by replacement of that hormone (Halaas et al., 1995; Maffei et al., 1995). Even before the discovery of leptin, over-weight had been declared to be a chronic disease by a National Institutes of Health consensus conference of 1985 (NIH, 1985). In the 20th century, bad eating habits were considered a primary cause for overweight. Because some bad habits can be behaviorally extinguished over a 12 week period of time, overweight medications approved before 1985 were approved for periods up to 12 weeks as an adjunct to a lifestyle change program. Equating overweight with bad habits and the stigmatization of obesity slowed the chronic use of overweight medications as is done with other chronic diseases (Puhl and

Brownell, 2003). With the recognition that longer-term therapy was needed, clinical trials have been extended in length, but since 1990 only three medications have been approved for the chronic treatment of overweight, and one of them, dexfenfluramine, was withdrawn 2 years later in 1997 (N. A., 1996; Putnam 1893).

USING THE CURRENTLY AVAILABLE DRUGS

This part reviews the field of drug therapy for the overweight patient. Table 1 lists the drugs that are available with whether they are approved by the US FDA for weight loss or not. For individuals desiring more detail or additional guidance in the use of medications to treat overweight, information can be found in a variety of sources (Bray and Greenway, 1999; Colman, 2005; Haddock et al., 2002; Kim et al., 2003; Li et al., 2005; National Institutes of Health et al., 2000; Padwal et al., 2004; Padwal et al., 2005; Snow et al., 2005; Vettor et al., 2005; Yanovski and Yanovski, 2002; Bray and Greenway, 2007).

As a guide for the use of medications, the algorithm that was described in Chapter 5 on evaluation of the overweight patient is used. The first step in this algorithm is to measure height, weight, and waist circumference to establish the body mass index (BMI) and central adiposity of the patient. If the BMI (weight in kg divided by the square of the height in meters [kg/m^2] or weight in pounds divided by square of the height {[inches] × 703}) is higher than 30 kg/m^2, the patient is by definition in the overweight class I category and can be considered for medications. Overweight individuals with a BMI above 25 may also be considered if they have diabetes, hypertension, sleep apnea, or another medical condition that would benefit from weight loss.

Waist circumference is also an important criterion to consider. The currently recommended upper limit for waist circumference is 102 cm (40 in.) for a man and 88 cm (35 in.) for a woman but, as noted in Chapter 1, other populations may need lower cut-points. The recent proposal from the International Diabetes Federation requires the presence of central adiposity to diagnose the metabolic syndrome, and uses values for waist circumference higher than 80 cm for females and 94 cm for males. Values above these numbers have the same meaning as a BMI higher than 30 kg/m^2.

Another important initial step is to assess the associated (comorbid) conditions by measuring blood pressure, glucose, lipids, and performing other tests when indicated. With this laboratory panel and the waist circumference, the presence of the metabolic syndrome can be diagnosed. This is best done with the criteria from the National Cholesterol Education Panel Adult Treatment III guidelines that were reviewed in Chapters 1 and 10.

Once it is established that the patient is an appropriate candidate to lose weight and that they are motivated to do so, the next step is to set a weight-loss goal. Most patients have an unrealistic view of how much weight they can lose. For them, a weight loss of less than 15% would often be viewed as a failure. In contrast, weight loss using monotherapy with the drugs that are currently available is not more than 10%. It is thus important for physician and patient alike to set a weight-loss goal for initial therapy that is not more than 10% and to set a lower limit for weight loss of less than 5%, which will suggest that an alternative strategy is needed.

The next step is to be certain that the patient is "ready" to lose weight. Using the ideas from psychology, the patient needs to be ready to work on weight loss as opposed to not

Table 1
Drugs approved by the US Food and Drug Administration That Produce Weight Loss

Generic name	Trade names	Usual dose	Comments
Drugs approved by the US FDA for the Long-term treatment of obesity			
Orlistat	Xenical	120 mg three times a day	May have gastrointestinal side effects
Sibutramine*	Meredia (US) Reductil (Rest of World)	5–15 mg once daily	Norepinephrine-serotonin reuptake inhibitor; May raise blood pressure
Rimonabant	Accomplia	20 mg once daily	
Drugs approved by the US FDA for short-term treatment of obesity			
Diethylpropion*			Sympathomimetic drugs; Approved for only a short time
Tablets	Tenuate	25 mg three times a day	
Extended release	Tenuate	75 mg in morning	
Phentermine HCl*			
Capsules	Phentridol Teramine Adipex-P	15–37.5 mg in the morning	
Tablets	Tetramine Adipex-P		
Extended release	Ionamin	15 or 30 mg/d in the morning	
Benzphetamine**	Didrex	25 to 150 mg/d in single or divided doses	
Phendimetrazine**			
Capsules - extended release	Adipost Bontril Melfial Prelu-2 X-trozine	105 mg once daily	
Tablets	Bontril Obezine	35 mg 2–3 times a day	
Drugs approved by the US FDA for purposes other than weight loss			
Bupropion			
Tablets and extended release	Wellbutrin Zyban (Anti-smoking)	300–400 mg/d	Anti-depressant; Smoking cessation
Topiramate	Topamax	25 mg/d titrated up to clinical effect	Anti-convulsant
Zonisamide	Zonergan	200 mg/d titrated up	Anti-convulsant
Metformin	Glucophage	500 mg twice daily up to maximal dose	Anti-diabetic drug used alone or in

(Continued)

Table 1 (*continued*)

Generic name	Trade names	Usual dose	Comments
		of 2500 mg	combination with other anti-diabetic drugs

Data from AHFS Drug Information 2005. Bethesda, MD:American Society of Health-System Pharmacists.
*Scheduled by the U.S. Drug Enforcement Agency as Schedule IV.
**Scheduled by the U.S. Drug Enforcement Agency as Schedule III.

yet thinking about the problem. Once the weight goal is established and the patient is prepared to take charge of their weight-loss program, the next steps are to help them develop lifestyle changes that will benefit their program. The most important of these are monitoring what they eat, where they eat it, and under what circumstances. A second element is to provide advice on diet and physical activity (*see* Chapters 6, 7 and 8). There are frozen foods, ready-to-make food items, and canned meal replacements that can be used for this purpose. The patient also needs more exercise. One strategy is to have them get a pedometer that records the number of steps taken, with the goal of gradually increasing it to 10,000 steps per day. In a review of lifestyle treatment used with pharmacotherapy in randomized clinical trials, Poston et al. (2001) found that balanced-deficit diets were used in 40.7%, low-calorie diets in 25%, and self-monitoring behavioral strategies in 23.1%.

When the patient returns, the physician establishes whether they have met their goals. If so, they continue as is. After 3 months, however, if they fail to meet their goals, medications may be considered. The next step is to discuss the pros and cons of medication with patients and have them sign a consent form for the use of medications to treat their overweight. An algorithm from the American College of Physicians (Snow et al., 2005) recommends six medications: orlistat, sibutramine, phentermine, diethylpropion, fluoxetine, and bupropion. The first four have been approved by the US FDA for treatment of overweight patients, but fluoxetine, sertraline, and bupropion have not, and they should not be used primarily for this purpose. In my view, fluoxetine and bupropion should only be used for weight loss in special situations. Fluoxetine is appropriate for the overweight patient who is depressed. Bupropion may also be helpful in reducing or preventing weight gain when people try to stop smoking and when they are depressed.

DRUGS APPROVED BY THE FDA FOR TREATMENT OF OVERWEIGHT

Drugs Approved for Long-Term Use

ORLISTAT

Mechanism of Action

Orlistat is a lipase inhibitor. In pharmacological studies, it was shown to be a potent selective inhibitor of pancreatic lipase that reduces the intestinal digestion of fat. The drug has a dose-dependent effect on fecal fat loss, increasing it to approximately 30% on a diet that has 30% of its energy as fat. Orlistat has little effect in subjects eating a low-fat diet, as might be anticipated from its mechanism of action.

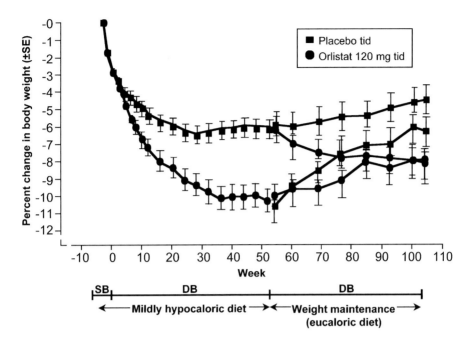

Fig. 1. Double-blind randomized clinical trial of orlistat versus placebo with a re-randomization of participants after the first year.

Long-Term Studies

A number of 1- to 2-year long-term clinical trials with orlistat have been published. The results of a 2-year trial are shown in Fig. 1 (Sjostrom et al., 1998). The trial consisted of two parts. In the first year, patients received a hypocaloric diet calculated to be 500 kcal per day less than the patient's requirements. During the second year, the diet was calculated to maintain body weight. By the end of year 1, the placebo-treated patients lost −6.1% of their initial body weight and the drug-treated patients lost −10.2%. The patients were randomized again at the end of year 1. Those switched from orlistat to placebo gained weight from −10 to −6% below baseline. Those switched from placebo to orlistat lost weight from −6% to −8.1% below baseline, which was essentially identical to the −7.9% loss in the patients treated with orlistat for the full 2 years.

In a second 2-year study, 892 patients were randomized to receive orlistat or placebo (Davidson et al., 1999). One group remained on placebo throughout the 2 years (97 patients), and a second group remained on orlistat (120 mg three times per day) for 2 years (109 patients). At the end of 1 year, two-thirds of the group (102 patients) treated with orlistat for 1 year were changed to orlistat (60 mg three times per day), and the others (95 patients) were switched to placebo (Davidson et al., 1999). After 1 year, the weight loss was 8.67 kg in the orlistat-treated group and 5.81 kg in the placebo group ($p < 0.001$). During the second year, those switched to placebo after 1 year reached the same weight as those treated with placebo for 2 years (−4.5% in those with placebo for 2 years and −4.2% in those switched to placebo during year 2).

In a third 2-year study, 783 patients remained in the placebo or orlistat-treated groups at 60 or 120 mg three times per day for the entire 2 years (Rossner et al., 2000). After

% Change

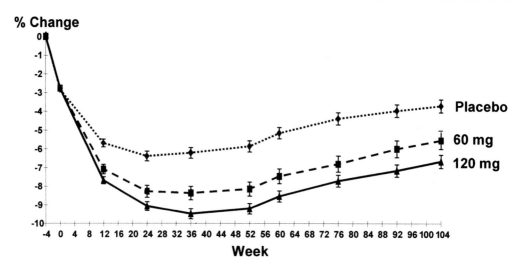

Fig. 2. Two year pooled data with orlistat (Figure provided by Dr. Jon Hauptman from the Files of Hoffmann LaRoche. Reproduced with permission.)

1 year with a weight-loss diet, the placebo group lost −7 kg, which was significantly less than the −9.6 kg lost by the group treated with orlistat (60 mg three times daily) or the −9.8 kg lost by the group treated with orlistat (120 mg three times daily). During the second year, when the diet was liberalized to a "weight maintenance" diet, all three groups regained some weight. At the end of 2 years, the patients in the placebo group were −4.3 kg below baseline, the patients treated with orlistat (60 mg three times daily) were −6.8 kg below baseline, and the patients who took orlistat (120 mg three times per day) were −7.6 kg below baseline.

The final 2-year trial evaluated 796 subjects in a general-practice setting (Hauptman, 2000). After 1 year of treatment with orlistat (120 mg three times per day), the orlistat-treated patients ($n = 117$) had lost −8.8 kg, compared with −4.3 kg in the placebo group ($n = 91$). During the second year, when the diet was liberalized to "maintain body weight," both groups regained some weight. At the end of 2 years, the orlistat group was −5.2 kg below their baseline weight, compared with −1.5 kg below baseline for the group treated with placebo.

The pooled 2-year data from these four studies in shown in Fig. 2. It contains information on both the 120 mg three times a day and the 60 mg three times a day dose. It is clear that there is a dose-response. The maximal weight loss was achieved between 6 and 9 months and then there was a slow regain in all of the groups during the rest of the study.

The results of a 4-year double-blind, randomized, placebo-controlled trial with orlistat have also been reported (Torgerson et al., 2004). A total of 3304 overweight patients, 21% of whom had impaired glucose tolerance, were included in this Swedish trial (Fig. 3). The lowest body weight was achieved during the first year: more than −11% below baseline in the orlistat-treated group and −6% below baseline in the placebo-treated group. Over the remaining 3 years of the trial, there was a small regain in weight, such that by the end of 4 years, the orlistat-treated patients were −6.9%

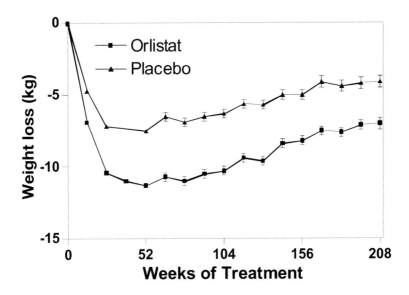

Fig. 3. Effect of orlistat on body weight in a 4-year randomized placebo-controlled clinical trial.

below baseline, compared with −4.1% for those receiving placebo. The trial also showed a 37% reduction in the conversion of patients from impaired glucose tolerance to diabetes; essentially all of this benefit occurred in the patients with impaired glucose tolerance at enrollment into the trial.

Weight maintenance with orlistat was evaluated in a 1-year study (Hill et al., 1999). Patients were enrolled if they had lost more than 8% of their body weight over 6 months while eating a 1000-kcal-per-day (4180-kJ/d) diet. The 729 patients were randomized to receive placebo or orlistat at 30, 60, or 120 mg three times daily for 12 months. At the end of this time, the placebo-treated patients had regained 56% of their body weight, compared with 32.4% in the group treated with the 120-mg dose of orlistat. The other two doses of orlistat were no different from placebo in preventing the regain of weight.

Studies in Special Populations

Studies in Diabetics. Patients with diabetes treated with orlistat, 120 mg three times daily for 1 year, lost more weight than the placebo-treated group (Hollander et al., 1998; Kelley et al., 2002; Miles et al., 2002). The subjects with diabetes also showed a significantly greater decrease in hemoglobin A1c levels. In another study of orlistat and weight loss, investigators pooled data on 675 subjects from three of the 2-year studies described previously in which glucose tolerance tests were available (Heymsfield et al., 2000). During treatment, 6.6% of the patients taking orlistat converted from a normal to an impaired glucose tolerance test, compared with 10.8% in the placebo-treated group. None of the orlistat-treated patients who originally had normal glucose tolerance developed diabetes, compared with 1.2% in the placebo-treated group. Of those who initially had normal glucose tolerance, 7.6% in the placebo group but only 3% in the orlistat-treated group developed diabetes. The effect of orlistat in preventing diabetes has been assessed in a 4-year study (Torgerson et al., 2004). In this trial, weight loss was reduced by 2.8 kg (95% confidence interval [CI] 1.1–4.5 kg) compared with

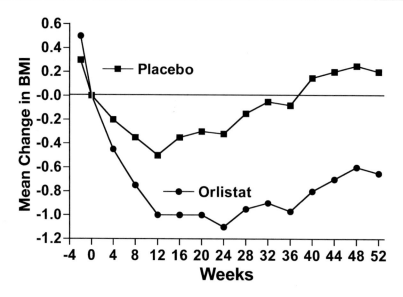

Fig. 4. Effect of orlistat on body mass index in a randomized placebo-controlled clinical trial of orlistat in adolescents. (Redrawn from Chaonoine et al., 2005.)

placebo, and the conversion rate of diabetes was reduced from 9 to 6% for a relative risk reduction of 0.63 (95% CI 0.46–0.86; Padwal et al., 2005).

Metabolic Syndrome and Lipids. In a further analysis, patients who had participated in previously reported studies were divided into the highest and lowest quintiles for triglyceride and high-density lipoprotein (HDL)-cholesterol levels (Reaven et al., 2001). Those with high triglyceride and low HDL-cholesterol levels were labeled "syndrome X," and those with the lowest triglyceride levels and highest HDL-cholesterol levels were the "nonsyndrome X" controls. In this classification, there were almost no men in the nonsyndrome X group, compared with an equal sex breakdown in the syndrome X group. In addition, the syndrome X group had slightly higher systolic blood pressure (SBP) and diastolic blood pressure (DBP) levels and a nearly twofold higher level of fasting insulin. Besides weight loss, the only difference between the placebo- and orlistat- treated patients was the decrease in low-density lipoprotein (LDL)-cholesterol levels in the patients treated with orlistat. However, the syndrome X subgroup showed a significantly greater decrease in triglyceride and insulin levels than those without syndrome X. Levels of HDL-cholesterol increased more in the syndrome X group, but LDL-cholesterol levels showed a smaller decrease than in the non-syndrome X group. All of the clinical studies with orlistat have shown significant decreases in serum cholesterol and LDL-cholesterol levels that usually are greater than can be accounted for by weight loss alone (Bray and Greenway, 1999). One study showed that orlistat reduces the absorption of cholesterol from the gastrointestinal (GI) tract, thus providing a mechanism for the clinical observations (Mittendorfer et al., 2001).

Studies in Children. A multicenter trial tested the effect of orlistat in 539 obese adolescents (Chanoine et al., 2005). Subjects were randomized to placebo or orlistat 120 mg three times a day and a mildly hypocaloric diet containing 30% fat. By the end of the study, BMI had decreased 0.55 kg/m^2 in the drug-treated group but had increased

Table 2
Meta-Analysis of Body Weight Change in Studies With Long-Term Use of Orlistat

Author (year)	Mean (95% confidence interval [CI])
Davidson et al. (1999)	–2.95 (95% CI –4.45 to –1.45)
Hauptman (2000)	–3.80 (95% CI –5.37 to –2.23)
Rossner et al. (2000)	–3.00 (95% CI –4.17 to –1.83)
Sjostrom et al. (1998)	–4.20 (95% CI –5.26 to –3.14)
Torgerson et al. (2004)	–4.17 (95% CI –4.60 to –3.74)

Adapted from Li et al., 2005.

Table 3
Meta-Analysis of Body Weight Change in Studies Using Orlistat

Author	Year	Treatment N	Treatment Mean SD	Placebo N	Placebo Mean SD	Wt %	WMD (95% confidence interval)
Sjostrom et al.	1998	343	–8.10 ± 8.21	340	–3.90 ± 7.02	11.1	–4.20 (–5.35 to –3.05)
Hollander et al.	1998	156	–3.84 ± 5.00	151	–1.43 ± 5.10	11.4	–2.41 (–3.54 to –1.29)
Davidson et al.	1999	657	–8.76 ± 9.48	223	–5.81 ± 10.01	6.5	–2.95 (–4.45 to –1.45)
Rossner et al.	2000	241	–8.13 ± 8.22	236	–5.23 ± 7.40	7.4	–2.90 (–4.30 to –1.50)
Hauptman	2000	210	–5.40 ± 7.44	212	–1.41 ± 6.31	8.4	–3.99 (–5.31 to –2.67)
Lindegarde	2000	190	–4.20 ± 7.03	186	–2.90 ± 6.74	7.5	–1.30 (–2.69 to 0.09)
Finer	2000	110	–3.29 ± 6.85	108	–1.31 ± 6.29	4.8	–1.98 (–3.73 to –0.23)
Broom	2002	259	–5.80 ± 8.50	163	–2.30 ± 6.40	8.7	–3.50 (–4.79 to –2.21)

Adapted from Avenell et al., 2004.
WMD, weighted mean difference.

0.31 kg/m^2 in the placebo group. By the end of the study, weight had increased by only 0.51 kg in the orlistat-treated group, compared with 3.14 kg in the placebo-treated group (Fig. 4). This difference resulted from differences in body fat. The side effects were GI in origin, as expected from the mode of action of orlistat. A second small 6-month randomized clinical trial from a single site failed to find a difference resulting from treatment with orlistat in a population of 40 adolescents (Maahs et al., 2006).

Meta-Analysis of Orlistat Studies

Several meta-analyses of orlistat have been published (Avenell et al., 2004b; Haddock et al., 2002; Li et al., 2005). By pooling six studies, Haddock et al. (2002) estimated the weight loss in patients treated with orlistat as –7.1 kg (range –4.0 to –10.3 kg) compared with –5.02 kg (range –3.0 to –6.1 kg) for the placebo-treated groups. In the meta-analysis of Li et al. (2005) the overall mean difference after 12 months of therapy in 22 studies was –2.70 kg (95% CI –3.79 to –1.61 kg). Because this analysis included subjects with and without diabetes, the data has been summarized from the five 2-year studies in non-diabetics (Table 2). In another meta-analysis of orlistat including 8-year-long studies, only one of which was in patients with diabetes, the overall effect of orlistat on weight loss at 12 months using the weighted mean difference (WMD) was −3.01 kg (95% CI −3.48 to −2.54 kg). This meta-analysis also examined the effects of weight loss at 1 and 2 years and on the various laboratory and clinical responses. The overall effect of orlistat on weight loss at 12 months using the WMD was −3.01 kg (95% CI −3.48 to −2.54 kg; Table 3). After 24 months, the overall effect of orlistat on weight loss was −3.26 kg (95% CI −4.15 to −2.37 kg). In terms of weight maintenance, the overall effect of orlistat after 12 months was −0.85 kg (95% CI −1.50 to −0.19 kg; Davidson et al., 1999; Hauptman, 2000; Hill et al., 1999; Rossner et al., 2000). Using the pooled data shows significant overall effects after 1 year of treatment on the change in cholesterol (−0.34 mmol/L [95% CI −0.41 to −0.027]; $N = 7$ studies), the change in LDL-cholesterol (−0.29 mmol/L [95% CI −0.34 to −0.24]; $N = 7$ studies), the change in HDL-cholesterol (−0.03 mmol/L [95% CI −0.05 to −0.01]; $N = 6$ studies), the change in triglycerides (0.03 mmol/L [95% CI −0.04 to 0.10]; $N = 6$ studies), the change in HbA1c (−0.17% [95% CI −0.24 to −0.10]; $N = 3$ studies; Broom et al., 2002; Hollander et al., 1998; Lindgarde, 2000), the change in SBP (−2.02 mmHg [95% CI −2.87 to −1.17]; $N = 7$ studies), and the change in DBP (−1.64 mmHg [95% CI −2.20 to −1.09]; $N = 7$ studies). In a meta-analysis focused on the use of orlistat in subjects with diabetes, Norris et al. (2004) reported a WMD in favor of orlistat of −2.6 kg (95% CI −3.2 to −2.1 kg) after 52 to 57 weeks of treatment.

Safety Considerations

Orlistat is not absorbed to any significant degree an its side effects are thus related to the blockade of triglyceride digestion in the intestine (Zhi et al., 1999). Fecal fat loss and related GI symptoms are common initially, but they subside as patients learn to use the drug (Bray and Greenway, 1999). The quality of life in patients treated with orlistat may improve despite concerns about GI symptoms. Orlistat can cause small but significant decreases in fat-soluble vitamins. Levels usually remain within the normal range, but a few patients may need vitamin supplementation. Because it is impossible to tell which patients need vitamins, it is wise to provide a multivitamin routinely with instructions to take it before bedtime. Orlistat does not seem to affect the absorption of other drugs, except cyclosporin.

SIBUTRAMINE

Mechanism of Action

Sibutramine is a highly selective inhibitor for the reuptake at nerve endings of norepinephrine, serotonin, and, to a lesser degree, dopamine. In experimental and clinical studies it reduces food intake. In a double-blind placebo-controlled 2-week trial, a 30 mg per day dose of sibutramine reduced food intake by 23% on day 7 and 26% on day 14 relative to placebo. A smaller dose of 10 mg also significantly reduced food intake at 14 days (Rolls et al., 1998). The effect of sibutramine on food intake has also been examined over a longer period of time (Barkeling et al., 2003). The first 2 weeks of this 10-month trial were conducted in a double-blind randomized placebo-controlled crossover design. Participants then entered a 10-month open-label trial with repeat food intake at the end. There was a 16% kcal reduction in energy intake at the test lunch in the first part of the study (after 2 weeks). Ten months later, there was still a 27% reduction when compared with their pre-weight-loss placebo-treated food intake. In animals, sibutramine also stimulates thermogenesis, but there is conflicting data in human beings (Hansen et al., 1998).

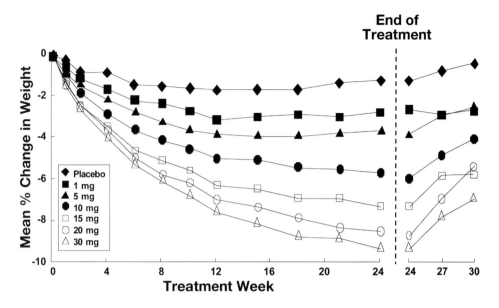

Fig. 5. Six-month randomized placebo-controlled dose-ranging trial with sibutramine at six doses and placebo. (Reproduced from Bray et al., 1999.)

Long-Term Studies

Sibutramine is approved by the US FDA for long-term use in treatment of overweight patients. Sibutramine has been evaluated extensively in several multicenter trials lasting 6 to 24 months. In a 6-month dose-ranging study of 1047 patients, 67% treated with sibutramine achieved a 5% weight loss from baseline, and 35% lost 10% or more (Bray et al., 1999). There was a clear dose–response effect in this 24-week trial, and patients regained weight when the drug was stopped, indicating that the drug remained effective when used. Data from this multicenter trial are shown in Fig. 5 (Bray et al., 1999).

In a 1-year trial of 456 patients who received sibutramine (10 or 15 mg per day) or placebo, 56% of those who stayed in the trial for 12 months lost at least 5% of their initial body weight, and 30% of the patients lost 10% of their initial body weight while taking the 10-mg dose (Smith et al., 2001).

Three trials have assessed the value of using sibutramine to prevent regain of body weight. The first was by Apfelbaum et al. (1999). In this multicenter trial, participants were initially given a VLCD for 6 weeks to induce weight loss. Of the initial 181 subjects enrolled, 142 were randomized to either 10 mg per day of sibutramine or placebo after losing −6 kg or more on the VLCD. After another 12 months, those receiving the drug had lost an additional −6.4 kg compared with a small weight gain of +0.2 kg for those receiving placebo. The authors concluded that sibutramine had effectively enhanced the initial weight loss and maintained it for an additional 12 months.

This was followed by the Sibutramine Trial of Obesity Reduction and Maintenance (STORM) trial, which lasted 2 years and provided evidence for weight maintenance (James et al., 2000). Seven centers participated in this trial, in which patients were initially enrolled in an open-label phase and treated with 10 mg per day of sibutramine for 6 months. Of the patients who lost more than −8 kg, two-thirds were then randomized

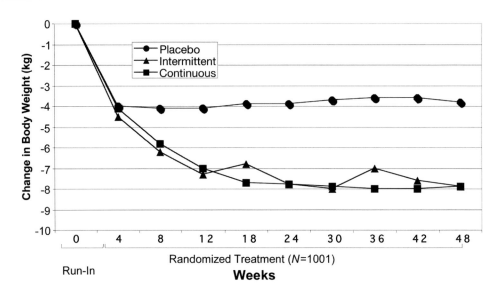

Fig. 6. Effect on body weight of continuous versus intermittent use of sibutramine in a randomized placebo-controlled clinical trial. (Adapted from Wirth and Krause, 2001.)

to sibutramine and one-third to placebo. During the 18-month double-blind phase of this trial, the placebo-treated patients steadily regained weight, maintaining only 20% of their weight loss at the end of the trial. In contrast, the subjects treated with sibutramine maintained their weight for 12 months and then regained an average of only 2 kg, thus maintaining 80% of their initial weight loss after 2 years (James et al., 2000). Despite the higher weight loss with sibutramine at the end of the 18 months of controlled observation, the blood pressure levels of the sibutramine-treated patients were still higher than in the patients treated with placebo.

The final trial for weight maintenance was a study conducted at eight hospitals in The Netherlands where patients were initially treated before referral to their primary care physicians. A total of 221 patients began the VLCD. Of these patients, 189 lost the required −10 kg or more during 3 months and were randomized to sibutramine 10 mg per day or placebo for the remaining 15 months. Mean weight loss during the VLCD period for the successful subjects was 14.5% from baseline. Following 2 additional months of treatment in the hospital clinic, the final 13 months were conducted in the general practitioners' offices. At 18 months, the odds ratio was 1.76 (95% CI 1.06, 2.93) favoring weight loss with sibutramine ($p = 0.03$). Using the intent to treat analysis, more than 80% of the weight loss at the end of the VLCD was maintained by 70, 51, and 30% of those on sibutramine at 6, 12, and 18 months compared with 48, 31, and 20% for those receiving placebo and these differences were significant at all time points ($p \leq 0.03$; Mathus-Vliegen, 2005).

The possibility of using sibutramine as intermittent therapy has been tested in a randomized, placebo-controlled trial lasting 52 weeks (Wirth and Krause, 2001; Fig. 6). The patients randomized to sibutramine received one of two regimens. One group received continuous treatment with 15 mg per day for 1 year, and the other had two 6-week periods when sibutramine was withdrawn. During the periods when the drug was replaced by placebo, there was a small regain in weight that was lost when the drug was resumed. At the end of the trial, the continuous- and intermittent-therapy groups had lost the same amount of weight.

Studies in Special Populations

Patients With Diabetes. A number of studies have examined the effect of sibutramine in patients with diabetes. In a 3-month (12-week) trial, patients with diabetes who were treated with 15 mg per day of sibutramine lost −2.4 kg (2.8%), compared with −0.1 kg (0.12%) in the placebo group (Fujioka et al., 2000). In this study, hemoglobin A1C levels decreased 0.3% in the drug-treated group and remained stable in the placebo group. Fasting glucose values decreased 0.3 mg/dL in the drug-treated patients and increased 1.4 mg/dL in the placebo-treated group. In a 24-week trial, the dose of sibutramine was increased from 5 to 20 mg per day over 6 weeks (Wadden et al., 2001). Among those who completed the treatment, weight loss was −4.3 kg (4.3%) in the sibutramine-treated patients, compared with −0.3 kg (0.3%) in placebo-treated patients. Hemoglobin A1C levels decreased 1.67% in the drug-treated group, compared with 0.53% in the placebo-treated group. These changes in glucose and hemoglobin A1C levels were expected from the amount of weight loss associated with drug treatment. In a 12-month multi-center, randomized placebo-controlled study (McNulty et al., 2003), 194 patients with diabetes receiving metformin were assigned to placebo ($N = 64$), sibutramine 15 mg per day ($N = 68$), or sibutramine 20 mg per day ($N = 62$). At 12 months, weight loss was 5.5 ± 0.6 kg in the 15 mg per day group, 8.0 ± 0.9 kg in the 20 mg per day group, and 0.2 ± 0.5 kg in the placebo group. Glycemic control improved in parallel with weight loss. Sibutramine raised sitting DBP by more than 5 mmHg in 43% of those receiving 15 mg per day of sibutramine compared with 25% in the placebo group ($P < 0.05$). Pulse rate increased more than 10 beats per minute (bpm) in 42% of those on sibutramine compared with 17% for those on placebo.

A meta-analysis has been done of eight studies in patients with diabetes receiving sibutramine (Vettor et al., 2005). In the meta-analysis, the changes in body weight, waist circumference, glucose, hemoglobin A1c, triglycerides, and HDL-cholesterol favored sibutramine. The mean weight loss was -5.53 ± 2.2 kg for those treated with sibutramine and -0.90 ± 0.17 kg for the placebo-treated patients. There was no significant change in SBP, but DBP was significantly higher in the sibutramine-treated patients (Vettor et al., 2005). In the meta-analysis by Norris et al. (2004) the net weight loss over 12 to 26 weeks in four trials including 391 patients with diabetes was −4.5 kg (95% CI −7.2 to −1.8 kg).

Patients With Hypertension. Some trials have reported the use of sibutramine to treat overweight patients with hypertension. In a 3-month trial, all patients were receiving β-blockers with or without thiazides for their hypertension (McMahon et al., 2000). The sibutramine-treated patients lost −4.2 kg (4.5%), compared with a loss of −0.3 kg (0.3%) in the placebo-treated group. Mean supine and standing DBP and SBP levels were not significantly different between drug- and placebo-treated patients. Heart rate, however, increased by 5.6 ± 8.25 bpm (mean ± standard deviation) in the sibutramine-treated patients, as compared with an increase of 2.2 ± 6.43 bpm in the placebo group. One 52-week trial involved patients with hypertension whose blood pressure levels were controlled with calcium channel blockers with or without β-blockers or thiazides (McMahon et al., 2000). Sibutramine doses were increased from 5 to 20 mg per day during the first 6 weeks. Weight loss was significantly greater in the sibutramine-treated patients, averaging −4.4 kg (4.7%), as compared with −0.5 kg (0.7%) in the placebo-treated group. DBP levels decreased 1.3 mmHg in the placebo-treated group and increased 2 mmHg in the sibutramine-treated group. The SBP levels increased 1.5 mmHg in the placebo-treated group and 2.7 mmHg in the sibutramine-treated group. Heart rate was unchanged in the placebo-treated patients, but increased by 4.9 bpm in the sibutramine-treated patients. The effects of sibutramine on blood pressure have been evaluated in a meta-analysis of 21 studies by Kim et al. (2003). Sibutramine produced a significant overall weight loss and significant increase in both SBP and DBP. In a subgroup analysis, they found the effect on SBP to be greater with higher doses of sibutramine in individuals weighing 92 kg or more and in younger individuals (<44 years of age). Body weights of 92 kg or more in older individuals also showed a greater rise in DBP. In another analysis of two studies using sibutramine for 48 weeks, Jordan et al. (2005) reported that sibutramine significantly reduced body weight but did not lead to a difference in SBP after 48 weeks (−0.1 ± 15.5 mmHg for placebo and −0.2 ± 1.52 mmHg for the sibutramine group). However, the change in DBP was statistically significant with a small rise of +0.3 ± 9.5 mmHg in the sibutramine group and −0.8 ± 9.2 mmHg in the placebo group ($p = 0.049$).

Sibutramine Plus Behavioral Weight Loss. Sibutramine has been studied as part of a behavioral weight-loss program in two reports (Wadden et al., 2005). With sibutramine alone and minimal behavioral intervention, the weight loss over 12 months was approximately −5.0 ± 7.4 kg (5%) over 12 months. Behavior modification alone produced a weight loss of −6.7 ± 7.9 kg. Adding a brief behavioral therapy session to a group that also received sibutramine produced a slightly larger weight loss of −5.0 ± 7.4 kg. When the intensive lifestyle intervention was combined with sibutramine, the weight loss increased to −12.1 ± 9.8 kg. When a structured meal plan was added to the medication and behavioral modification in one of these studies (Wadden et al., 2005) the weight loss increased further to 15 kg (Wadden et al., 2001). Completing the food intake records was a strong predictor of success (Wadden et al., 2005). Those in the combined therapy group receiving intensive lifestyle and sibutramine who were in the highest third for record keeping lost −18.1 ± 9.8 compared to −7.7 ± 7.5 kg in the lowest third for record keeping (Fig. 7).

Studies in Children. Sibutramine has also been used in children and adolescents (Berkowitz et al., 2003; Berkowitz et al., 2006; Godoy-Matos et al., 2005). The trial by Berkowitz et al. included 85 adolescents 13 to 17 years of age with a BMI of 32 to 44 kg/m^2 who were treated for 6 months. Weight loss in the drug-treated group was −7.8 kg, for an 8.5% reduction in BMI, compared with −3.2 kg for the placebo group, for a 4.0% reduction in BMI. When the placebo group was switched to sibutramine after 6 months, there was an additional significant weight loss in this group. In a 12-month multicenter, randomized, placebo-controlled trial, 498 adolescents aged 12 to 16 were treated with sibutramine or placebo (Berkowitz et al., 2006). The dose of sibutramine was 10 mg per day for 6 months and then increased to 15 mg per day in those who had not lost more than 10% of their baseline BMI. After 12 months, the mean absolute change in BMI was −2.9 kg/m^2 (−8.2%) in the sibutramine group compared with −0.3 kg/m^2 (−0.8%) in the placebo group ($p < 0.001$). Triglycerides,

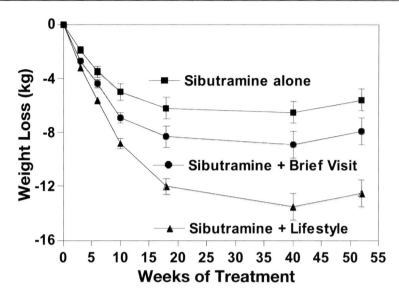

Fig. 7. Effect on body weight loss of sibutramine alone or with additional supplementary behavior therapies. (Adapted from Wadden et al., 2005.)

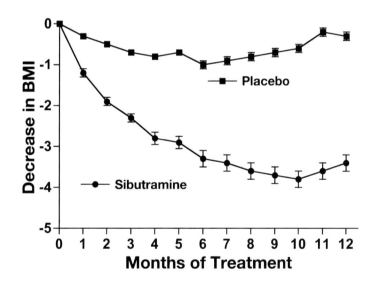

Fig. 8. Effect on body mass index of sibutramine in a randomized placebo-controlled multi-center clinical trial in adolescents. (Adapted from Berkowitz et al., 2006.)

HDL-cholesterol, and insulin sensitivity improved, and there was no significant difference in the changes in either SBP or DBP (Fig. 8).

Meta-Analysis

Several meta-analyses of sibutramine have been published (Avenell et al., 2004b; Haddock et al., 2002; Li et al., 2005). By pooling four studies, Haddock et al. (2002)

Table 4
Effect of Sibutramine Versus Placebo and Diet at 12 Months

Author	Year	N	Treatment Mean SD	N	Control Mean SD	Wt %	WMD (95% confidence interval)
Apfelbaum et al.	1999	81	−5.20 ± 7.50	78	0.50 ± 5.70	17.14	−5.70 (−7.77 to −3.63)
McMahon et al.	2000	142	−4.40 ± 7.16	69	−0.50 ± 6.06	21.32	−3.90 (−5.75 to −2.05)
Smith	2001	154	−4.40 ± 7.16	157	−1.60 ± 6.37	32.20	−2.80 (−4.31 to −1.29)
Smith	2001	153	−6.40 ± 7.73	157	−1.60 ± 6.37	29.34	−4.32 (−6.38 to −3.22)

Adapted from Avenell et al., 2004 a,b.
WMD, weighted mean difference.

estimated the weight loss in patients treated with sibutramine as −5.3 kg (range 4.0–7.3 kg) compared with −1.8 kg (range 0.8–3.3 kg) for the placebo-treated groups. In the meta-analysis of Li et al. (2005), the overall mean difference after 12 months of therapy in five studies was −4.45 kg (95% CI −5.29 to −3.62 kg). In the study by Avenell et al. (2004b) the overall effect of sibutramine at 12 months was −4.12 kg (95% CI −4.97 to −3.26 kg). Table 4 is a summary for each of the trials that had data for 12 months with sibutramine (Avenell et al., 2004b). After an additional interval in the weight maintenance studies, the data showed a −3.70-kg loss at 15 months (95% CI −5.71 to −1.69 kg; Apfelbaum et al., 1999) and a −3.40-kg loss at 18 months (95% CI −4.45 to −2.35 kg; James et al., 2000).

Combining Sibutramine and Orlistat

Because sibutramine works on noradrenergic and serotonergic reuptake mechanisms in the brain, and orlistat works peripherally to reduce triglyceride digestion in the GI tract, their mechanisms of action do not overlap and combining them might provide additive weight loss (Wadden et al., 2000). To test this possibility, researchers randomly assigned patients to orlistat or placebo after 1 year of treatment with sibutramine (Fig. 9; Wadden et al., 2000). During the additional 4 months of treatment, the two groups lost no significant amount of weight and adding orlistat had no detectable effect.

In an open-label, randomized 12 week study, 86 overweight patients were assigned to treatment with either orlistat 120 mg three times daily, sibutramine 10 mg daily, a combination of orlistat and sibutramine, or to a diet group. During the 12 weeks, sibutramine produced more weight loss than orlistat alone. Adding orlistat to sibutramine did not significantly enhance weight loss, confirming the observations of Wadden et al. (Kaya et al., 2004; Wadden et al., 2000).

Safety Considerations

Sibutramine is available in 5-, 10-, and 15-mg doses; 10 mg per day as a single dose is the recommended starting level, with titration up or down depending on response. Doses higher than 15 mg per day are not recommended. Of the patients who lost 2 kg (4 lb.) in the first 4 weeks of treatment, 60% achieved a weight loss of more than 5%,

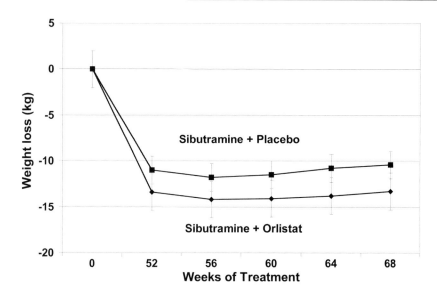

Fig. 9. Effect on weight loss of adding orlistat or placebo after a 1-year treatment with sibutramine.

compared with less than 10% of those who did not lose 2 kg (4 lb.) in 4 weeks. Combining data from the 11 studies on sibutramine showed a reduction in triglyceride, total cholesterol, and LDL-cholesterol levels and an increase in HDL-cholesterol levels that were related to the magnitude of the weight loss.

RIMONABANT

Mechanism of Action

There are two cannabinoid receptors, CB-1 (470 amino acids in length) and CB-2 (360 amino acids in length). The CB-1 receptor has almost all the amino acids that comprise the CB-2 receptor and additional amino acids at both ends. CB-1 receptors are distributed throughout the brain in the areas related to feeding, on fat cells, in the GI tract, and on immune cells. Marijuana and tetrahydrocannabinol, which stimulate the CB-1 receptor, increase high-fat and sweet food intake, and fasting increases the levels of endocannabinoids. The rewarding properties of cannabinoid agonists are mediated through the meso-limbic dopaminergic system. Rimonabant is a specific antagonist of the CB-1 receptor, and inhibits sweet food intake in marmosets as well as high-fat food intake in rats but not in rats fed standard chow. In addition to being specific in inhibiting highly palatable food intake, pair feeding experiments in diet-induced obese rats show that the rimonabant-treated animals lost 21% of their body weight compared with 14% in the pair-fed controls. This suggests, at least in rodents, that rimonabant increases energy expenditure in addition to reducing food intake. CB-1 knockout mice are lean and resistant to diet-induced overweight. CB-1 receptors are upregulated on adipocytes in diet-induced obese mice, and rimonabant increases adiponectin, a fat cell hormone associated with insulin sensitivity (Bensaid et al., 2003; Juan-Pico et al., 2006; Kirkham, 2005; Pagotto et al., 2006).

Long-Term Clinical Studies

The results of four phase III trials of rimonabant for the treatment of overweight have been published. The first trial, called the Rimonabant in Obesity (RIO)-Europe trial was reported in 2005 (Van Gaal et al., 2005) and was intended to be conducted in Europe, but slow recruitment led to inclusion of 276 subjects from the United States. This was a 2-year trial with 1-year results reported in this paper. A total of 1057 patients with a BMI higher than 30 kg/m^2 without comorbidities or higher than 27 kg/m^2 with hypertension or dyslipidemia were stratified on whether they lost more or less than 2 kg during run-in and then randomized in a ratio of 1:2:2 to receive placebo, rimonabant 5 mg per day, or rimonabant 20 mg per day. The energy content of the diet was calculated by subtracting 600 kcal per day from the energy requirements calculated from the Harris-Benedict equation. The trial consisted of a 4-week run-in period followed by 52 weeks of treatment. Of those who started, 61% (920) completed the first year. Weight loss was 2% in the placebo group and 8.5% in the 20-mg rimonabant group. Baseline weight was between 98.5 (placebo group) and 102.0 kg (for the rimonabant 20-mg dose). During run-in, there was a mean −1.9 kg weight loss. From baseline at the end of run-in, the placebo group that completed the trial lost an additional −2.3 kg, the low-dose rimonabant group lost −3.6 kg, and the high-dose group lost −8.6 kg. On an intent-to-treat basis, these numbers were a weight loss of −1.8 kg for the placebo group, −3.4 kg for the low-dose rimonabant group, and −6.6 kg for the high-dose rimonabant group. Expressing the data as a responder analysis, the authors reported that 30.5% of the placebo group lost 5% or more, compared with 44.2% for the low-dose rimonabant group and 67.4% for the high-dose rimonabant group. When a weight loss of 10% or more was considered, the numbers were 12.4% for the placebo group, 15.3% for the low-dose rimonabant group, and 39% for the high-dose rimonabant group. Waist circumference was also reduced by treatment. With the intent-to-treat analysis, waist declined 2.4 cm in the placebo group, 3.9 cm in the low-dose rimonabant group, and 6.5 cm in the high-dose rimonabant group. Triglycerides were reduced by 6.8% in the high-dose rimonabant group compared with a rise of 8.3% in the placebo group. HDL-cholesterol was improved. It increased by 22.3% compared with 13.4% in the placebo group. These changes in metabolic parameters were reflected in a change in the prevalence of the metabolic syndrome. Among the completers, there was a 33.9% reduction in the prevalence of the metabolic syndrome, compared with 34.8% in the low-dose rimonabant group and 64.8% in the high-dose rimonabant group. In the high-dose rimonabant group, the LDL particle size increased, adiponectin increased, glucose decreased, insulin decreased, C-reactive protein decreased, and the metabolic syndrome prevalence was cut in half. There was no significant change in blood pressure or pulse between groups.

The second study was in patients with dyslipidemia and is called the RIO-Lipids study (Despres et al., 2005). This was a 12-month randomized, double-blind, placebo-controlled trial of rimonabant at two doses versus placebo in overweight subjects eating a 600-kcal-per-day deficit diet. It was conducted at 67 sites in 8 countries. As a lipids trial, the inclusion criteria were a BMI of 27 to 40 kg/m^2, elevated fasting triglycerides (150–700 mg/dL), ratio of cholesterol to HDL-cholesterol more than 5 in men and more than 4.5 in women and no more than 5 kg variation in body weight in the previous 3 months. Subjects were stratified at run-in by triglycerides below or above

400 mg/dL and at the end of run-in by a weight loss of more or less than 2 kg. Randomization was on a 1:1:1 basis of placebo: 5 mg per day rimonabant to 20 mg per day rimonabant. Following the end of the 4-week run-in, participants were randomized and treated for 12 months. The dropout rate was about 40% by the end of 12 months. Weight losses in this trial were almost identical to those in the Rio-Europe trial. After an approximate 2-kg weight loss during run-in, the placebo-treated patients in the completers group lost an additional −2.3 kg, compared with −4.2 kg in the low-dose rimonabant group and −8.8 kg in the high-dose rimonabant group. Waist circumference also showed a dose-dependent reduction by 3.4 cm in the placebo group, 4.9 cm in the low-dose rimonabant group, and 9.1 cm in the high-dose rimonabant group. A number of other metabolic parameters also responded to the drug or weight loss. They included a decrease in triglycerides, an increase in HDL-cholesterol, a decrease in peak size of LDL-cholesterol particles, an increase in adiponectin, a decline in fasting insulin, a fall in leptin, and a decrease in C-reactive protein. Several liver enzymes fell with treatment, suggesting improvement in non-alcoholic steatosis. Blood pressure decreased significantly in RIO-Lipids in contrast with RIO-Europe. As might be expected from these metabolic changes, the prevalence of the metabolic syndrome in those who met the Adult Treatment Panel III criteria at randomization fell to 25.8% in the high-dose rimonabant group, 40.0% in the low-dose rimonabant group, and 41.0% in the placebo group.

The third randomized, double-blind, placebo-controlled study called RIO-North America, was also a 2-year study that randomized 3045 overweight subjects with a BMI higher than 30 kg/m^2 or with a BMI higher than 27 kg/m^2 with treated or untreated hypertension or dyslipidemia and without diabetes to placebo, 5 mg rimonabant, or 20 mg rimonabant. Participants were instructed in a 600-kcal-per-day deficit diet. Randomization and baseline occurred after a 4 week run-in period when subjects had lost an average of 1.9 kg. They were thus stratified by whether they lost more or less than 2 kg during run-in. At 1 year, half of the patients in each drug group were switched to placebo based on their initial randomization. The trial was conducted at 64 American and 8 Canadian centers. At 1 year, completion rates were 51 to 55% for the three arms. During the first year, weight loss was −2.8 kg in the placebo group and −8.6 kg in the 20-mg rimonabant group (Fig. 10). Weight loss declined steadily until week 36, after which it plateaued. For the second year, those individuals who were switched from rimonabant to placebo regained weight at almost the mirror image of the rate at which they lost it during the first year. At the end of the study, they were still slightly lighter but no different from the group treated with placebo for the full 2 years. Waist circumference decreased, and the percentage with the metabolic syndrome decreased from 34.8 to 21.2% compared with a change from 31.7 to 29.2% in the placebo-treated group. HDL-cholesterol rose more in the rimonabant group treated with 20 mg per day than placebo, and triglycerides fell more in the participants receiving the higher dose of rimonabant. Patients with depression were not included in this study. Adverse events leading to discontinuation of the study were higher in the rimonabant- than in the placebo-treated participants. This said, the profile and effectiveness of this agent appear very promising for treatment of obesity and the physical and laboratory findings that make up the metabolic syndrome.

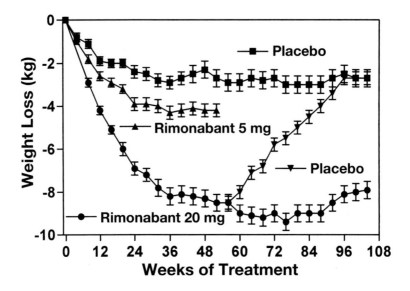

Fig. 10. Effect on body weight of a rimonabant in a 2-year, randomized, placebo-controlled clinical trial. (Adapted from Pi-Sunyer et al., 2006.)

Studies in Special Populations

Patients With Diabetes. The fourth study, RIO-Diabetes, randomized 1045 subjects in 151 centers in 11 countries to treatment who already had diabetes treated with diet, metformin, or sulfonylurea drugs to 1 year of treatment with rimonabant 5 or 20 mg per day (Scheen et al., 2007). Weight loss in the placebo group was −1.4 kg, compared with −2.3 kg in the 5-mg group and −5.3 kg in the 20-mg group. Triglycerides and blood pressure declined more in the subjects treated with 20 mg per day of rimonabant. Of completers, 55.9% lost more than 5% of body weight during treatment with 20 mg per day of rimonabant compared with 19.5% in the placebo-treated group.

Safety Considerations

Discontinuation for adverse events was similar, but the reasons were different. Among placebo-treated patients, it was for lack of weight loss. With the higher dose of rimonabant (20 mg/d) depressed mood disorders, nausea, vomiting, diarrhea, headache, dizziness, and anxiety were all more common in than in the placebo group. The Hamilton Depression scales were not significantly different between treatment groups.

The patients withdrawing for drug-related adverse events was slightly higher in the low-dose rimonabant group and even higher in the high-dose rimonabant group. The major reasons for withdrawal were psychiatric, nervous system, and GI track symptoms. The complaints, which occurred with more than 5% frequency in the drug-treated patients, included upper respiratory tract infection, naospharyngitis, nausea, influenza, diarrhea, arthralgia, anxiety, insomnia, viral gastroenteritis, dizziness, depressed mood, and fatigue in the high-dose rimonabant group (Pi-Sunyer et al., 2006).

Drugs Approved by the FDA for Short-Term Treatment of Overweight Patients
PHENTERMINE AND DIETHYLPROPION: SYMPATHOMIMETIC DRUGS APPROVED FOR SHORT-TERM USE

Mechanism of Action

Phentermine and diethylpropion behave in many ways like the adrenergic neuro-transmitters and are thus called "sympathomimetic amines." They were originally thought to "release" norepinephrine from vesicular stores, but more recent data would suggest that they act primarily to inhibit reuptake of norepinephrine and dopamine at nerve endings.

Clinical Studies

Most of the data on phentermine, diethylpropion, benzphetamine, and phendimetrazine come from short-term trials (Bray and Greenway, 1999; 2007). One of the longest of these clinical trials lasted 36 weeks and compared placebo treatment with continuous or intermittent phentermine (Munro et al., 1968). Both continuous and intermittent phentermine therapy produced more weight loss than placebo. In the drug-free periods, the patients treated intermittently slowed their weight loss, only to lose more rapidly when the drug was reinstituted. In their analysis of pharmacotherapy for treatment of the overweight patient, Haddock et al. (2002) compiled data on both phentermine and diethylpropion. They found that in six studies, phentermine produced a mean weight loss of −6.3 kg (range −3.6 to −8.8 kg) compared with a placebo-induced weight loss of −2.8 kg (range −1.5 to −5.2 kg). For diethylpropion, the mean weight loss in nine studies was −6.5 kg (range −1.9 to −13.1 kg) and for the placebo group it was −3.5 kg (range −0.4 to −10.5 kg). Similar data for benzphetamine is −4.03 kg (range −1.6 to −7.3 kg) and for placebo −0.73 kg (range −1.3 to −2.0 kg).

Phentermine and diethylpropion are classified by the US Drug Enforcement Agency as schedule IV drugs; benzphetamine and phendimetrazine are schedule III drugs. This regulatory classification indicates the government's belief that they have the potential for abuse, although this potential appears to be very low. Phentermine and diethylpropion are approved for only a "few weeks," which usually is interpreted as up to 12 weeks. Weight loss with phentermine and diethylpropion persists for the duration of treatment, suggesting that tolerance does not develop to these drugs. If tolerance were to develop, the drugs would be expected to lose their effectiveness, and patients would require increased amounts of the drug to maintain weight loss. This does not occur.

ANTIDEPRESSANT AND ANTI-EPILEPTIC DRUGS THAT PRODUCE WEIGHT LOSS BUT ARE NOT APPROVED BY THE FDA FOR WEIGHT LOSS

Fluoxetine and Sertraline
MECHANISM OF ACTION

Fluoxetine and sertraline are both selective serotonin reuptake inhibitors that block the transporters that remove serotonin from the neuronal cleft into the pre-synaptic

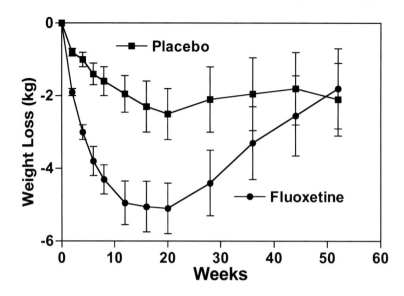

Fig. 11. Effect on body weight of fluoxetine from pooled data of randomized placebo-controlled clinical trials. (Redrawn from Goldstein et al., 1995.)

space for metabolism by the monoamine oxidase or storage in granules. It also reduces food intake. In a 2-week placebo-controlled trial, fluoxetine at a dose of 60 mg per day produced a 27% decrease in food intake (Lawton et al., 1995).

CLINICAL TRIALS

Both fluoxetine and sertraline are approved by the FDA for treatment of depression. In clinical trials in patients with depression lasting 8 to 16 weeks, sertraline gave an average weight loss of −0.45 to −0.91 kg. Fluoxetine at a dose of 60 mg per day (three times the usual dose for treatment of depression) was evaluated in clinical trials for the treatment of overweight patients by the Eli Lilly Company. A meta-analysis of six studies showed a wide range of results with a mean weight loss in one study of −14.5 kg and a weight gain of +0.40 kg in another (Li et al., 2005). In the meta-analysis by Avenell et al. (2004b), the weight loss at 12 months was −0.33 kg (95% CI −1.49 to 0.82 kg). Goldstein et al. (1995) reviewed the trials with fluoxetine that included one 36-week trial in subjects with type 2 diabetes, a 52-week trial in subjects with uncomplicated overweight, and two 60-week trials in subjects with dyslipidemia, diabetes, or both. A total of 1441 subjects were randomized to fluoxetine (719) or placebo (722). Five hundred twenty-two subjects on fluoxetine and 504 subjects on placebo completed 6 months of treatment. Weight loss in the placebo and fluoxetine groups at 6 months and 1 year were −2.2 and −4.8 kg and −1.8 and −2.4 kg, respectively (Fig. 11). The regain of 50% of the lost weight during the second 6 months of treatment with fluoxetine makes it inappropriate for the long-term treatment of overweight that requires chronic treatment. Fluoxetine and sertraline, although not good anti-overweight drugs, may be preferred in the obese patient with depression over some of the tricyclic antidepressants that are associated with significant weight gain.

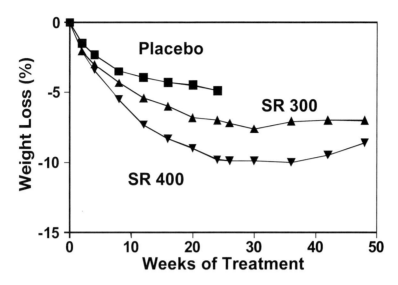

Fig. 12. Effect on body weight of bupropion in a randomized placebo-controlled clinical trial. (Adapted from Anderson et al., 2002.)

Bupropion

MECHANISM OF ACTION

Bupropion is a norepinephrine and dopamine reuptake inhibitor that is approved for the treatment of depression and for smoking cessation.

CLINICAL STUDIES OF WEIGHT LOSS

One clinical use for bupropion has been to prevent the weight gain following cessation of smoking. It was thus a potential drug for treatment of overweight patients. In one clinical trial, 50 overweight subjects were randomized to bupropion or placebo for 8 weeks with a blinded extension for responders to 24 weeks. The dose of bupropion was increased to a maximum of 200 mg twice daily in conjunction with a calorie-restricted diet. At 8 weeks, 18 subjects in the bupropion group lost −6.2 ± 3.1% of body weight compared with −1.6 ± 2.9% for the 13 subjects in the placebo group ($p < 0.0001$). After 24 weeks, the 14 responders to bupropion lost −12.9 ± 5.6% of initial body weight, of which 75% was fat as derermined by dual-energy X-ray absorptiometry (Gadde et al., 2001).

Two multicenter clinical trials, one in obese subjects with depressive symptoms and one in uncomplicated overweight patients, followed this study. In the study of overweight patients with depressive symptom ratings of 10 to 30 on a Beck Depression Inventory, 213 patients were randomized to 400 mg of bupropion per day and 209 subjects to placebo for 24 weeks. The 121 subjects in the bupropion group that completed the trial lost −6.0 ± 0.5% of initial body weight compared with −2.8 ± 0.5 % in the 108 subjects in the placebo group ($p < 0.0001$; Jain et al., 2002). The study in uncomplicated overweight subjects randomized 327 subjects to bupropion 300 mg per day, bupropion 400 mg per day, or placebo in equal proportions. At 24 weeks, 69% of those randomized remained in the study and the percent losses of initial body weight were −5 ± 1%, −7.2 ± 1%, and −10.1 ± 1% for the placebo,

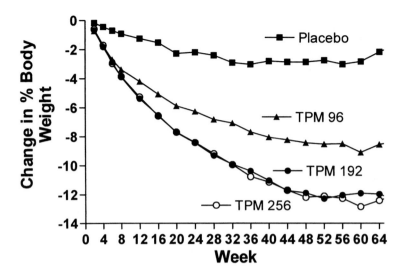

Fig. 13. Effect on body weight of topiramate in a double-blind, randomized, placebo-controlled, dose-ranging clinical trial. (Adapted from Bray et al., 2003.)

bupropion 300 mg, and bupropion 400 mg groups respectively ($p < 0.0001$). The placebo group was randomized to the 300-mg or 400-mg group at 24 weeks and the trial was extended to week 48. By the end of the trial, the dropout rate was 41% and the weight loss in the bupropion 300 mg and bupropion 400 mg groups were $-6.2 \pm 1.25\%$ and $-7.2 \pm 1.5\%$ of initial body weight, respectively (Anderson et al., 2002). Thus, it appears that subjects without depression may respond to bupropion with weight loss to a greater extent than those with depressive symptoms (Fig. 12).

Topiramate

MECHANISM OF ACTION

Topiramate is a novel neurotherapeutic agent that is approved for treatment of selected seizure disorders. It is a weak carbonic anhydrase inhibitor, exhibiting selectivity for carbonic anhydrase isoforms II and IV. Topiramate also modulates the effects at receptors for the γ-aminobutyric acid receptor and the α-amino-3-hydroxy-5-methyl-4-isoxazolepropionic acid/kainate subtype of the glutamate receptor. This drug also exhibits state-dependent blockade of voltage-dependent Na^+ or Ca^{2+} channels. These mechanisms are believed to contribute to its anti-epileptic properties. The modulation of γ-aminobutyric acid receptors may provide one potential mechanism to reduce food intake, although other mechanisms, yet to be described, may be more important in defining its effects on body weight (Astrup and Toubro, 2004).

CLINICAL STUDIES FOR WEIGHT LOSS

Topiramate is an anti-epileptic drug that was discovered to give weight loss in the clinical trials for epilepsy. Weight losses of -3.9% of initial weight were seen at 3 months and losses of -7.3% of initial weight were seen at 1 year (Ben-Menachem et al., 2003). Bray et al. reported a 6-month, placebo-controlled, dose-ranging study.

Three hundred eighty-five obese subjects were randomized to placebo or topiramate at 64, 96, 192, or 384 mg per day. These doses were gradually reached by a tapering increase and were reduced in a similar manner at the end of the trial. Weight loss from baseline to 24 weeks was −2.6, −5, −4.8, −6.3, and 6.3% in the placebo, 64-mg, 96-mg, 192-mg, and 384-mg groups, respectively. The most frequent adverse events were paresthesias, somnolence, and difficulty with concentration, memory, and attention (Bray et al., 2003) (Fig. 13). This trial was followed by two multicenter trials. The first trial randomized 1289 obese subjects to topiramate 89, 192, or 256 mg per day. This trial was terminated early because of the sponsor's decision to pursue a time-release form of the drug. The 854 subjects who completed 1 year of the trial before it was terminated by the sponsor lost −1.7, −7, −9.1, and −9.7% of their initial body weight in the placebo, 89-mg, 192-mg, and 256-mg groups, respectively. Subjects in the topiramate groups had significant improvement in blood pressure and glucose tolerance (Wilding et al., 2004). The second trial enrolled 701 subjects who were treated with a VLCD to induce an 8% loss of initial body weight. The 560 subjects who achieved an 8% weight loss were randomized to topiramate 96 mg per day, 192 mg per day, or placebo. The sponsor terminated this study early too. At the time of early termination, 293 had subjects completed 44 weeks. The topiramate groups lost 15.4 and 16.5% of their baseline weight, while the placebo group lost 8.9% (Astrup et al., 2004). Although topiramate is still available as an anti-epileptic drug, the development program to obtain an indication for overweight was terminated by the sponsor because of the associated adverse events.

SPECIAL SITUATIONS

Topiramate has also been evaluated in the treatment of binge-eating disorder. Thirteen women with binge-eating disorder were treated with a mean dose of 492 mg per day of topiramate. The binge-eating disorder symptoms improved and weight loss was observed (Shapira et al., 2000). This open-label study was followed by a 14-week randomized controlled trial in subjects with binge-eating disorder. Sixty-one subjects were randomized to 25 to 600 mg per day of topiramate or placebo in a 1:1 ratio. The topiramate group had improvement in binge-eating symptoms and lost −5.9 kg at an average topiramate dose of 212 mg per day (McElroy et al., 2003). The 35 completers of this trial were given the opportunity to participate in an open-label extension. The topiramate-treated subjects continued to maintain improvement in binge-eating symptoms and weight (McElroy et al., 2004b).

Topiramate has also been used to treat patients with Prader-Willi syndrome. Three subjects with Prader-Willi syndrome were treated with topiramate and had a reduction in the self-injurious behavior that is associated with this uncommon genetic disease (Shapira et al., 2002). A second study in seven additional subjects confirmed these findings (Smathers et al., 2003). A third study evaluated appetite, food intake, and weight. Although the self-injurious behavior improved, there was no effect on these other parameters (Shapira et al., 2004). Topiramate was also used to treat two subjects with nocturnal eating syndrome and two subjects with sleep-related eating disorders. There was an improvement in all subjects and an 11-kg weight loss over 8.5 months with an average topiramate dose of 218 mg per day (Winkelman, 2003).

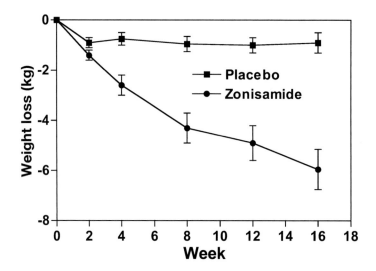

Fig. 14. Effect on body weight of zonisamide in a randomized placebo-controlled clinical trial. (Redrawn from Gadde et al., 2003.)

Zonisamide

MECHANISM OF ACTION

Zonisamide is an anti-epileptic drug that has serotonergic and dopaminergic activity in addition to inhibiting sodium and calcium channels.

CLINICAL STUDIES FOR WEIGHT LOSS

Weight loss was noted in the clinical trials for the treatment of epilepsy, again suggesting a potential agent for weight loss. Gadde et al. tested this possibility by performing a 16-week randomized control trial in 60 obese subjects. Subjects were placed on a calorie-restricted diet and randomized to zonisamide or placebo (Fig. 14). The zonisamide was started at 100 mg per day and increased to 400 mg per day. At 12 weeks, those subjects who had not lost 5% of initial body weight were increased to 600 mg per day. The zonisamide group lost −6.6% of initial body weight at 16 weeks compared with −1% in the placebo group. Thirty-seven subjects (20 in the zonisamide group and 17 in the placebo group) completing the 16-week trial elected to continue to week 32. At the end of 32 weeks, the 19 subjects in the zonisamide group lost 9.6% of their initial body weight compared with 1.6% for the 17 subjects in the placebo group (Gadde et al., 2003).

McElroy et al. evaluated zonisamide in an open-label prospective trial in subjects with binge-eating disorder. Fifteen subjects were treated with doses of 100 to 600 mg per day for 12 weeks. The eight subjects who completed the trial with an average dose of 513 mg per day experienced an improvement in their binge-eating symptoms and lost a significant amount weight (McElroy et al., 2004a).

Lamotrigine

MECHANISM OF ACTION

Lamotrogine is an anti-epileptic drug that does not produce weight gain (Devinsky et al., 2000).

CLINICAL STUDIES

A recent double-blind, randomized, placebo-controlled trial examined the effects of lamotrigine escalated from 25 to 200 mg per day over 6 weeks on weight loss against placebo treatment for 26 weeks in 40 healthy overweight (BMI 30–40 kg/m^2) adults over 18 years of age. At the end of the trial, body weight was marginally lower ($p = 0.062$) in the lamotrigine-treated group (–6.4 kg) than in the placebo-treated group (–1.2 kg; Merideth, 2006).

DRUGS APPROVED BY THE FDA
FOR USES OTHER THAN OVERWEIGHT

Metformin

MECHANISM OF ACTION

Metformin is a biguanide that is approved for the treatment of diabetes mellitus, a disease that is exacerbated by overweight and weight gain. This drug reduces hepatic glucose production, decreases intestinal absorption from the GI tract, and enhances insulin sensitivity.

CLINICAL TRIALS

In clinical trials in which metformin was compared with sulfonylureas, it produced weight loss (Bray and Greenway, 1999). In one French trial, BIGPRO, metformin was compared to placebo in a 1-year multicenter study in 324 middle-aged subjects with upper body adiposity and the insulin resistance syndrome (metabolic syndrome). The subjects on metformin lost significantly more weight (1–2 kg) than the placebo group, and the study concluded that metformin may have a role in the primary prevention of type 2 diabetes (Fontbonne et al., 1996). In a meta-analysis of three of these studies Avenell et al. (2004b) reported a weight loss at 12 months of –1.09 kg (95% CI –2.29 to 0.11 kg).

The best trial of metformin, however, is the DPP study of individuals with impaired glucose tolerance. The main part of this study included three treatment arms to which participants were randomly assigned, if they were over 25 years of age, had a BMI above 24 kg/m^2 (except Asian-Americans who only needed a BMI $\geq$ 22 kg/m^2), and had impaired glucose tolerance. The three primary arms included lifestyle ($N = 1079$ participants), metformin ($N = 1073$), and placebo ($N = 1082$). At the end of 2.8 years on average, the Data Safety Monitoring Board terminated the trial because the advantages of lifestyle and metformin were clearly superior to placebo. During this time the metformin-treated group lost 2.5% of their body weight ($P < 0.001$ compared with placebo), and the conversion from impaired glucose tolerance to diabetes was reduced by 31% compared with placebo (Fig. 15). In the DPP trial, metformin was more effective in reducing the development of diabetes in the subgroup that was most overweight and in the younger members of the cohort (Knowler et al., 2002). Although metformin does not produce enough weight loss (5%) to qualify as a weight-loss drug using the FDA criteria, it would appear to be a very useful choice for overweight individuals who have or are at high risk for diabetes. One area in which metformin has found use is in treating women with the polycystic ovarian syndrome, in which modest weight loss may contribute increased fertility and reduced insulin resistance (Ortega-Gonzalez et al., 2005; Fig. 15).

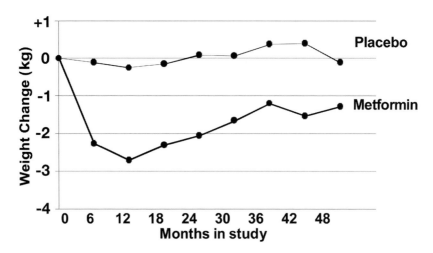

Fig. 15. Effect on body weight of metformin in a double-blind placebo- controlled randomized trial from the Diabetes Prevention Program. (Adapted from Knowler et al., 2002.)

Pramlintide

MECHANISM OF ACTION

Amylin is peptide found in the beta-cell of the pancreas. It is secreted along with insulin, and circulates in the blood. Amylin is deficient in type 1 diabetes in which beta-cells are immunologically destroyed. Pramlintide, a synthetic amylin analog, has a prolonged biological half-life (Riddle and Drucker, 2006).

CLINICAL STUDIES

Pramlintide was approved by the FDA in 2005 for the treatment of diabetes. Unlike insulin and many other diabetes medications, pramlintide is associated with weight loss. In a study in which 651 subjects with type 1 diabetes were randomized to placebo or subcutaneous pramlintide 60 µg three or four times a day along with an insulin injection, the hemoglobin A1c decreased 0.29 to 0.34% and weight decreased −1.2 kg relative to placebo (Ratner et al., 2004). Maggs et al. (2003) analyzed the data from two 1-year studies in subjects with insulin-treated type 2 diabetes randomized to pramlintide 120 µg twice a day or 150 µg three times a day. Weight decreased by −2.6 kg and hemoglobin A1c decreased 0.5%. When weight loss was then analyzed by ethnic group, African Americans lost −4 kg, Caucasians lost −2.4 kg, and Hispanics lost −2.3 kg. The improvement in diabetes correlated with the weight loss, suggesting that pramlintide is effective in ethnic groups with the greatest burden from overweight. The most common adverse event was nausea, which was usually mild and confined to the first 4 weeks of therapy.

Exenatide

MECHANISM OF ACTION

Glucagon-like peptide (GLP)-1 is derived from the processing of the proglucagon peptide, which is secreted by L-cells in the terminal ileum in response to a meal.

Increased GLP-1 inhibits glucagon secretion, stimulates insulin secretion, stimulates gluconeogenesis, and delays gastric emptying (Patriti et al., 2004). It has been postulated to be responsible for the superior weight loss and superior improvement in diabetes seen after gastric bypass surgery for overweight (Greenway et al., 2002; Small and Bloom, 2004). GLP-1 is rapidly degraded by dipeptidyl peptidase-IV, an enzyme that is elevated in the obese. Bypass operations for overweight increase GLP-1, but do not change the levels of dipeptidyl peptidase-IV (Lugari et al., 2004; Riddle and Drucker, 2006).

Exenatide (Exendin-4) is a 39-amino-acid peptide that is produced in the salivary gland of the Gila monster lizard. It has 53% homology with GLP-1, but it has a much longer half-life. Exenatide decreases food intake and body weight gain in Zucker rats while lowering HgbA1c (Szayna et al., 2000). It also increases beta-cell mass to a greater extent than would be expected for the degree of insulin resistance (Gedulin et al., 2005). Exendin-4 induces satiety and weight loss in Zucker rats with peripheral administration and crosses the blood–brain barrier to act in the central nervous system (Kastin and Akerstrom, 2003; Rodriquez de Fonseca et al., 2000). Exenatide has been approved by the FDA for treatment of people with type 2 diabetes who are inadequately controlled while being treated with either metformin or sulfonylureas.

CLINICAL STUDIES WITH WEIGHT LOSS AS A COMPONENT

In humans, exenatide reduces fasting and post-prandial glucose levels, slows gastric emptying, and decreases food intake by 19% (Edwards et al., 2001). The side effects of exenatide in humans are headache, nausea, and vomiting that are lessened by gradual dose escalation (Fineman et al., 2004). Several clinical trials of 30 weeks duration have been reported using exenatide at 10 µg subcutaneously per day or a placebo (Buse et al., 2004; DeFronzo et al., 2005; Kendall et al., 2005). In one trial with 377 subjects with type 2 diabetes who were failing maximal sulfonylurea therapy, exenatide produced a fall of 0.74% more in HgbA1c than placebo. Fasting glucose also decreased and there was a progressive weight loss of 1.6 kg (Buse et al., 2004). The interesting feature of this weight loss is that it occurred without lifestyle changes, diet, or exercise (Fig. 16). In a 26-week randomized control trial, exenatide produced a 2.3-kg weight loss compared with a gain of 1.8 kg in the group receiving insulin glargine (Heine et al., 2005).

Somatostatin

MECHANISM OF ACTION

Somatostatin is a small peptide that is released in the GI track and the brain. It inhibits the release of most peptides, including insulin, glucagon, and growth hormone (GH), among others.

CLINICAL STUDIES FOR WEIGHT LOSS

Overweight resulting from hypothalamic injury has been associated with insulin hypersecretion (Bray and Gallagher, 1975). Lustig treated eight children with overweight

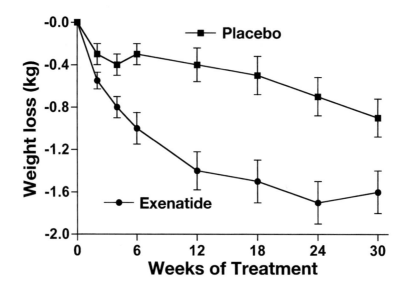

Fig. 16. Effect on body weight of exenatide in a randomized placebo-controlled clinical trial. (Adapted from Kendall et al., 2005.)

resulting from hypothalamic damage with octreotide injections to decrease insulin hypersecretion. These children gained 6 kg in the 6 months before octreotide treatment and lost −4.8 kg in the 6 months on octreotide, an analog of somatostatin. The weight loss was correlated with the reduction of insulin secretion on a glucose tolerance test (Lustig et al., 1999). This open-label trial was followed by a randomized controlled trial of octreotide treatment in children with hypothalamic overweight. The subjects received octreotide 5 to 15 µ/kg per day or placebo for 6 months. The children on octreotide gained 1.6 kg compared with 9.1 kg for those in the placebo group (Lustig et al., 2003b). This same group of investigators postulated that there might be a subset of obese subjects who were insulin hypersecretors and that these subjects would respond with weight loss to treatment with octreotide. Following an oral glucose tolerance test in which glucose and insulin were measured, 44 subjects were treated with octreotide-LAR 40 mg per month for 6 months. These subjects lost weight and reduced food and carbohydrate intake. Weight loss was greatest in those with insulin hypersecretion and the amount of weight loss was correlated with the reduction in insulin hypersecretion (Velasquez-Mieyer et al., 2003). In a multicenter randomized controlled trial, 172 obese subjects (144 women and 28 men) who had insulin hypersecretion during a glucose tolerance test at screening received octreotide-LAR in doses of 20, 40, or 60 mg per month or placebo for 6 months. The greatest weight loss was 3.5 to 3.8% of initial body weight in the two higher-dose groups, an amount that was statistically significant, but not enough to meet the criteria for approval by the FDA (Lustig et al., 2003a; Lustig et al., 2006).

Octreotide has been shown to decrease gastric emptying (Foxx-Orenstein et al., 2003). Treatment of patients with Prader-Willi syndrome who have an elevated ghrelin does not cause weight loss but ghrelin levels are normalized. The reason for the lack of weight loss was postulated to be the reduction of PYY, a satiating GI hormone that also decreased (Tan et al., 2004).

GH and GH Fragment

Mechanism of Action

GH is a pituitary peptide that is essential for the adolescent growth spurt. Bioengineered GH is widely used to treat short stature as well as GH deficiency in adults (Hoffman et al., 2004) and has been used by athletes to build muscle, because one of its effects is to enhance protein accretion. GH has been consistently shown to increase body protein and to reduce total body fat and particularly visceral fat, making it a potential agent for the overweight patient.

Clinical Trials

In a small clinical trial, 18 newly diagnosed overweight patients with diabetes were randomly assigned to placebo or GH injection along with dietary restriction in a double-blind study (Nam et al., 2001). They found a greater decrease in visceral fat, an increase in lean body mass, and improved insulin sensitivity during this 12-week trial. In a 12-month randomized double-blind, placebo-controlled clinical trial, 40 postmenopausal women were assigned to daily placebo injections or injections of GH (0.67 mg/d). After 1 year, Franco et al. (2005) reported that the women had significantly reduced their abdominal and visceral adiposity, had improved their insulin sensitivity and total and LDL-cholesterol concentrations.

A group working in Australia has identified a fragment of GH that is lipolytic. This compound, called AOD9604 is a modified fragment of the amino acids in GH from 177 to 191, and is orally active. It is said to bind to the fat cell stimulating lipolysis and inhibiting re-esterification without stimulating growth. A 12-week multicenter trial randomized 300 obese subjects to one of five daily doses (1, 5, 10, 20, and 30 mg) of AOD9604 or placebo. The 1-mg dose was the most effective for weight loss. Subjects on the 1-mg dose lost 2.6 kg compared with 0.8 kg in the placebo group and the rate of weight loss was constant throughout the trial (N. A., 2004). Phase III trials are evidently in the planning stages.

DRUGS IN CLINICAL TRIALS

Leptin

Mechanism of Action

The lack of leptin, a hormone derived from the fat cell, causes massive overweight in animals and man. Its placement reverses the overweight associated with the deficiency state. The discovery of leptin generated hope that leptin would be an effective treatment for overweight.

Clinical Trials

Leptin at subcutaneous doses of 0, 0.01, 0.05, 0.1, and 0.3 mg/kg daily was tested in lean (Hukshorn et al., 2003) and obese (Hukshorn et al., 2000, Heymsfield 1999) humans of both sexes. Lean subjects were treated for 4 weeks and lost −0.4 to −1.9 kg. Obese subjects were treated for 24 weeks and a dose–response relationship for weight loss was seen with the 0.3 mg/kg group, which lost −7.1 kg (Heymsfield et al., 1999). Pegylated leptin allows for weekly, rather than daily, injections. Although pegylated leptin at 20 and 60 mg per week in obese subjects over 8 to 12 weeks did not give any weight loss above placebo, pegylated leptin at 80 mg weekly combined with a VLCD for 46 days gave 2.8 kg more weight loss in 12 subjects randomized to leptin compared with the 10 randomized to placebo ($p < 0.03$; Hukshorn et al., 2003).

Leptin has been found to ameliorate many of the symptoms of lipodystrophy (Oral et al., 2002). Nine female patients with lipodystrophy and a serum leptin level of less than 4 ng/mL were treated with recombinant methionyl human leptin for 4 months. Eight of the women had diabetes. During treatment with leptin, glycosylated hemoglobin decreased an average of 1.9%. During the 4 months of therapy, triglyceride levels decreased by 60%. Liver volume was also reduced by an average of 28% and resting metabolic rate decreased significantly with therapy. A reduction in body weight produced by eating a low-calorie diet is associated with decreased 24-hour energy expenditure and decreased leptin and thyroid hormone levels. When body weight was reduced by 10%, circulating T3, T4, and leptin concentrations were decreased. All of these endocrine changes were reversed by administration of "replacement" doses of recombinant human methiony-leptin (Rosenbaum et al., 2002). Total energy expenditure increased in all subjects during treatment with leptin, indicating that decreased leptin may account for some aspects of the endocrine adaptations to weight loss.

Axokine

MECHANISM OF ACTION

Axokine is a pegylated derivative of cilliary neurotrophic factor that, like leptin, acts through the STAT signaling pathway in the brain (Anderson et al., 2003).

CLINICAL TRIALS

Axokine has been tested in two phase II studies, one in overweight patients and one in subjects with diabetes, and a phase III study in overweight patients. The first multicenter 12-week phase II study randomized 170 obese subjects with a BMI between 35 and 50 kg/m^2. The optimal dose was 1 µg/kg, and this group lost –4.6 kg compared with a weight gain of +0.6 kg in the placebo group (Ettinger et al., 2003). The second 12-week phase II study randomized 107 overweight and obese subjects with type 2 diabetes and a BMI between 35 and 50 kg/m^2 (Website). Those subjects treated with the 1.0-µg/kg dose of axokine lost –3.2 kg compared with –1.2 kg in the placebo group ($p < 0.01$).

The 1-year phase III trial with a 1-year open label extension randomized 501 subjects to placebo and 1467 subjects to axokine at a dose of 1 µg/kg per day (Ettinger et al., 2003). Subjects had a BMI between 30 and 55 kg/m^2, if their overweight was uncomplicated, or between 27 and 55 kg/m^2, if their overweight was complicated by hypertension or dyslipidemia. At the end of 1 year, the axokine group lost –3.6 kg compared with –2.0 kg in the placebo group ($p < 0.001$), a difference that does not meet the FDA efficacy criteria for approval. The most common adverse events were mild and included injection site reactions, nausea, and cough. The most concerning finding, however, was that two-thirds of those receiving axokine developed antibodies after 3 months that limited weight loss, and there was no way to predict prospectively those who would develop antibodies. Development of axokine has been terminated.

Neuropeptide-Y Receptor Antagonists

MECHANISM OF ACTION

Neuropeptide Y (NPY) is a widely distributed neuropeptide that has five receptors: Y-1, Y-2, Y-4, Y-5, and Y-6. NPY stimulates food intake, inhibits energy expenditure,

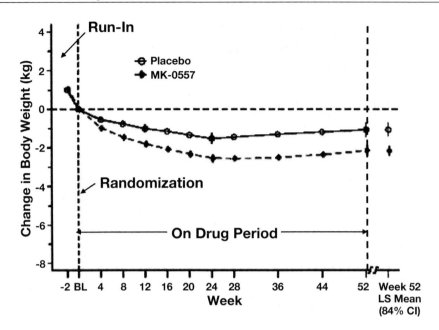

Fig. 17. Effect of an antagonist to the Neuropeptide-Y5 receptor on body weight in a 1-year randomized, double-blind controlled trial. (Erondu et al., 2006.)

and increases body weight by activating Y-1 and Y-5 receptors in the hypothalamus (Parker et al., 2002). Levels of NPY in the hypothalamus are temporally related to food intake and are elevated with energy depletion. Surprisingly, NPY knockout mice have no phenotype. NPY-5 receptor antagonists fall into two categories, those that reduce food intake and those that do not, but those that do seem to do so through a mechanism separate from Y-5. Thus, Y-5 receptor antagonists do not appear promising as anti-overweight agents (Levens and Della-Zuana, 2003). Y-1 receptor antagonists appear to have greater potential as anti-overweight agents. A dihydropyridine NPY-1 antagonist inhibited NPY-induced feeding in satiated rats (Poindexter et al., 2002). Another Y-1 receptor antagonist, J-104870, suppressed food intake when given orally to Zucker rats (Kanatani et al., 2001).

CLINICAL TRIALS

A study measuring NPY in obese humans casts doubt on the importance of the NPY antagonists in the treatment of overweight in man. Obese women had lower NPY levels than lean women and weight loss with a 400-kcal-per-day diet and adrenergic agonists (caffeine and ephedrine or caffeine, ephedrine, and yohimbine) did not change NPY levels at rest or after exercise (Zahorska-Markiewicz et al., 2001).

Several clinical trials with a selective Y-5 receptor anatagonist have been completed. The first was a 2-year randomized, placebo-controlled trial. It included two doses (Fig. 17).

The effect of a NPY-5 receptor antagonist has been tested in two clinical trials. In the positron emission tomography (PET) study done as part of the drug trial, a dose of 1 mg appeared adequate to completely block binding to the NPY-5 receptor. A 12-week proof of concept and dose-ranging study suggested that MK-0557 could produce weight loss in obese adults. A multicenter, randomized, double blind, placebo-controlled parallel-group trial involved 1667 overweight and obese patients who were treated with MK-0557 1 mg/day or placebo in addition to a prescribed dietary deficit of 500 kcal/day and exercise regimen. After 52 weeks, the mean (95% CI) difference in weight loss in the Modified Intention-to-Treat (MITT) population between MK-0557 and placebo was −1.1 (−1.7, −0.5) kg ($p < 0.001$) (Erondu et al., 2006).

To test the effect of MK-0557 in maintaining weight loss, participants were treated with a very low calorie diet for 6 weeks and those who lost more than 6% of body weight were enrolled. The average weight loss with the VLCD diet alone was 9.1 kg. After 12 weeks of double-blind treatment, weight began to gradually increase for both placebo- and MK-0557-treated patients. Among all patients, the least squares mean weight change (95% CI) from baseline (end of VLCD) to week 52 was +3.1 (2.1, 4.0) and +1.5 (0.5, 2.4) kg for patients treated with placebo and MK-0557, respectively. The difference of 1.6 kg between the two groups was significant ($p = 0.014$) (Erondu et al., 2007).

Although the differences in weight loss and in weight regain between placebo- and MK-0557-treated patients were statistically significant, the magnitude of the effect was small and not clinically significant. Antagonism of the NPY5R is not an efficacious treatment strategy for producing weight loss or maintaining it.

Serotonin 2C Receptor Agonists

MECHANISM OF ACTION

Mice lacking the 5HT-2c receptor have increased food intake, because they take longer to be satiated. These mice also are resistant to fenfluramine, a serotonin agonist that causes weight loss. A human mutation of the 5HT-2c receptor has been identified that is associated with early-onset human overweight (Gibson et al., 2004; Nilsson, 2006). The precursor of serotonin, 5-hydroxytryptophan, reduces food intake and body weight in clinical studies (Cangiano et al., 1992; Cangiano et al., 1998). Fenfluramine (Foltin et al., 1996; Rogers and Blundell, 1979) and dexfenfluramine (Drent et al., 1995), two drugs that act on the serotonin system, but were withdrawn from the market in 1997 because of cardiovascular side effects, also reduce food intake in human studies. Meta-chlorophenylpiperazine, a direct serotonin agonist, reduces food intake by 28% in women and 20% in men (Cowen et al., 1995). Another serotoninergic drug, sumatriptan, which acts on the 5-HT1B/1D receptor, also reduced food intake in human subjects (Boeles et al., 1997). Because of the robust effects of agonists toward the HT-2C receptors in suppressing food intake, a number of new agents are now under development. Only one of these has advanced to formal clinical trials.

CLINICAL TRIALS

The results of a phase II dose-ranging study for (APD356) Loreasern have been presented (Smith et al., 2006). A total of 459 male and female subjects with a BMI between 29 and 46 kg/m^2 with an average weight of 100 kg were enrolled in a randomized, double-blind controlled trial comparing placebo with 10 and 15 mg given once daily and 10 mg given twice daily (20 mg/d). Over 12 weeks, the placebo group lost −0.32 kg ($N = 88$ completers) compared with −1.8 kg in the group receiving 10 mg per day twice daily ($N = 86$), −2.6 kg in the group receiving 15mg per day

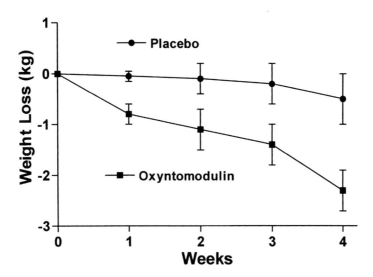

Fig. 18. Effect of oxyntomodulin on body weight in a 4-week trial. (Redrawn from Wynne et al., 2005.)

($N = 82$ completers) and -3.6 kg in the group receiving 10 mg twice daily (20 mg total; $N = 77$ completers). Side effects that were higher in the active treatment groups than the placebo group were headache, nausea, dizziness, vomiting, and dry mouth. No cardiac valvular changes were noted (Smith et al., 2006). Additional clinical trials are being planned.

PYY 3-36

MECHANISM OF ACTION

PYY is a hormone produced by the L-cells in the GI tract and is secreted in proportion to the caloric content of a meal. PYY 3-36 levels are lower fasting and after a meal in the overweight subjects compared with lean subjects. Development of a nasal spray formulation for PYY 3-36 has undergone a Phase I clinical trial. Based on the review of this trial, Merck severed its commercial relationship with Nastech on March 1, 2006. Nastech, the developer of the nasal formulation, plans to continue developing this product.

CLINICAL TRIALS

Thrice daily nasal administration over 6 days was well-tolerated and reduced caloric intake by about 30% while giving 0.6 kg weight loss (VBrandt et al., 2004). Caloric intake at a lunch buffet was reduced by 30% in 12 obese subjects and by 29% in 12 lean subjects after 2 hours of PYY 3-36 infused intravenously (Batterham et al., 2003; Fig. 18).

The effect of intranasal administration of PYY 3-36 was investigated in a double-blind, randomized, placebo-controlled trial lasting 12 weeks. A total of 133 obese patients were enrolled and took an intranasal spray of peptide 200 or 600 µg or placebo 20 minutes before each main meal. Drop-outs were high in the highest dose group. The difference in weight between placebo and PYY 3-36 at the end of the trial was -0.9 kg, which was not statistically significant. Thus, the intranasal route with this preparation is ineffective in aiding weight loss (Gantz et al., 2007).

Oxyntomodulin

MECHANISM OF ACTION

Oxyntomodulin is a GI peptide produced in the L-cells of the intestine that is released in response to food. Animals injected with oxyntomodulin have a reduction in body fat and food intake.

CLINICAL TRIALS

In a short-term clinical study, it was reported to reduce food intake by 19.3% compared with a placebo infusion. In a 4-week randomized, double-blind, placebo-controlled trial, overweight volunteers injected oxyntomodulin subcutaneously three times a day 30 minutes before meals. Body weight was reduced −2.3 ± 0.4 kg in the group receiving oxyntomodulin compared with −0.5 ± 0.5 kg in the placebo group. Serum leptin decreased and adiponectin increased in the group receiving oxyntomodulin. Energy intake in the treated group decreased by 170 ± 37 kcal (25 ± 5%) at the beginning study meal and by 250 ± 63 kcal (35 ± 9%) at the final meal (Wynne et al., 2005). Further studies on this intriguing peptide are awaited.

Cholecystokinin

Cholecystokinin decreases food intake by causing subjects to stop eating sooner (Pi-Sunyer et al., 1982). Although the relationship between cholecystokinin and satiety has been known for many years, development as a weight-loss agent has been slow because of concerns regarding pancreatitis. Because the human pancreas has no cholecystokinin-A receptors, an orally active compound that is a selective agonist of the cholecystokinin-A receptor is being evaluated in clinical trials, but no reports of those trials have yet appeared.

Oleoylestrone

Oleoylestrone is a weakly estrogenic compound that is produced in fat cells, carried in the blood on HDL particles, and fed back to the central nervous system to reduce food intake while maintaining energy expenditure. Oleoylestrone is orally active and has been used to treat one morbidly obese male without an accompanying weight-loss program. Oleoylestrone was given in doses of 150-300 μmol per day in 10 consecutive 10-day courses of treatment separated by at least 2 months. Weight dropped 38.5 kg and BMI dropped from 51.9 to 40.5 kg/m^2 over 27 months, and weight was still declining at the time of the report (Alemany et al., 2003). Oleoylestrone was well tolerated and there were no estrogenic side effects observed. Pharmaceutical company-sponsored phase I trials are presently in progress.

DRUGS IN THE EARLY PHASES OF DEVELOPMENT

Melanin Concentrating Hormone Receptor-1 Antagonist

Melanin concentrating hormone and α-melanocyte-stimulating hormone have opposite effects on skin coloration in fish, and excess melanin concentrating hormone blocks the effects of α-melanocyte-stimulating hormone when both are injected into the cerebral ventricles of rats (Ludwig et al., 1998). Melanin concentrating hormone has two receptors, MCH-1 and MCH-2. Mice without the MCH-1 receptor have increased activity, increased temperature, and increased sympathetic tone (Astrand et al., 2004). Overexpression of the MCH-1 receptor and chronic infusion of an MCH-1 agonist cause enhanced feeding, caloric efficiency, and weight gain, whereas an MCH-1 antagonist reduces food intake and body weight gain without an effect on lean tissue (Shearman et al., 2003). MCH-1 antagonists reduce food intake by decreasing meal size and also act as antidepressants and anxiolytics (Borowsky et al., 2002; Kowalski et al., 2004). An orally active MCH-1 receptor antagonist that has good plasma levels and central nervous system exposure induced weight loss in obese mice with chronic treatment (Souers et al., 2005). A number of other MCH-1 antagonists reduce food intake and body weight in experimental animals (Handlon and Zhou, 2006). No human studies have been reported.

Pancreatic Lipase Inhibitor

Although orlistat, a lipase inhibitor, is already approved for the treatment of overweight, cetilistat (ATL-962), another GI lipase inhibitor, is also in development. A 5-day trial of cetilistat in 90 normal volunteers was conducted in an inpatient unit. There was a 3.7-fold increase in fecal fat that was dose-dependent, but only 11% of subjects had more than one oily stool. It was suggested that this lipase inhibitor may have fewer GI adverse events than with orlistat (Dunk et al., 2002).

Cetilistat has been evaluated in a double-blind, placebo-controlled, 12-week clinical trial involving 442 patients who received a 500 kcal/day deficit diet. Weight loss with the three doses of cetilistat was similar. The placebo group lost just over 2 kg and the weight loss with cetilistat was just over 4 kg. The discontinuations relative to placebo were similar in all groups (Kopelman et al., 2007).

Ghrelin Antagonists

Ghrelin is a small peptide synthesized in the stomach. Its active form contains an octanoate on the third amino acid. The level rises with fasting and declines after eating, suggesting it may be a satiety signal. Chronic administration produces hyperphagia and weight gain in animals. Moreover, overweight subjects have lower levels than normal-weight individuals.

Ghrelin acts at the GH secretogogue receptor to produce its effects. A group of GH-stimulating peptides that also act on the GH secretogogue receptor are known to increase food intake in human subjects (Laferrere et al., 2005). Antagonists to this receptor might thus be useful drugs for treating overweight patients. This is supported by suppression of food intake and attenuated weight regain in diet-induced obese mice treated with such drugs.

Angiogenesis Antagonists and Fat Cell Antibodies

Formation of an enlarging fat organ requires new blood vessels, and the concept of inhibiting the growth of these vessels and thus showing fat cell growth is an intriguing possibility. Experimental studies in mice have shown that an antagonist of angiogenesis can inhibit fat cell development in ob/ob mice (Brakenhielm et al., 2004; Rupnick et al., 2002). The discovery that fumagillin, isolated from the fungus *Aspergillus fumigatus*, inhibits blood vessel growth has provided a platform for developing new drugs. Fumagillol had provided one derivative TNP-470 that has been tested by Rupnick et al. (2002), who showed that it reduces body weight and slightly decreases food intake in animal models of obesity.

DRUGS AND HERBAL MEDICATIONS
NO LONGER UNDER INVESTIGATION OR WITHDRAWN

Ephedra

Ephedrine combined with methylxantines were used in the treatment of asthma for decades. A physician in Denmark noted weight loss in his patients taking this combination drug for asthma. The combination of caffeine 200 mg and ephedrine 20 mg given three times a day was subsequently approved as a prescription medication for overweight in Denmark where it enjoyed commercial success for more than a decade (Greenway, 2001). In 1994, legislation in the United States declared ephedra and caffeine to be foods, eligible to be sold as dietary herbal supplements. The use of this combination as an unregulated dietary supplement for the treatment of overweight was accompanied by reports of cardiovascular and neuropsychiatric adverse events, which led the FDA to declare ephedra, the herbal form of ephedrine, an adulterant (Shekelle et al., 2003). Recently, courts in the United States have overturned the FDA decision to withdraw ephedra from the herbal market, at least in regard to ephedra doses of 10 mg or less. The implications this legal decision may have on the availability of ephedra in the herbal dietary supplement market remains to be determined.

β-3 Adrenergic Agonists

In the early 1980s, the β-3 adrenergic receptor was identified and shown, when stimulated, to increase lipolysis, fat oxidation, energy expenditure, and insulin action. Selective β-adrenergic agonists based on the rodent β-3 adrenergic receptor were not selective in humans, and the human β-3 adrenergic receptor was subsequently cloned and found to be only 60% homologous with rodents (de Souza and Burkey, 2001). A β-3 adrenergic agonist selective for the human β-3 receptor, L-796568, increased lipolysis and energy expenditure when given as a single 1000-mg dose to overweight men without significant stimulation of the β-2 adrenergic receptor (van Baak et al., 2002). A 28-day study with the same compound at 375 mg per day versus a placebo in obese men gave no significant increase in energy expenditure, reduction in respiratory quotient, or changes in glucose tolerance. There was a significant reduction of triglycerides, however. This lack of a chronic effect was interpreted as either a lack of recruitment of β-3 responsive tissues, a downregulation of β-3 receptors or both (Larsen et al., 2002). Thus, despite encouraging results from rodent trials, human trials of selective β-3 agonists have been disappointing.

Bromocriptine

Hibernating and migratory animals change their ability to store and burn fat based on circadian rhythms, which are controlled by prolactin secretion. It has been postulated that overweight and diabetic individuals have abnormal circadian rhythms. These abnormal rhythms favor fat storage and insulin resistance. Rapid-release bromocriptine (Ergocet®), given at 8:00 a.m., has been postulated to reverse this abnormal circadian rhythm and effectively treat diabetes and overweight. An uncontrolled trial of quick-release bromocriptine given orally for 8 weeks significantly decreased 24-hr plasma glucose, free fatty acid, and triglyceride levels from baseline (Kamath et al., 1997). This was followed by a controlled trial in which 22 subjects with diabetes were randomized to quick-release bromocriptine or placebo. The hemoglobin A1c fell from 8.7 to 8.1% in the bromocriptine group and rose from 8.5 to 9.1% in the placebo group, a statistically significant difference (Pijl et al., 2000). In an uncontrolled trial, 33 overweight post-menopausal women reduced their body fat by 11.7% measured by skinfold thickness over 6 weeks of treatment with quick-release bromocriptine (Meier et al., 1992). This was followed by a controlled trial in which 17 overweight subjects were randomized to rapid-release bromocriptine (1.6–2.4 mg/d) or a placebo for 18 weeks. The bromocriptine group lost significantly more weight (6.3 versus 0.9 kg) and more fat as measured by skinfolds (5.4 versus 1.5 kg; Cincotta and Meier, 1996). The company developing Ergocet received approval from the FDA for quick-release bromocriptine to treat diabetes, but was asked to do additional safety studies. These studies were never performed, and the overweight development program proceeded no further.

Ecopipam

Ecopipam is a dopamine 1 and 5 receptor antagonist that was originally studied for the treatment of cocaine addiction (Nann-Vernotica et al., 2001). Ecopipam was in development as a drug to treat overweight but its development was recently terminated (Bays and Dujovne, 2002).

OVER-THE-COUNTER MEDICATIONS

Orlistat

Orlistat at a dose of 60 mg per day is approved as an over-the-counter preparation for overweight individuals.

Phenylpropanolamine

Short-term studies with phenylpropanolamine were reviewed in 1992, and weight loss was similar to the short-term weight loss seen with prescription drugs for overweight (Greenway, 1992). The longest study of phenylpropanolamine lasted 20 weeks. There was a 5.1 kg weight loss in the drug group and 0.4 kg weight loss in the placebo group, meeting the FDA criteria for a prescription weight-loss drug of a greater than 5% weight loss compared with placebo (Schteingart, 1992). Although phenylpropanolamine had a long history of safety in clinical trials dating to the 1930s, it was taken off the market because of an association with hemorrhagic stroke in women (Kernan et al., 2000).

COMPLEMENTARY AND HERBAL MEDICINE

Two recent reviews and commentary have examined randomized clinical trials for complementary therapies for reducing body weight (Dwyer et al., 2005; Pittler and Ernst, 2005).

Interventions Requiring Special Training

ACUPUNCTURE/ACCUPRESSURE

Acupuncture consists of placing needles at key points controlling neural connections for relief of pain and other clinical purposes. Pittler and Ernst (2005) identified four randomized controlled trials in which sham treatments were used. Two of the randomized trials of acupuncture reported a reduction in hunger, whereas two others showed no differences in body weight. Overall the evidence does not support a specific acupuncture procedure that works.

HOMEOPATHY

Two different preparations have been used in homeopathic doses to treat overweight and they were reflected in two randomized controlled trials. Helianthus tuberoses D1 was investigated for 3 months in one trial in which those receiving the active ingredient lost 7.1 kg, which was significantly more than in the placebo group. In a second trial, a single dose of Thyroidinum 30cH was given to fasting patients, but it was no more effective than placebo.

HYPONOTHERAPY

Hyponotherapy has been examined in six randomized controlled trials that compared hypotherapy plus cognitive behavior therapy with cognitive behavior therapy alone. The addition of hyponotherapy to cognitive behavior therapy adds a small, but significant weight loss to the cognitive behavior therapy (Pittler and Ernst, 2005).

Minerals and Metabolites

CHROMIUM PICOLINATE

Chromium is a trace mineral and a co-factor to insulin. It has been claimed that chromium can cause weight and fat loss while increasing lean body mass. A recent meta-analysis of 10 double-blind randomized controlled trials in participants with a BMI between 28 and 33 kg/m^2, showed a statistically significant weight loss of 1.1 to 1.2 kg over a 6- to 14-week treatment period. There were no adverse events, but the authors pointed out that this weight loss, although statistically significant was not clinically significant (Pittler and Ernst, 2004). This data has to be interpreted cautiously, because it relies heavily on one robust study. In a review of the field, Cefalu et al. (2002) showed that chromium picolinate may have a significant effect in preventing weight regain. Dwyer et al. (2005) conclude that there is little evidence of benefit and few or no adverse events.

HYDROXYMETHYL BUTYRATE

β-hydroxy-β-methylbutyrate is a metabolite of leucine. It acts in vivo to inhibit the breakdown of protein. The literature review by Pittler and Ernst (2005) found two randomized controlled trials that reported significant differences in fat mass reduction and at least a trend toward an increase in lean body mass. Further studies are clearly needed.

PYRUVATE

Pyruvate is an intermediary in the metabolism of glucose, and also serves as a hydrogen shuttle between liver and muscle. It has been suggested to improve exercise performance and body composition. Pittler and Ernst (2005) identified two randomized controlled trials that included subjects with a BMI of 25 kg/m^2 or higher. There were no significant effects on body weight reduction compared with placebo. They conclude that the case for pyruvate is weak.

CONJUGATED LINOLEIC ACID

The word "conjugated" in linoleic acid refers to the position of the double bond between carbons 9 to 11 or 10 to12. There are differences in effects of each of the isomeric combinations. In an analysis of 13 randomized, controlled trials lasting 6 months or less, Larsen et al. (2003) reported that there was little evidence that conjugated linoleic acid produced weight loss in human beings, although one report suggests it lowers body fat without effect on body weight (Riserus et al., 2004). There is also concern about liver toxicity from the *trans*-10, *cis*-12 isomer. Dwyer et al. (2005) conclude that there is little evidence of benefit.

CALCIUM

The relationship of calcium and body weight is the most confusing, because there is a patent issued for the effects of dairy products for producing weight loss issued to one of the proponents of this approach. Such a relationship where monetary gain is associated with publication of positive studies raises concerns when reading the published studies. Moreover, there is inconsistency in both the animal and human studies. In one small clinical trial increasing dietary intake of calcium by adding 800 mg per day of supplemental calcium to a diet containing 400 to 500 mg per day was claimed to augment weight and fat loss on reducing diets (Zemel et al., 2004). In two small studies in African-American adults, Zemel et al. (2005b) claimed that substitution of calcium-rich foods in isocaloric diets reduced adiposity and improved metabolic profiles during a 24-week trial. In another small study, Zemel et al. randomized 34 subjects to receive a control calcium diet with 400 to 500 mg per day ($N = 16$) or a yogurt-supplemented diet ($N = 18$) for 12 weeks. In this small, short duration study, fat loss was greater on the yogurt diet (−4.43 kg) than the control diet (−2.75 kg). Based on this data they claim that yogurt enhances central fat loss (Zemel et al., 2005a). In a large multicenter trial that enrolled nearly 100 subjects, the same authors claim that a hypocaloric diet with calcium supplemented to the level of 1400 mg per day did not significantly improve weight loss or body composition when compared with a diet with lower calcium intake (600 mg/d), whereas a diet with three servings per day of dairy products augmented weight and fat loss (Zemel et al., 2005a).

Two other studies, however, failed to find any effect of calcium supplementation on body weight or body fat (Barr, 2003; Shapses et al., 2004). Dwyer et al. (2005) conclude that the evidence of benefit is equivocal and limited to small trials, but there are no major concerns regarding adverse events.

Herbal Dietary Supplements

EPHEDRA SINICA

Ephedra sinica is an evergreen that grows in central Asia, and its principal ingredient is ephedrine. Ephedrine with caffeine has been shown to produce weight loss in randomized, placebo-controlled clinical trials (Astrup et al., 1992). The ephedra alkaloids from Ma huang contain ephedrine, and two randomized placebo-controlled clinical trials, one for 3 months and one for 6 months, showed significantly greater weight loss than with placebo (Boozer et al., 2001). The ephedra-containing herbal preparations were pulled from the market by the US FDA in April 2004 because of alleged harmful cardiovascular side effects (Shekelle et al., 2003), but this, as stated previously, has recently been reversed.

GARCINIA CAMBOGIA

Garcinia cambobia contains hydroxycitric acid, an inhibitor of citrate cleavage enzyme (ATP;citrate lyase) that inhibits fatty acid synthesis from carbohydrate. Hydroxycitrate was studied by Roche in the 1970s and was shown to reduce food intake and cause weight loss in rodents (Sullivan and Triscari, 1977). Although there have been reports of successful weight loss with small studies in humans, some of which combined other herbs, the largest and best designed placebo-controlled study demonstrated no difference in weight loss compared with placebo (Heymsfield et al., 1998; Pittler and Ernst, 2004). Thus, there is no evidence for efficacy.

YOHIMBINE FROM *PAUSINYSTALIA YOHIMBE*

Yohimbine is an α_2-adrenergic receptor antagonist that is isolated from *Pausinystalia yohimbe*. The three randomized clinical trials that Pittler and Ernst (2005) identified give conflicting results as to whether there is significant weight loss with this plant extract compared with placebo.

HOODIA

Hoodia gordonii is a cactus that grows in Africa. It has been eaten by Bushmen to decrease appetite and thirst on long treks across the desert. The active ingredient is steroidal glycoside, called P57AS3 or just P57. P57 injected into the third ventricle of animals increases the ATP content of hypothalamic tissue by 50 to 150% and decreases food intake by 40 to 60% over 24 hours (N. A., 2001). Phytopharm is developing P57 in partnership with Unilever. Information on the Phytopharm Website describes a double-blind 15-day trial in which 19 overweight males were randomized to P57 or placebo. Nine subjects in each group completed the study. There was a statistically significant decrease in calorie intake and body fat with good safety. Because Hoodia is a rare cactus in the wild and cultivation is difficult, it is not clear what the dietary herbal supplements claiming to contain Hoodia actually contain or if they are effective in causing weight loss.

CITRUS AURANTIUM (BITTER ORANGE)

Since the withdrawal of ephedra from the dietary herbal supplement market, manufacturers of dietary herbal supplements for weight loss have turned to citrus aurantium, which contains phenylephrine. A recent systematic review found only one randomized, placebo-controlled trial involving 20 subjects treated with citrus aurantium for 6 weeks. This trial demonstrated no statistically significant benefit for weight loss (Bent et al., 2004). There have been reports of cardiovascular events associated with the use of citrus aurantium, including a prolonged QT interval with syncope and an acute myocardial infarction (Nasir et al., 2004; Nykamp et al., 2004). Thus, there is no evidence for efficacy of citrus aurantium in the treatment of overweight, but concern does exist regarding its safety. Dwyer et al. (2005) conclude that there is no adequate evidence for efficacy and that there are safety concerns.

AYURVEDIC PREPARATIONS

Ayurvedic medicine is the traditional medicine of India. Ayurvedic herbal preparations containing Triphala guggul have been assessed in one randomized clinical trial (Pittler and Ernst, 2005). Patients in the treated group lost between 7.9 and 8.2 kg, which was significantly greater than placebo (Paranjpe et al., 1990).

Fibers

The possibility that fiber might be useful in maintaining lower weight comes from epidemiological studies. A recent re-examination of data from the Seven Countries studies has shown that the fiber intake within each of the participating country was inversely related to the body weight. Men eating more fiber had lower body weight. Epidemiological data suggests that countries that have higher fiber consumption have a lower prevalence of overweight (Kromhout et al., 2001). Fiber intake may also be related to the development of heart disease (Wolk et al., 1999) and diabetes (Salmeron et al., 1997).

CHITOSAN

Chitosan, or acetylated chitin, is a dietary fiber derived from crustaceans that has been advocated as a weight-loss agent. A recent systematic review of the randomized clinical trials of chitosan concluded, based on 14 trials longer than 4 weeks involving 1071 subjects, that chitosan gives 1.7-kg weight loss that is statistically significant (Mhurchu et al., 2005). This degree of weight loss falls far short of the 5 kg felt to be clinically significant, however. Dwyer et al. (2005) conclude that there is little evidence of benefit and some adverse GI symptoms.

GLUCOMANNAN

Glucomannan is derived from the root of the *Amorphophallus konjac* plant. Its chemical structure is similar to that of galactomannan in guar gum. They are both polysaccharide changes of glucose and mannose and serve as water soluble fibers. In one randomized controlled trial identified by Pittler and Ernst (2005), the subjects were 20% or more overweight and those on the glucomannan lost more weight than the placebo group.

GUAR GUM

Guar gum is an extract from *Cyamopsis tetragonolobus*. It is the most widely studied of the compounds in this group with 20 randomized placebo-controlled trials. In a meta-analysis of 11 of these trials, the data show that guar gum is no more effective than placebo (Pittler and Ernst, 2005).

PLANTAGO PSYLLIUM

The psyllium extract from the seeds of *Plantago psyllium* is a water-soluble fiber. In one randomized placebo-controlled trial identified by Pittler and Ernst (2005), there was no significant change in body weight in either the treatment or placebo group.

Sweeteners

STEVIA

Stevia rebaudiana is a South American plant that contains stevosides, which act as non-caloric sweeteners. In fact, Stevia has been used as a sweetener in Brazil and Japan for more than 20 years. Stevia is sold as a dietary herbal supplement and has been said

Table 5
Net Effect of Drug Trials for Anti-Obesity Drugs

Drug	Duration of studies	Weight loss (mean and 95% confidence interval)	FDA approval for obesity	Drug enforcement agency schedule
Orlistat	52 weeks	−2.75 (−3.32 to −2.20)	Yes	None
Sibutramine	52 weeks	−4.45 (−5.29 to − 3.62)	Yes	IV
Phentermine	2 to 24 weeks	−3.6 (−6.0 to −0.6)	Yes	III
Diethylpropion	6 to 52 weeks	−3.0 (−11.5 to 1.6)	Yes	III
Fluoxetine	52 weeks	−14.5 to + 0.4	No	None
Sertraline	26 weeks	Maintenance trial	No	None
Bupropion	24 to 52 weeks	−2.77 (−4.5 to −1.0)	No	None
Topiramate	24 weeks	6.5% more than placebo	No	None
Zonisamide	16 weeks	5% more than placebo	No	None

Adapted from L. et al., 2005.

to be useful in the treatment of overweight (N. A. Stevia Extract and Stevia Tea). There are three clinical trials testing stevia. The first was a randomized multicenter, placebo-controlled trial that treated 106 subjects with hypertension for 1 year. Subjects took stevoside 250 mg three times a day or a placebo. By 3 months, the SBP dropped from 166 to 153 mmHg and the DBP fell from 105 to 90 mmHg, and subjects maintained this statistically significant reduction for the rest of the year-long trial (Chan et al., 2000). The second trial enrolled 12 subjects with diabetes in a cross-over design. Glucose and insulin were measured around a standard meal. Stevioside 1 g or corn starch 1 g was given just before the meal. There was a statistically significant 18% reduction in the glucose area under the curve and an increase in insulin sensitivity (Gregersen et al., 2004). The third trial randomized 174 subjects with hypertension to stevioside 500 mg three times a day or placebo for 2 years. The SBP fell from 150 to 140 mmHg and the DBP fell from 95 to 89 mmHg by the end of the first week and this statistically significant difference persisted for the rest of the 2-year study. The stevoside group was protected from left ventricular hypertrophy, and like the other two trials, there were no adverse events or laboratory abnormalities (Hsieh et al., 2003). There was no weight loss in this 2-year trial. Thus, stevia does not appear to give weight loss, but may be useful in the treatment of the metabolic syndrome.

CONCLUSIONS

The drugs presently available for the treatment of overweight are few in number. The relative efficacy from a meta-analysis of many of the drugs I have discussed is shown in Table 5. The range of weight changes are quite small. In contrast the pipeline for overweight drug development is very rich. Because drug development is more sophisticated today than in the past, the development of safe and effective drugs for the treatment of overweight is anticipated to proceed at a more rapid pace than was the case for other chronic diseases that presently have safe and effective medications, such as hypertension and diabetes.

ACKNOWLEDGMENT

Some of the content for this chapter was prepared in collaboration with Dr. Frank L. Greenway.

REFERENCES

(1985). NIH Consensus Conference. Health implications of obesity. Ann Intern Med 103:1973–1977.

Alemany, M., et al. (2003). Weight loss in a patient with morbid obesity under treatment with oleoyl-estrone. Med Clin (Barc) 121(13):496–499.

Anderson, J. W., et al. (2002). Bupropion SR enhances weight loss: a 48-week double-blind, placebo-controlled trial. Obes Res 10(7):633–641.

Anderson, K. D., et al. (2003). Activation of the hypothalamic arcuate nucleus predicts the anorectic actions of ciliary neurotrophic factor and leptin in intact and gold thioglucose-lesioned mice. J Neuroendocrinol 15(7):649–660.

Apfelbaum, M., et al. (1999). Long-term maintenance of weight loss after a very-low-calorie diet: a randomized blinded trial of the efficacy and tolerability of sibutramine. Am J Med 106(2):179–184.

Astrand, A., et al. (2004). Mice lacking melanin-concentrating hormone receptor 1 demonstrate increased heart rate associated with altered autonomic activity. Am J Physiol Regul Integr Comp Physiol 287(4):R749–R758.

Astrup, A., et al. (1992). The effect and safety of an ephedrine/caffeine compound compared to ephedrine, caffeine and placebo in obese subjects on an energy restricted diet. A double blind trial. Int J Obes Relat Metab Disord 16(4):269–277.

Astrup, A., et al. (2004). Topiramate: long-term maintenance of weight loss induced by a low-calorie diet in obese subjects. Obes Res 12(10):1658–1669.

Astrup, A. and Toubro, S. (2004). Topiramate: a new potential pharmacological treatment for obesity. Obes Res 12(Suppl):167S–173S.

Avenell, A, et al. (2004a). Systematic review of the long-term effects and economic consequences of treatments for obesity and implication for health improvement. Health Technol Assess 8(21):i–x;1–458.

Avenell, A., et al. (2004b). What interventions should we add to weight reducing diets in adults with obesity? A systematic review of randomized controlled trials of adding drug therapy, exercise, behaviour therapy or combinations of these interventions. J Hum Nutr Diet 17(4):293–316.

Barkeling, B., et al. (2003). Short-term effects of sibutramine (Reductil) on appetite and eating behaviour and the long-term therapeutic outcome. Int J Obes Relat Metab Disord 27(6):693–700.

Barr, S. I. (2003). Increased dairy product or calcium intake: is body weight or composition affected in humans? J Nutr 133(1):245S–248S.

Batterham, R. L., et al. (2003). Inhibition of food intake in obese subjects by peptide YY3-36. N Engl J Med 349(10):941–948.

Bays, H. and Dujovne, C. (2002). Anti-obesity drug development. Expert Opin Investig Drugs 11(9):1189–1204.

Ben-Menachem, E., et al. (2003). Predictors of weight loss in adults with topiramate-treated epilepsy. Obes Res 11(4):556–562.

Bensaid, M., et al. (2003). The cannabinoid CB1 receptor antagonist SR141716 increases Acrp30 mRNA expression in adipose tissue of obese fa/fa rats and in cultured adipocyte cells. Mol Pharmacol 63(4):908–914.

Bent, S., et al. (2004). Safety and efficacy of citrus aurantium for weight loss. Am J Cardiol 94(10):1359–1361.

Berkowitz, R., et al. (2006). Effects of sibutramine treatment in obese adolescents: a randomized trial. Ann Intern Med 145(2):81–90.

Berkowitz, R. I., et al. (2003). Behavior therapy and sibutramine for the treatment of adolescent obesity: a randomized controlled trial. JAMA 289(14):1805–1812.

Boeles, S., et al. (1997). Sumatriptan decreases food intake and increases plasma growth hormone in healthy women. Psychopharmacology (Berl) 129(2):179–182.

Boozer, C. N., et al. (2001). An herbal supplement containing Ma Huang-Guarana for weight loss: a randomized, double-blind trial. Int J Obes Relat Metab Disord 25(3):316–324.

Borowsky, B., et al. (2002). Antidepressant, anxiolytic and anorectic effects of a melanin-concentrating hormone-1 receptor antagonist. Nat Med 8(8):825–830.

Brakenhielm, E., et al. (2004). Angiogenesis inhibitor, TNP-470, prevents diet-induced and genetic obesity in mice. Circ Res 94(12):1579–1588.

Bray, G. A., et al. (1999). Sibutramine produces dose-related weight loss. Obes Res 7(2):189–198.

Bray, G. A., et al. (2003). A 6-month randomized, placebo-controlled, dose-ranging trial of topiramate for weight loss in obesity. Obes Res 11(6):722–733.

Bray, G. A. and Gallagher, T. F. Jr. (1975). Manifestations of hypothalamic obesity in man: a comprehensive investigation of eight patients and a review of the literature. Medicine (Baltimore) 54(4):301–330.

Bray, G. A. and Greenway, F. L. (1999). Current and potential drugs for treatment of obesity. Endocr Rev 20(6):805–875.

Broom, I., et al. (2002). Randomised trial of the effect of orlistat on body weight and cardiovascular disease risk profile in obese patients: UK Multimorbidity Study. Int J Clin Pract 56(7):494–499.

Buse, J. B., et al. (2004). Effects of exenatide (exendin-4) on glycemic control over 30 weeks in sulfonyl-urea-treated patients with type 2 diabetes. Diabetes Care 27(11):2628–2635.

Cangiano, C., et al. (1992). Eating behavior and adherence to dietary prescriptions in obese adult subjects treated with 5-hydroxytryptophan. Am J Clin Nutr 56(5):863–867.

Cangiano, C., et al. (1998). Effects of oral 5-hydroxy-tryptophan on energy intake and macronutrient selection in non-insulin dependent diabetic patients. Int J Obes Relat Metab Disord 22(7): 648–654.

Cefalu, W. T., et al. (2002). Oral chromium picolinate improves carbohydrate and lipid metabolism and enhances skeletal muscle Glut-4 translocation in obese, hyperinsulinemic (JCR-LA corpulent) rats. J Nutr 132(6):1107–1114.

Chan, P., et al. (2000). A double-blind placebo-controlled study of the effectiveness and tolerability of oral stevioside in human hypertension. Br J Clin Pharmacol 50(3):215–220.

Chanoine, J. P., et al. (2005). Effect of orlistat on weight and body composition in obese adolescents: a randomized controlled trial. JAMA 293(23):2873–2883.

Cincotta, A. H. and Meier, A. H. (1996). Bromocriptine (Ergoset) reduces body weight and improves glucose tolerance in obese subjects. Diabetes Care 19(6):667–670.

Colman, E. (2005). Anorectics on trial: a half century of federal regulation of prescription appetite suppressants. Ann Intern Med 143(5):380–385.

Cowen, P. J., et al. (1995). Hypophagic, endocrine and subjective responses to m-chlorophenylpiperazine in healthy men and women. Hum Psychopharmacol 10:385–391.

Davidson, M. H., et al. (1999). Weight control and risk factor reduction in obese subjects treated for 2 years with orlistat: a randomized controlled trial. JAMA 281(3):235–242.

Davies, K. M., et al. (2000). Calcium intake and body weight. J Clin Endocrinol Metab 85(12):4635–4638.

de Souza, C. J. and Burkey, B. F. (2001). Beta 3-adrenoceptor agonists as anti-diabetic and anti-obesity drugs in humans. Curr Pharm Des 7(14):1433–1449.

DeFronzo, R. A., et al. (2005). Effects of exenatide (exendin-4) on glycemic control and weight over 30 weeks in metformin-treated patients with type 2 diabetes. Diabetes Care 28(5):1092–1100.

Despres, J. P., et al. (2005). Effects of rimonabant on metabolic risk factors in overweight patients with dyslipidemia. N Engl J Med 353(20):2121–2134.

Devinsky, O., et al. (2000). Stable weight during lamotrigine therapy: a review of 32 studies. Neurology 54(4):973–975.

Drent, M. L., et al. (1995). The effect of dexfenfluramine on eating habits in a Dutch ambulatory android overweight population with an overconsumption of snacks. Int J Obes Relat Metab Disord 19(5):299–304.

Dunk, C., et al. (2002). Increased fecal fat excretion in normal volunteers treated with lipase inhibitor ATL-962. Int J Obes Relat Metab Disord 26(Suppl):S135.

Dwyer, J. T., et al. (2005). Dietary supplements in weight reduction. J Am Diet Assoc 105(5 Suppl 1):S80–S86.

Edwards, C. M., et al. (2001). Exendin-4 reduces fasting and postprandial glucose and decreases energy intake in healthy volunteers. Am J Physiol Endocrinol Metab 281(1):E155–E161.

Erondu, N., et al. (2006). Neuropeptide is receptor antagonism does not induce clinically meaningful weight loss in overweight and obese adults. Cell Metab 4(4):275–282.

Erondu, N., Wadden, T., Gantz, I., et al. (2007). Effect of NPY5R antagonist MK-0558 on weight regain after very-low-calorie diet-induced weight loss. Obesity 15:895–905.

Ettinger, M. P., et al. (2003). Recombinant variant of ciliary neurotrophic factor for weight loss in obese adults: a randomized, dose-ranging study. JAMA 289(14):1826–1832.

Fineman, M. S., et al. (2004). Effectiveness of progressive dose-escalation of exenatide (exendin-4) in reducing dose-limiting side effects in subjects with type 2 diabetes. Diabetes Metab Res Rev 20(5):411–417.

Finer, N., et al. (2000). One-year treatment of obesity: a randomized, double-blind, placebo-controlled, multicentre study of orlistat, a gastrointestinal lipase inhibitor. Int J Obes Relat Metab Disord 24(3):306–313.

Foltin, R. W., et al. (1996). Effect of fenfluramine on food intake, mood, and performance of humans living in a residential laboratory. Physiol Behav 59(2):295–305.

Fontbonne, A., et al. (1996). The effect of metformin on the metabolic abnormalities associated with upper-body fat distribution. BIGPRO Study Group. Diabetes Care 19(9):920–926.

Foxx-Orenstein, A., et al. (2003). Effect of a somatostatin analogue on gastric motor and sensory functions in healthy humans. Gut 52(11):1555–1561.

Franco, C., et al. (2005). Growth hormone treatment reduces abdominal visceral fat in postmenopausal women with abdominal obesity: a 12-month placebo-controlled trial. J Clin Endocrinol Metab 90(3):1466–1474.

Fujioka, K., et al. (2000). Weight loss with sibutramine improves glycaemic control and other metabolic parameters in obese patients with type 2 diabetes mellitus. Diabetes Obes Metab 2(3):175–187.

Gadde, K. M., et al. (2001). Bupropion for weight loss: an investigation of efficacy and tolerability in overweight and obese women. Obes Res 9(9):544–551.

Gadde, K. M., et al. (2003). Zonisamide for weight loss in obese adults: a randomized controlled trial. JAMA 289(14):1820–1825.

Gantz, I., Erondu, N., Mallick, M., et al. (2007). Efficacy and safety of intranasal peptide YY3-36 for weight reduction in obese adults. J Clin Endocrinol Metab. E-Pub March 6.

Gedulin, B. R., et al. (2005). Exenatide (exendin-4) improves insulin sensitivity and {beta}-cell mass in insulin-resistant obese fa/fa Zucker rats independent of glycemia and body weight. Endocrinology 146(4):2069–2076.

Gibson, W. T., et al. (2004). Mutational analysis of the serotonin receptor 5HT2c in severe early-onset human obesity. Can J Physiol Pharmacol 82(6):426–429.

Godoy-Matos, A., et al. (2005). Treatment of obese adolescents with sibutramine: a randomized, double-blind, controlled study. J Clin Endocrinol Metab 90(3):1460–1465.

Goldstein, D. J., et al. (1995). Efficacy and safety of long-term fluoxetine treatment of obesity—maximizing success. Obes Res 3(Suppl 4):481S–490S.

Greenway, F. L. (1992). Clinical studies with phenylpropanolamine: a metaanalysis. Am J Clin Nutr 55(1 Suppl):203S–205S.

Greenway, F. L. (2001). The safety and efficacy of pharmaceutical and herbal caffeine and ephedrine use as a weight loss agent. Obes Rev 2(3):199–211.

Greenway, S. E., et al. (2002). Effects of obesity surgery on non-insulin-dependent diabetes mellitus. Arch Surg 137(10):1109–1117.

Gregersen, S., et al. (2004). Antihyperglycemic effects of stevioside in type 2 diabetic subjects. Metabolism 53(1):73–76.

Haddock, C. K., et al. (2002). Pharmacotherapy for obesity: a quantitative analysis of four decades of published randomized clinical trials. Int J Obes Relat Metab Disord 26(2):262–273.

Halaas, J. L., et al. (1995). Weight-reducing effects of the plasma protein encoded by the obese gene. Science 269(5223):543–546.

Handlon, A. and Zhou, H. (2006). Melanin-concentrating hormone-1 receptor antagonists for the treatment of obesity. J Med Chem 49(14):4017–4022.

Hansen, D. L., et al. (1998). Thermogenic effects of sibutramine in humans. Am J Clin Nutr 68(6):1180–1186.

Hauptman, J. (2000). Orlistat: selective inhibition of caloric absorption can affect long-term body weight. Endocrine 13(2):201–206.

Heine, R. J., et al. (2005). Exenatide versus insulin glargine in patients with suboptimally controlled type 2 diabetes: a randomized trial. Ann Intern Med 143(8):559–569.

Heymsfield, S. B., et al. (1998). Garcinia cambogia (hydroxycitric acid) as a potential antiobesity agent: a randomized controlled trial. JAMA 280(18):1596–1600.

Heymsfield, S. B., et al. (1999). Recombinant leptin for weight loss in obese and lean adults: a randomized, controlled, dose-escalation trial. JAMA 282(16):1568–1575.

Heymsfield, S. B., et al. (2000). Effects of weight loss with orlistat on glucose tolerance and progression to type 2 diabetes in obese adults. Arch Intern Med 160(9):1321–1326.

Hill, J. O., et al. (1999). Orlistat, a lipase inhibitor, for weight maintenance after conventional dieting: a 1-y study. Am J Clin Nutr 69(6):1108–1116.

Hoffman, A. R., et al. (2004). Growth hormone (GH) replacement therapy in adult-onset gh deficiency: effects on body composition in men and women in a double-blind, randomized, placebo-controlled trial. J Clin Endocrinol Metab 89(5):2048–2056.

Hollander, P. A., et al. (1998). Role of orlistat in the treatment of obese patients with type 2 diabetes. A 1-year randomized double-blind study. Diabetes Care 21(8):1288–1294.

Hsieh, M. H., et al. (2003). Efficacy and tolerability of oral stevioside in patients with mild essential hypertension: a two-year, randomized, placebo-controlled study. Clin Ther 25(11):2797–2808.

Hukshorn, C. J., et al. (2000). Weekly subcutaneous pegylated recombinant native human leptin (PEG-OB) administration in obese men. J Clin Endocrinol Metab 85(11):4003–4009.

Hukshorn, C. J., et al. (2003). Pegylated human recombinant leptin (PEG-OB) causes additional weight loss in severely energy-restricted, overweight men. Am J Clin Nutr 77(4):771–776.

Jain, A. K., et al. (2002). Bupropion SR vs. placebo for weight loss in obese patients with depressive symptoms. Obes Res 10(10):1049–1056.

James, W. P., et al. (2000). Effect of sibutramine on weight maintenance after weight loss: a randomised trial. STORM Study Group. Sibutramine Trial of Obesity Reduction and Maintenance. Lancet 356(9248):2119–2125.

Jordan, J., et al. (2005). Influence of Sibutramine on blood pressure: evidence from placebo-controlled trials. Int J Obes (Lond) 29(5):509–516.

Juan-Pico, P., et al. (2006). Cannabinoid receptors regulate Ca(2+) signals and insulin secretion in pancreatic beta-cell. Cell Calcium 39(2):155–162.

Kamath, V., et al. (1997). Effects of a quick-release form of bromocriptine (Ergoset) on fasting and postprandial plasma glucose, insulin, lipid, and lipoprotein concentrations in obese nondiabetic hyperinsulinemic women. Diabetes Care 20(11):1697–1701.

Kanatani, A., et al. (2001). A typical Y1 receptor regulates feeding behaviors: effects of a potent and selective Y1 antagonist, J-115814. Mol Pharmacol 59(3):501–505.

Kastin, A. J. and Akerstrom, V. (2003). Entry of exendin-4 into brain is rapid but may be limited at high doses. Int J Obes Relat Metab Disord 27(3):313–318.

Kaya, A., et al. (2004). Efficacy of sibutramine, orlistat and combination therapy on short-term weight management in obese patients. Biomed Pharmacother 58(10):582–587.

Kelley, D. E., et al. (2002). Clinical efficacy of orlistat therapy in overweight and obese patients with insulin-treated type 2 diabetes: A 1-year randomized controlled trial. Diabetes Care 25(6):1033–1041.

Kendall, D. M., et al. (2005). Effects of exenatide (exendin-4) on glycemic control over 30 weeks in patients with type 2 diabetes treated with metformin and a sulfonylurea. Diabetes Care 28(5):1083–1091.

Kernan, W. N., et al. (2000). Phenylpropanolamine and the risk of hemorrhagic stroke. N Engl J Med 343(25):1826–1832.

Kim, S. H., et al. (2003). Effect of sibutramine on weight loss and blood pressure: a meta-analysis of controlled trials. Obes Res 11(9):1116–1123.

Kirkham, T. C. (2005). Endocannabinoids in the regulation of appetite and body weight. Behav Pharmacol 16(5–6):297–313.

Knowler, W. C., et al. (2002). Reduction in the incidence of type 2 diabetes with lifestyle intervention or metformin. N Engl J Med 346(6):393–403.

Kopelman, P., Bryson, A., Hickling, R., et al. (2007). Cetilistat (ATL-962), a novel lipase inhibitor: a 12 week randomized, placebo-controlled study of weight reduction in obese patients. Intern J Obes 31:494–499.

Kowalski, T. J., et al. (2004). Melanin-concentrating hormone-1 receptor antagonism decreases feeding by reducing meal size. Eur J Pharmacol 497(1):41–47.

Kromhout, D., et al. (2001). Physical activity and dietary fiber determine population body fat levels: the Seven Countries Study. Int J Obes Relat Metab Disord 25(3):301–306.

Laferrere, B., et al. (2005). Growth hormone releasing peptide-2 (GHRP-2), like ghrelin, increases food intake in healthy men. J Clin Endocrinol Metab 90(2):611–614.

Larsen, T. M., et al. (2002). Effect of a 28-d treatment with L-796568, a novel beta(3)-adrenergic receptor agonist, on energy expenditure and body composition in obese men. Am J Clin Nutr 76(4):780–788.

Larsen, T. M., et al. (2003). Efficacy and safety of dietary supplements containing CLA for the treatment of obesity: evidence from animal and human studies. J Lipid Res 44(12):2234–2241.

Lawton, C. L., et al. (1995). Serotoninergic manipulation, meal-induced satiety and eating pattern: effect of fluoxetine in obese female subjects. Obes Res 3(4):345–356.

Levens, N. R. and Della-Zuana, O. (2003). Neuropeptide Y Y5 receptor antagonists as anti-obesity drugs. Curr Opin Investig Drugs 4(10):1198–1204.

Li, Z., et al. (2005). Meta-analysis: pharmacologic treatment of obesity. Ann Intern Med 142(7):532–546.

Lindgarde, F. (2000). The effect of orlistat on body weight and coronary heart disease risk profile in obese patients: the Swedish Multimorbidity Study. J Intern Med 248(3):245–254.

Ludwig, D. S., et al. (1998). Melanin-concentrating hormone: a functional melanocortin antagonist in the hypothalamus. Am J Physiol 274(4 Pt 1):E627–E633.

Lugari, R., et al. (2004). Glucagon-like peptide 1 (GLP-1) secretion and plasma dipeptidyl peptidase IV (DPP-IV) activity in morbidly obese patients undergoing biliopancreatic diversion. Horm Metab Res 36(2):111–115.

Lustig, R. H., et al. (1999). Hypothalamic obesity caused by cranial insult in children: altered glucose and insulin dynamics and reversal by a somatostatin agonist. J Pediatr 135(2 Pt 1):162–168.

Lustig, R., et al. (2003a). Weight loss in obese adults with insulin hypersecretion treated with Sandostatin LAR Depot. Obes Res 11(Suppl):A25.

Lustig, R. H., et al. (2003b). Octreotide therapy of pediatric hypothalamic obesity: a double-blind, placebo-controlled trial. J Clin Endocrinol Metab 88(6):2586–2592.

Lustig, R. H., et al. (2006). A multicenter, randomized, double-blind, placebo-controlled, dose-finding trial of a long-acting formulation of octreotide in promoting weight loss in obese adults with insulin hypersecretion. Int J Obes (Lond) 30(2):331–341.

Maahs, D., et al. (2006). Randomized, double-blind, placebo-controlled trial of orlistat for weight loss in adolescents. Endocr Pract 12(1):18–28.

Maffei, M., et al. (1995). Increased expression in adipocytes of ob RNA in mice with lesions of the hypothalamus and with mutations at the db locus. Proc Natl Acad Sci USA 92(15):6957–6960.

Maggs, D., et al. (2003). Effect of pramlintide on A1C and body weight in insulin-treated African Americans and Hispanics with type 2 diabetes: a pooled post hoc analysis. Metabolism 52(12):1638–1642.

Mathus-Vliegen, E. M. (2005). Long-term maintenance of weight loss with sibutramine in a GP setting following a specialist guided very-low-calorie diet: a double-blind, placebo-controlled, parallel group study. Eur J Clin Nutr 59(Suppl 1):S31–S38; discussion S39.

McElroy, S. L., et al. (2003). Topiramate in the treatment of binge eating disorder associated with obesity: a randomized, placebo-controlled trial. Am J Psychiatry 160(2):255–261.

McElroy, S. L., et al. (2004a). Zonisamide in the treatment of binge-eating disorder: an open-label, prospective trial. J Clin Psychiatry 65(1):50–56.

McElroy, S. L., et al. (2004b). Topiramate in the long-term treatment of binge-eating disorder associated with obesity. J Clin Psychiatry 65(11):1463–1469.

McMahon, F. G., et al. (2000). Efficacy and safety of sibutramine in obese white and African American patients with hypertension: a 1-year, double-blind, placebo-controlled, multicenter trial. Arch Intern Med 160(14):2185–2191.

McNulty, S. J., et al. (2003). A randomized trial of sibutramine in the management of obese type 2 diabetic patients treated with metformin. Diabetes Care 26(1):125–131.

Meier, A. H., et al. (1992). Timed bromocriptine administration reduces body fat stores in obese subjects and hyperglycemia in type II diabetics. Experientia 48(3):248–253.

Merideth, C. H. (2006). A single-center, double-blind, placebo-controlled, evaluation of lamotrigine in the treatment of obesity in adults. J Clin Psychiatry 67(2):258–262.

Mhurchu, C. N., et al. (2005). Effect of chitosan on weight loss in overweight and obese individuals: a systematic review of randomized controlled trials. Obes Rev 6(1):35–42.

Miles, J. M., et al. (2002). Effect of orlistat in overweight and obese patients with type 2 diabetes treated with metformin. Diabetes Care 25(7):1123–1128.

Mittendorfer, B., et al. (2001). Orlistat inhibits dietary cholesterol absorption. Obes Res 9(10):599–604.

Munro, J., et al. (1968). Comparison of continuous and intermittent anorectic therapy in obesity. BMJ 1: 352–354.

N. A. Stevia Extract and Stevia Tea. Available from: http://www.primalnature.com/stevia.html.

N. A. (1996). Dexfenfluramine for obesity. Med Lett Drugs Ther 38(979):64–65.

N. A. (2001). Phytopharm plc Successful Completion of Proof of Principle Clinical Study of P57 for Obesity. Available from: http://www.metabolic.com.au/files/T5SH4035T6/ASX_%20 AOD9604_result%20announcement.pdf.

N. A. (2004). AOD9604 Phase 2b Clinical Trial Successful. Available from: http://www.phytopharm.co.uk/ press/P57%20Third%20Stage%20final.htm.

Nam, S. Y., et al. (2001). Low-dose growth hormone treatment combined with diet restriction decreases insulin resistance by reducing visceral fat and increasing muscle mass in obese type 2 diabetic patients. Int J Obes Relat Metab Disord 25(8):1101–1107.

Nann-Vernotica, E., et al. (2001). Repeated administration of the D1/5 antagonist ecopipam fails to attenuate the subjective effects of cocaine. Psychopharmacology (Berl) 155(4):338–347.

Nasir, J. M., et al. (2004). Exercise-induced syncope associated with QT prolongation and ephedra-free Xenadrine. Mayo Clin Proc 79(8):1059–1062.

National Institutes of Health, National Heart, Lung, and Blood Institute, et al. (2000). The practical guide: identification, evaluation and treatment of overweight and obesity in adults. National Institutes of Health. Available from: http://www.nhlbi.nih.gov/guidelines/obesity/prctgd_c.pdf

Nilsson, B. M. (2006) 5-Hydroxytryptamine 2C (5-HT2C) receptor agonists as potential antiobesity angents. J Med Chem 49(14):4023–4034.

Norris, S. L., et al. (2004). Efficacy of pharmacotherapy for weight loss in adults with type 2 diabetes mellitus: a meta-analysis. Arch Intern Med 164(13):1395–1404.

Nykamp, D. L., et al. (2004). Possible association of acute lateral-wall myocardial infarction and bitter orange supplement. Ann Pharmacother 38(5):812–816.

Oral, E. A., et al. (2002). Leptin-replacement therapy for lipodystrophy. N Engl J Med 346(8):570–578.

Ortega-Gonzalez, C., et al. (2005). Responses of serum androgen and insulin resistance to metformin and pioglitazone in obese, insulin-resistant women with polycystic ovary syndrome. J Clin Endocrinol Metab 90(3):1360–1365.

Padwal, R., et al. (2004). Long-term pharmacotherapy for obesity and overweight. Cochrane Database Syst Rev (3):CD004094.

Padwal, R., et al. (2005). A systematic review of drug therapy to delay or prevent type 2 diabetes. Diabetes Care 28(3):736–744.

Pagotto, U., et al. (2006). The emerging role of the endocannabinoid system in endocrine regulation and energy balance. Endocr Rev 27(1):73–100.

Paranjpe, P., et al. (1990). Ayurvedic treatment of obesity: a randomised double-blind, placebo-controlled clinical trial. J Ethnopharmacol 29(1):1–11.

Parker, E., et al. (2002). Neuropeptide Y receptors as targets for anti-obesity drug development: perspective and current status. Eur J Pharmacol 440(2-3):173–187.

Patriti, A., et al. (2004). The enteroinsular axis and the recovery from type 2 diabetes after bariatric surgery. Obes Surg 14(6):840–848.

Pi-Sunyer, F. X., et al. (2006). Effect of rimonabant, a cannabinoid-1 receptor blocker, on weight and cardiometabolic risk factors in overweight or obese patients: RIO-North America: a randomized controlled trial. JAMA 295(7):761–775.

Pi-Sunyer, X., et al. (1982). C-terminal octapeptide of cholecystokinin decreases food intake in obese men. Physiol Behav 29(4):627–630.

Pijl, H., et al. (2000). Bromocriptine: a novel approach to the treatment of type 2 diabetes. Diabetes Care 23(8):1154–1161.

Pittler, M. H. and Ernst, E. (2004). Dietary supplements for body-weight reduction: a systematic review. Am J Clin Nutr 79(4):529–536.

Pittler, M. H. and Ernst, E. (2005). Complementary therapies for reducing body weight: a systematic review. Int J Obes (Lond) 29(9):1030–1038.

Poindexter, G. S., et al. (2002). Dihydropyridine neuropeptide Y Y(1) receptor antagonists. Bioorg Med Chem Lett 12(3):379–382.

Poston, W. S., et al. (2001). Lifestyle treatments in randomized clinical trials of pharmacotherapies for obesity. Obes Res 9(9):552–563.

Puhl, R. M. and Brownell, K. D. (2003). Psychosocial origins of obesity stigma: toward changing a powerful and pervasive bias. Obes Rev 4(4):213–227.

Putnam, J. (1893). Cases of myxedema and acromegalia treated with benefit by sheep's thyroids: recent observations respecting the pathology of the cachexias following disease of the thyroid; clinical relationships of grave's disease and acromegalia. Am J Med Sci 106:125–148.

Ratner, R. E., et al. (2004). Amylin replacement with pramlintide as an adjunct to insulin therapy improves long-term glycaemic and weight control in Type 1 diabetes mellitus: a 1-year, randomized controlled trial. Diabet Med 21(11):1204–1212.

Reaven, G., et al. (2001). Effect of orlistat-assisted weight loss in decreasing coronary heart disease risk in patients with syndrome X. Am J Cardiol 87(7):827–831.

Riddle, M. C. and Drucker, D. J. (2006). Emerging therapies mimicking the effects of amylin and glucagon-like peptide 1. Diabetes Care 29(2):435–449.

Riserus, U., et al. (2004). Metabolic effects of conjugated linoleic acid in humans: the Swedish experience. Am J Clin Nutr 79(6 Suppl):1146S–1148S.

Rodriquez de Fonseca, F., et al. (2000). Peripheral versus central effects of glucagon-like peptide-1 receptor agonists on satiety and body weight loss in Zucker obese rats. Metabolism 49(6):709–717.

Rogers, P. J. and Blundell, J. E. (1979). Effect of anorexic drugs on food intake and the micro-structure of eating in human subjects. Psychopharmacology (Berl) 66(2):159–165.

Rolls, B. J., et al. (1998). Sibutramine reduces food intake in non-dieting women with obesity. Obes Res 6(1):1–11.

Rosenbaum, M., et al. (2002). Low dose leptin administration reverses effects of sustained weight-reduction on energy expenditure and circulating concentrations of thyroid hormones. J Clin Endocrinol Metab 87(5):2391–2394.

Rossner, S., et al. (2000). Weight loss, weight maintenance, and improved cardiovascular risk factors after 2 years treatment with orlistat for obesity. European Orlistat Obesity Study Group. Obes Res 8(1):49–61.

Rupnick, M. A., et al. (2002). Adipose tissue mass can be regulated through the vasculature. Proc Natl Acad Sci USA 99(16):10,730–10,735.

Salmeron, J., et al. (1997). Dietary fiber, glycemic load, and risk of non-insulin-dependent diabetes mellitus in women. JAMA 277(6):472–477.

Scheen, A. J., Finer, N., Hollander, P., Jensen, M. D., Van Gaal, L. P., RIO-Diabetes Study Group. (2006). Efficacy and tolerability of rimonabant in overweight or obese patients with type 2 diabetes: a randomised controlled study. Lancet 368:1660–1672.

Schteingart, D. E. (1992). Effectiveness of phenylpropanolamine in the management of moderate obesity. Int J Obes Relat Metab Disord 16(7):487–493.

Shapira, N. A., et al. (2000). Treatment of binge-eating disorder with topiramate: a clinical case series. J Clin Psychiatry 61(5):368–372.

Shapira, N. A., et al. (2002). Topiramate attenuates self-injurious behaviour in Prader-Willi Syndrome. Int J Neuropsychopharmacol 5(2):141–145.

Shapira, N. A., et al. (2004). Effects of topiramate in adults with Prader-Willi syndrome. Am J Ment Retard 109(4):301–309.

Shapses, S. A., et al. (2001). Bone turnover and density in obese premenopausal women during moderate weight loss and calcium supplementation. J Bone Miner Res 16(7):1329–1336.

Shapses, S. A., et al. (2004). Effect of calcium supplementation on weight and fat loss in women. J Clin Endocrinol Metab 89(2):632–637.

Shearman, L. P., et al. (2003). Chronic MCH-1 receptor modulation alters appetite, body weight and adiposity in rats. Eur J Pharmacol 475(1–3):37–47.

Shekelle, P. G., et al. (2003). Efficacy and safety of ephedra and ephedrine for weight loss and athletic performance: a meta-analysis. JAMA 289(12):1537–1545.

Sjostrom, L., et al. (1998). Randomised placebo-controlled trial of orlistat for weight loss and prevention of weight regain in obese patients. European Multicentre Orlistat Study Group. Lancet 352(9123): 167–172.

Sjostrom, L., et al. (2004). Lifestyle, diabetes, and cardiovascular risk factors 10 years after bariatric surgery. N Engl J Med 351(26):2683–2693.

Small, C. J. and Bloom, S. R. (2004). Gut hormones as peripheral anti obesity targets. Curr Drug Targets CNS Neurol Disord 3(5):379–388.

Smathers, S. A., et al. (2003). Topiramate effectiveness in Prader-Willi syndrome. Pediatr Neurol 28(2): 130–133.

Smith, S. R., et al. (2006). APD356, an orally-active selective 5HT2C agoinst reduces body weight in obese men and women. Diabetes and metabolism 55(Suppl 1):A80.

Smith, I. G., et al. (2001). Randomized placebo-controlled trial of long-term treatment with sibutramine in mild to moderate obesity. J Fam Pract 50(6):505–512.

Snow, V., et al. (2005). Pharmacologic and surgical management of obesity in primary care: a clinical practice guideline from the American College of Physicians. Ann Intern Med 142(7):525–531.

Souers, A. J., et al. (2005). Identification of 2-(4-benzyloxyphenyl)-N-[1-(2-pyrrolidin-1-yl-ethyl)-1H-indazol-6-yl]acetamide, an orally efficacious melanin-concentrating hormone receptor 1 antagonist for the treatment of obesity. J Med Chem 48(5):1318–1321.

Sullivan, C. and Triscari, J. (1977). Metabolic regulation as a control for lipid disorders. I. Influence of (−)-hydroxycitrate on experimentally induced obesity in the rodent. Am J Clin Nutr 30(5):767–776.

Szayna, M., et al. (2000). Exendin-4 decelerates food intake, weight gain, and fat deposition in Zucker rats. Endocrinology 141(6):1936–1941.

Tan, T. M., et al. (2004). Somatostatin infusion lowers plasma ghrelin without reducing appetite in adults with Prader-Willi syndrome. J Clin Endocrinol Metab 89(8):4162–4165.

Torgerson, J. S., et al. (2004). XENical in the prevention of diabetes in obese subjects (XENDOS) study: a randomized study of orlistat as an adjunct to lifestyle changes for the prevention of type 2 diabetes in obese patients. Diabetes Care 27(1):155–161.

van Baak, M. A., et al. (2002). Acute effect of L-796568, a novel beta 3-adrenergic receptor agonist, on energy expenditure in obese men. Clin Pharmacol Ther 71(4):272–279.

Van Gaal, L. F., et al. (2005). Effects of the cannabinoid-1 receptor blocker rimonabant on weight reduction and cardiovascular risk factors in overweight patients: 1-year experience from the RIO-Europe study. Lancet 365(9468):1389–1397.

VBrandt, G., et al. (2004). Intranasal peptide YY 3-36: phase 1 dose ranging and dose sequencing studies. Obes Res 12(Suppl):A28.

Velasquez-Mieyer, P. A., et al. (2003). Suppression of insulin secretion is associated with weight loss and altered macronutrient intake and preference in a subset of obese adults. Int J Obes Relat Metab Disord 27(2):219–226.

Vettor, R., et al. (2005). Effect of sibutramine on weight management and metabolic control in type 2 diabetes: a meta-analysis of clinical studies. Diabetes Care 28(4):942–949.

Wadden, T. A., et al. (2000). Effects of sibutramine plus orlistat in obese women following 1 year of treatment by sibutramine alone: a placebo-controlled trial. Obes Res 8(6):431–437.

Wadden, T. A., et al. (2001). Benefits of lifestyle modification in the pharmacologic treatment of obesity: a randomized trial. Arch Intern Med 161(2):218–227.

Wadden, T. A., et al. (2005). Randomized trial of lifestyle modification and pharmacotherapy for obesity. N Engl J Med 353(20):2111–2120.

Website http://www.clinicaltrials.gov/t/show/NCT00104507?order=1.

Website http://www.regeneron.com/. Last accessed April 5, 2007.

Wilding, J., et al. (2004). A randomized double-blind placebo-controlled study of the long-term efficacy and safety of topiramate in the treatment of obese subjects. Int J Obes Relat Metab Disord 28(11): 1399–1410.

Winkelman, J. W. (2003). Treatment of nocturnal eating syndrome and sleep-related eating disorder with topiramate. Sleep Med 4(3):243–246.

Wirth, A. and Krause, J. (2001). Long-term weight loss with sibutramine: a randomized controlled trial. JAMA 286(11):1331–1339.

Wolk, A., et al. (1999). Long-term intake of dietary fiber and decreased risk of coronary heart disease among women. JAMA 281(21):1998–2004.

Wynne, K., et al. (2005). Subcutaneous oxyntomodulin reduces body weight in overweight and obese subjects: a double-blind, randomized, controlled trial. Diabetes 54(8):2390–2395.

Yanovski, S. Z. and Yanovski, J. A. (2002). Obesity. N Engl J Med 346(8):591–602.

Zahorska-Markiewicz, B., et al. (2001). Neuropeptide Y in obese women during treatment with adrenergic modulation drugs. Med Sci Monit 7(3):403–408.

Zemel, M. B., et al. (2000). Regulation of adiposity by dietary calcium. FASEB J 14(9):1132–1138.

Zemel, M. B., et al. (2004). Calcium and dairy acceleration of weight and fat loss during energy restriction in obese adults. Obes Res 12(4):582–590.

Zemel, M. B., et al. (2005a). Dairy augmentation of total and central fat loss in obese subjects. Int J Obes (Lond) 29(4):391–397.

Zemel, M. B., et al. (2005b). Effects of calcium and dairy on body composition and weight loss in African-American adults. Obes Res 13(7):1218–1225.

Zhi, J., et al. (1999). Long-term systemic exposure of orlistat, a lipase inhibitor, and its metabolites in obese patients. J Clin Pharmacol 39(1):41–46.

10   Should We Treat the Metabolic Syndrome or Its Components?

KEY POINTS

- Weight reduction reduces the prevalence of all components of the metabolic syndrome.
- If weight loss fails to lower blood pressure to satisfactory levels, then anti-hypertensive drugs should be used.
- If weight loss fails to improve blood lipids sufficiently, then medication and diet aimed at these abnormalities should be considered.
- If blood glucose is impaired, weight loss or metformin can both reduce the risk of developing diabetes.

INTRODUCTION

The metabolic syndrome is a collection of physical signs and laboratory measurements that often cluster together with central adiposity and insulin resistance. The more of these diagnostic features that are present, the higher the predictive power for development of future diabetes or cardiovascular disease. The observation that an increasing number of risk factors increases the prediction of cardiovascular disease has been made many times (Stamler et al., 1986; Wilson et al., 1987; Wilson et al., 2005; Yusuf et al., 2005). The value of this syndrome in predicting either heart disease or diabetes depends on which factors are present. When impaired fasting glucose (IFG) is present, the risk of diabetes is significantly increased. This should not be surprising because IFG has long been known to be a predictor of diabetes. Similarly, when hypertension or atherogenic dyslipidemia (i.e., low high-density lipoprotein [HDL]-cholesterol or high triglycerides), is present, the prediction of cardiovascular disease is significantly increased. Because diagnosis of the metabolic syndrome using the criteria proposed by either the National

From: *The Metabolic Syndrome and Obesity*
By: G. A. Bray © Humana Press Inc., Totowa, NJ

Table 1
**Diagnostic Criteria for the Metabolic Syndrome According
to the WHO, ATP III, and the IDF**

	WHO	*ATP-III-revised*	*IDF*
Definition	Diabetes, or impaired fasting glucose, or impaired glucose tolerance, or insulin resistance (assessed by euglycemic clamp) plus two or more of the following:	Three or more of the following:	Central adiposity (criteria below are for Europid men and women; other waist criteria needed in other populations)
Adiposity level	Waist-to-hip ratio	Waist circumference	Waist circumference
Female	>0.85	>88 cm	>80 cm
Male	>0.90	>102 cm	>90 cm in europid female and male
	BMI > 30 kg/m^2		
Fasting glucose		≥100 mg/dL^a	≥100 mg/dL or diagnosed diabetes
Microalbuminuria	≥20 ug/min or albumin/creatinine ratio 30 mg/g		
Triglycerides	≥150 mg/dL	≥150 mg/dL	≥150 mg/dL or treatment for this lipid abnormality
HDL-cholesterol			
Female	<39 mg/dL	<50 mg/dL	<50 mg/dL
Male	<35 mg/dL	<40 mg/dL	<40 mg/dL
Blood pressure	≥140/90 mmHg	≥135/85 mg/dL	≥135/85 mmHg or treatment for this abnormality

[a]Revised ATP-III criteria lowered this from 110 mg/dL to 100 mg/dL.
WHO, World Health Organization; ATP, Adult Treatment Panel; IDF, International Diabetes Federation.

Cholesterol Education Program Adult Treatment Panel (ATP) III or the International Diabetes Federation are clinically feasible, the evaluation was useful in alerting the physician to potential cardiovascular disease or diabetes. A recent detailed critique of the metabolic syndrome concludes that the compilation of factors is not better than the individual components. However, the constellation remains clinically useful, despite a publication to the contrary (Kahn et al., 2005). A comparison of the criteria for the metabolic syndrome is provided again in Table 1. The National Cholesterol Education Program ATP III have recently been modified by lowering the fasting glucose level of 100 mg/dL (5.6 mmol/L).

The next question that naturally arises is: how do we treat the metabolic syndrome? It is clear from the earlier discussion in Chapters 6 to 9 that weight loss alone will improve all components of the metabolic syndrome. Alternatively, we could treat individual components of this syndrome, because the treatment options are often better for each component than the syndrome as a whole. This chapter reviews treatments for the individual components of the metabolic syndrome.

TREATMENT OF CENTRAL ADIPOSITY AND VISCERAL FAT

Diet

The effects of weight loss on visceral fat are proportionately greater than on total fat (Smith and Zachwieja, 1999). In the Diabetes Prevention Program (DPP), a multi-center study of weight loss on the development of diabetes in individuals with impaired glucose tolerance (IGT; Fujimoto, 2000), 745 participants had a computed tomography (CT) scan at baseline and 1 year. Weight loss for men in the lifestyle intervention group was -8.5 ± 0.8 kg (m $\pm$ SD); for women, it was -7.0 ± 7.1 (m $\pm$ SD). The visceral adipose tissue (VAT) at the L4–L5 cross-sectional area decreased by 48 cm^2 or 26% after a weight loss of 7% of body weight. Subcutaneous adipose decreased by 58 cm^2 or 17%, which was significantly less than the VAT. Thus, relatively, the VAT was more responsive to weight loss than the subcutaneous fat.

There is now abundant evidence that weight loss is associated with a decrease in visceral fat, and that a decrease in visceral fat will improve most of the features of the metabolic syndrome (Knowler et al., 2002; Tuomilehto et al., 2001). Convincing evidence for this proposition is found in the DPP (Orchard et al., 2005). A total of 1711 of the 3234 participants (53%) had the metabolic syndrome at randomization (Table 2). This is comparable with the data for this age group provided by the National Center for Health Statistics (Ford and Giles, 2003). The prevalence did not vary by gender or age groups (<45; 45–60; >60). However, ethnicity did affect the prevalence, which was lowest in Asians (41%) and highest in whites (57%). Among African Americans, triglycerides were elevated in only 20.6%, compared with 47 to 53% for the Caucasian, Hispanic, Asian, and Native Americans. Among Native Americans, the prevalence of hypertension and IFG was lower than in the other groups. Approximately half of those with IGT had the metabolic syndrome with little difference by age, but differences by component. Treatment reversed the metabolic syndrome in the DPP. Lifestyle and metformin both reduced the incidence of new cases of the metabolic syndrome, but lifestyle was more effective than metformin in this regard. After 3.2 years, the prevalence of the metabolic syndrome was 61% in the placebo group, a 6% increase from baseline. In the lifestyle group, 42% still had the metabolic syndrome, a 9% decline from baseline. In addition, 38% had reversed the metabolic syndrome (Table 3).

Loss of body weight and subcutaneous fat, without a corresponding loss of visceral fat does not improve the cardiovascular risk factors. This was shown clearly in a study of liposuction. The effect of removing of subcutaneous fat by liposuction on the cardiovascular risk factors was measured in a group of 15 women, 7 of whom had diabetes (Klein et al., 2004) (Chapter 11). Three months following liposuction body weight had decreased −6.3 kg and body fat (determined by dual energy X-ray absorptiometry) had decreased by −9.1 kg with 6.3% of total body fat being removed. From the CT scan, this reduction was almost entirely the subcutaneous fat with little change in visceral fat. When the components of the metabolic syndrome (glucose, insulin, HDL-cholesterol, triglycerides, and blood pressure [BP]) were measured at baseline and follow-up, there was no significant change in any of these variables, in spite of a significant decrease in subcutaneous body fat. This study implies that it is the reduction in visceral fat that is important for improvement in the cardiovascular risk factors.

Table 2
Prevalence (n [%]) of the Metabolic Syndrome (NCEP ATP III Criteria)
and Its Components by Age and Gender in the Diabetes Prevention Program

| | Total | Age (years) | | | Gender | |
		<45	45–59	60+	Men	Women
Number of participants	3234	1000	1586	648	1043	2191
Metabolic syndrome	1711 (53%)	521 (52%)	868 (55%)	322 (50%)	550 (53%)	1161 (53%)
Waist circumference[a,b]	2532 (78%)	818 (82%)	1240 (78%)	474 (73%)	656 (63%)	1876 (86%)
Low HDL-cholesterol[a,b]	1838 (57%)	698 (70%)	883 (56%)	257 (40%)	529 (51%)	1309 (60%)
High triglycerides or Rx[b]	1472 (46%)	423 (42%)	764 (48%)	285 (44%)	522 (50%)	950 (43%)
High FPG[a,b]	1060 (33%)	307 (31%)	526 (33%)	227 (35%)	435 (42%)	625 (28%)
High blood pressure[a]	1460 (45%)	310 (31%)	740 (47%)	410 (63%)	569 (55%)	891 (41%)

NCEP ATP, National Cholesterol Education Program Adult Treatment Panel; HDL, high-density lipoprotein; FPG, Fasting plasma glucose.
[a]$p < 0.05$ comparing across all age groups.
[b]p across all gender groups.

Table 3
Development and Reversal of the Metabolic Syndrome in the DPP

Overall prevalence at 3.2 years		
Placebo	61%	+6% from baseline
Metformin	55%	+2% from baseline
Lifestyle	42%	−9% from baseline
Reversal at 3.2 years		
Placebo	18%	
Metformin	23%	
Lifestyle	38%	

Source: Orchard et al., 2005.

Omentectomy produces the opposite effect (Chapter 11). This procedure directly removes intra-abdominal fat by surgical means. In a randomized controlled trial of this procedure in 50 overweight subjects, omentectomy with a lap-band was compared with a lap-band alone (Thorne et al., 2002). Of the original 50 patients, 37 were re-evaluated 2 years after the surgery. The reduction in body weight was 27 kg in the lap-band group and 36 kg in the lap-band plus omentectomy group ($p = 0.07$). Both glucose and insulin improved more in the subjects with omentectomy than in those without it. This study complements the one by Klein et al. (2004) described earlier by showing that removal of extra visceral fat can have a small but significant effect, while decreasing subcutaneous fat alone has little impact.

Twins with Negative Energy Balance by Exercise

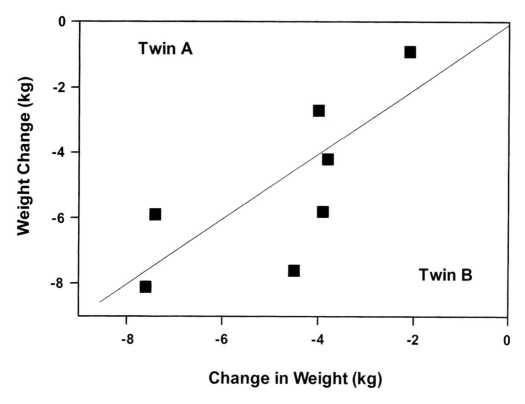

Fig. 1. Weight loss induced by increasing physical activity in 7 pairs of identical twins. (Adapted from Bouchard et al., 1994.)

The effectiveness of weight-loss programs for overweight patients with the metabolic syndrome is often deemed inadequate. The question thus arises as to whether it is better to treat the metabolic syndrome as a whole by trying to induce and maintain significant loss of weight and visceral fat, or whether it is better to treat the components of the syndrome separately. We will evaluate the effects of treatment for the various components of the ATP III metabolic syndrome as defined by these criteria.

Exercise

Exercise decreases VAT and there is a genetic component to the response. A group of 12 overweight identical male twins were recruited to lose body weight and fat by exercise (Fig. 1). Five pairs discontinued the study before it was completed. Among the other seven pairs who completed the study, there was a correlation of $r = 0.84$ in the decrease in visceral between the two pairs of twins. The decrease in visceral fat within pairs of twins was more closely related than between them, indicating that exercise decreases visceral fat, and that there is a significant genetic component to this effect (Bouchard et al., 1994).

Table 4
Effect of Diet and Exercise on Plasma Lipids During 1 Year
of Adherence to a Diet or Exercise Program

Change from baseline	Control	Diet	Exercise
Weight (kg)	+0.6	−9.3	−4.1
Triglyceride	+0.08	−0.27	−0.17
LDL-cholesterol	−0.21	−0.31	−0.25
HDL-cholesterol	−0.03	+0.24	+0.21

Source: Wood et al., 1989.
LDL, low-density lipoprotein; HDL, high-density lipoprotein.

Chapter 8 discussed the effectiveness of exercise programs on change in body weight. Data on effects of a long-term study of exercise on components of the metabolic syndrome is shown in Table 4. In this 1-year study, subjects were randomized to a control, diet, or exercise group. There was very little effect over one year on body weight (+0.6kg) or lipids in the control group. The diet group lost a little more than twice as much weight as the exercise group (−9.3 kg versus −4.1 kg) and there were correspondingly greater decreases in low-density lipoprotein (LDL)-cholesterol and triglycerides, and an increase in HDL cholesterol. Thus, either a vigorous exercise program with weight loss or a diet-induced weight loss can significantly improve the metabolic syndrome.

Growth Hormone, Cortisol, and Androgens

GROWTH HORMONE

Several hormones directly affect visceral fat. They include growth hormone (GH), cortisol, testosterone and dehydroepiandrosterone (DHEA). Chronic treatment with GH reduces the visceral fat compartment more than the subcutaneous one (Franco et al., 2005; Hoffman et al., 2004; Nam et al., 2001). In a 1-year study, body weight decreased −1.2 kg in the GH-treated group compared and −0.9 kg in the placebo-treated group (Franco et al., 2005). This was accompanied by a decrease of −1.5 kg of body fat in the GH-treated subjects compared with −1.0 kg in the placebo group. Subcutanoeus adipose tissue (SAT) increased 1.8 cm^2 and VAT decreased −6.6 cm^2 in the GH-treated group compared with a decrease of −0.4 cm^2 in SAT and an increase of 11 cm^2 in the VAT compartment in the placebo group. This differential effect on VAT and SAT suggests that these two compartments have different hormonal controls for maintaining their mass.

Conversely, treatment of acromegaly will increase visceral and subcutaneous fat. Acromegaly results from a pituitary tumor that secretes excessive quantities of GH. Among other things, this GH reduces subcutaneous and visceral fat. When acromegaly is effectively treated, the effects of excess GH are reversed. This leads to accumulation of both subcutaneous and visceral fat, with a greater proportional increase in the visceral compartment.

CORTISOL

Cortisol also affects visceral fat. Following treatment of Cushing's disease, a disease that results from excess secretion of cortisol from the adrenal gland, VAT decreased by 37% and SAT by 33% (Lonn et al., 1994).

Testosterone Cream

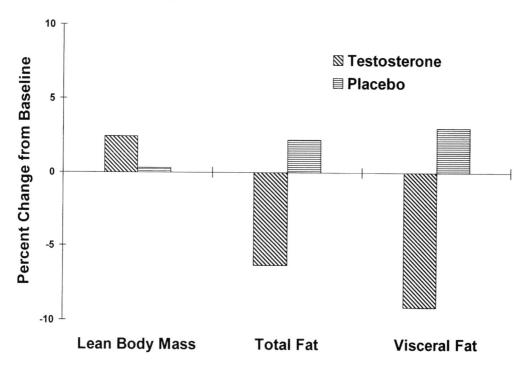

Fig. 2. Effect of testerone by subcutaneous patch on visaral fat and total body fat. (Adapted from Marin et al., 1993.)

In experimental animals, manipulation of the genes that metabolize cortisol has significant effects on VAT. This evidence suggests that increasing visceral fat may reflect altered metabolism of cortisol by visceral fat cells. When 11-β-hydroxysteroid dehydrogenase type 1 is overexpressed in the visceral fat of mice, the rate of conversion from the inactive steroid cortisone to the active cortisol form is increased (Masuzaki et al., 2001), and this is accompanied by an increase in VAT in these animals. Overactivity of the enzyme that produces cortisol has been suggested as a cause of centrally deposited fat in human beings.

TESTOSTERONE AND ANABOLIC STEROIDS

Testosterone, anabolic steroids, and dehydroandrosterone all affect visceral fat as much or more than subcutaneous fat. In a study of older men with low levels of testosterone, Marin et al. (1993) applied testosterone, dihydrotesterone, or placebo cream to the arms of overweight men for 9 months and measured their visceral fat by CT before and after treatment (Fig. 2). The placebo- and dihydrotestosterone-treated groups showed no change in body weight and a small increase in visceral and subcutaneous fat. In contrast, visceral fat was significantly reduced in the testosterone-treated group by –9.3% and subcutaneous fat by –6.1%. The men treated with testosterone also showed an improvement in insulin sensitivity using the glucose-clamp technique (Marin et al., 1993).

A second study using anabolic steroids in a weight-loss study reached similar conclusions (Lovejoy et al., 1995).

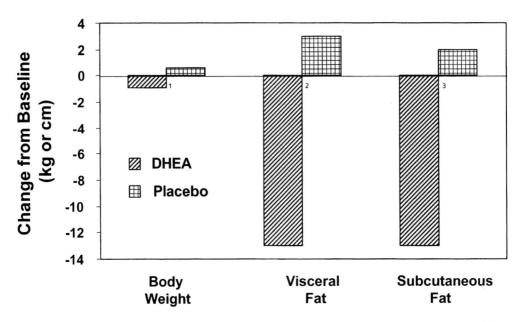

Fig. 3. Effect of DHEA and body weight and visceral fat in elderly men and women. (Adapted from Villareal and Holloszy, 2004.)

DEHYDROEPIANDROSTERONE

Dehydroepiandrosterone (DHEA) also reduces visceral fat. In a study with DHEA, 56 elderly men and women aged 65 to 78 years were randomly assigned to either placebo or 50 mg/day of DHEA for 6 months. Compliance with the intervention was 97%. After 6 months of treatment, body weight declined by −0.9 kg in the DHEA-treated group compared with a small gain of 0.6 kg in the placebo-treated group (Fig. 3). Visceral fat decreased by −13 cm^2 in the DHEA-treated group corresponding to 10.2% reduction for women and 7.4% for men, compared with a small gain of +0.3 cm^2 ($p < 0.001$) in the placebo-treated group. There were similar changes in subcutaneous fat (−13 cm^2 in the DHEA group and +2 cm^2 in the placebo group, $p < 0.003$). The insulin response after an oral glucose tolerance test was improved in the DHEA-treated group and glucose response was unchanged, indicating improved insulin sensitivity after treatment with DHEA (Villareal and Holloszy, 2004).Thus, DHEA can have significant effects on visceral fat.

Smoking

Smokers have a higher amount of visceral fat than nonsmokers (Shimokata et al., 1989). Using the waist to hip ratio, Shimokata et al. (1989) found that as smoking increased the visceral fat increased, and that in former smokers the waist to hip ratio had returned to nearly normal levels.

Table 5
Diagnosis of Diabetes: Plasma Glucose Cutoff Points

Category	FPG		2-Hour on OGTT	
	mg/dL	*mmol/L*	*mg/dL*	*mmol/L*
Normal	<100	<5.5	<140	<7.8
Impaired fasting glucose	100 to 126	5.5 to 6.9	—	—
Impaired glucose tolerance	—	—	140 to <200	7.8 to <11.1
Diabetes	≥126	≥7.0	≥200	≥11.1

Data from the expert committee on the diagnosis and classification of diabetes mellitus. (1997) Diabetes Care 20:1183–1197.

Medication

Several clinical trials with weight-loss medications also show a reversal of the metabolic syndrome (Chapter 9). The prevalence of the metabolic syndrome was about 50% in the subjects in several clinical trials with rimonabant. In the placebo groups, the metabolic syndrome was still present in 53% of the subjects after 1 year of treatment in the Rimonabant in Obesity (RIO)-Europe study (Van Gaal et al., 2005), 51% of those in the RIO-Lipids study (Despres et al., 2005), and 38% of those in the RIO-North America study (Pi-Sunyer et al., 2006). Substantial decreases occurred in the rimonabant treatment groups. For the RIO-Europe and RIO-Lipids groups only 21% still had the metabolic syndrome, a 60% decrease. For the RIO-North America group, it was 7.9%, a decrease of almost 60% (Despres et al., 2005; Pi-Sunyer et al., 2006; Van Gaal et al., 2005).

TREATMENT OF IMPAIRED FASTING GLUCOSE AND IMPAIRED GLUCOSE TOLERANCE

Diet and Exercise

IFG can be defined from the ATP III criteria for the metabolic syndrome (Table 1). A glucose tolerance test is used in the diagnosis of IGT. The current values for fasting glucose and 2-hour glucose after a 75 g oral glucose load that are diagnostic for IFG, IGT, and diabetes are shown in Table 5.

It is clear that weight loss and exercise will delay the onset of diabetes in individuals with IGT (Knowler et al., 2002; Tuomilehto et al., 2001). The largest and most clear-cut study to reach this conclusion is the DPP. This is a multicenter trial that recruited nearly 4000 individuals with IGT from a broad range of ethnic groups in the United States. Participants were randomized to one of four treatment arms: placebo, metformin, intensive lifestyle, or troglitazone. The troglitazone arm was discontinued after the first year of the trial due to withdrawal of the drug by the Food and Drug Administration. After the trial had been underway for 2.8 years, the double-blind part of the trial was terminated because the beneficial effects of the intensive lifestyle program were significantly better than the other two. During this interval, the conversion to diabetes was reduced by 58% in those assigned to the intensive lifestyle group (Knowler et al., 2002). The significant components of this trial were the diet and its reduction in dietary fat and implementation of an exercise program (Wing et al., 2004; *see* Fig. 2 in Chapter 7).

Medications

METFORMIN

Metformin is also successful in treating IGT. In the DPP, individuals randomly assigned to metformin lost a small amount of weight—about 2.5%, most of which was maintained for the duration of treatment—and reduced the risk of developing diabetes by 31% (Knowler et al., 2002). This was significantly greater than in the subjects receiving placebo. In the individuals receiving metformin, weight loss was the major factor associated with their reduced conversion rate to diabetes (*see* Figure 15 in Chapter 9).

GLITAZONES

Thiazolidinediones (pioglitazone and rosiglitazone) are activators of the peroxisome proliferator-activated receptor (PPAR)-γ. They significantly improve insulin sensitivity and produce weight gain (Smith et al., 2005). The increase in body weight is almost entirely fat, and the increase in fat is almost entirely in the subcutaneous compartment with no significant change to the visceral fat compartment. Some of the clinical studies show that the degree of improvement in hemoglobin A1c is related to the degree of weight gain. In the DPP (Knowler et al., 2002), 544 participants were randomized to receive troglitazone, a PPAR-γ activator. During the average of 9 months of treatment with this drug, the conversion to diabetes was reduced by 75% compared with placebo. The effect was significantly greater than metformin, but not different from lifestyle. Clinical trials to test the effect of the newer glitazones as potential agents to slow the development of diabetes in high risk subjects are currently underway.

TREATMENT OF ATHEROGENIC DYSLIPIDEMIA (LOW HDL-CHOLESTEROL AND HIGH TRIGLYCERIDES)

Diet and Exercise

As with the other components of the metabolic syndrome, dyslipidemia is responsive to both diet and exercise. The effect of diet can be seen in the responses from the lifestyle arm of the DPP. This group lost an average of 7% of their body weight during the first 6 months of the trial and maintained it for the next 6 months. Triglyceride levels fell significantly more in the intensive lifestyle group than in the other groups as anticipated from the greater weight loss (−25.4 mg/dL versus. −7.4 mg/dL in the lifestyle and placebo groups, respectively; $p = 0.001$). The intensive lifestyle group also demonstrated a greater increase in HDL-cholesterol than the placebo group (+1.0 mg/dL versus. −0.1 mg/dL, respectively; $p = 0.002$). Furthermore, intensive lifestyle favorably altered the LDL phenotype, with a reduction in the incidence of phenotype B, representing a smaller, denser, more atherogenic LDL particle.

The effect of exercise and diet is shown further in a year-long study. Wood et al. (1988) reported a decrease of −9.3 kg in body weight in the group receiving the dietary prescription and a decrease of −4.1 kg in body weight of the group participating in the exercise intervention (*see* Table 4).

Table 6
LDL-Cholesterol Goals and Thresholds

Risk category	LDL-cholesterol goal (mg/dL)	Initiate therapeutic lifestyle changes (mg/dL)	Consider drug Rx
CHD or risk equivalent (10-year risk>20%)	<100	≥100	≥130 (100–129 optional)
2 or more risk factors (10-year risk≤20%)	<130	≥130	≥130(10-year risk 10–20%,≥130; 10-year risk<10%, ≥160)
0 to 1 risk factor	<160	≥160	≥190(160–189 drug Rx optional)

In both cases, there was a decrease in LDL-cholesterol and triglycerides and an increase in HDL-cholesterol. These effects occurred in both men and women. In a meta-analysis of changes in lipids with diet and exercise, Dattillo et al. (1992) found that for each decrease of 1 kg in body weight there was a decrease of –0.75 mg/dL in total cholesterol and 0.6 mg/dL in triglycerides, and a change in HDL-cholesterol that depended on whether body weight was stable or body weight was still declining. If it was stable, HDL-cholesterol increased +0.35 mg/dL, but if weight loss was still occurring HDL-cholesterol was –0.25 mg/dL lower.

Use of natural products is another dietary approach to reducing cholesterol. Plant stanols have been incorporated into spreads for bread that can be used in place of margarine. These stanols have a small but significant effect in lowering plasma cholesterol by competing with absorption of cholesterol from the gastrointestinal track.

Medication

STATIN DRUGS

Elevated serum cholesterol, especially in LDL-cholesterol, is considered one of the major cardiovascular risk factors. The goals and thresholds for treatment of dyslipidemia are shown in Table 6. The criteria tend to be even more stringent for individuals with diabetes, because it is considered a cardiovascular risk, equivalent to having a prior heart attack. When cholesterol is high, both therapeutic lifestyle changes and medications are to be considered and this table describes the criteria based on laboratory tests and clinical information.

There are now a number of statin drugs that act by inhibiting the rate-limiting step in the biosynthesis of cholesterol. In clinical trials with statins, the reduction in cholesterol varies (Collins et al., 2003). In the Heart Protection Study, the overall risk reduction was 25%, and this was sufficient to reduce significantly the risk of heart attack. The statin drugs also reduce C-reactive protein, a marker for inflammation. In the Scandinavian Simvastatin Study, called the 4S study, patients with high LDL who had already had a myocardial infarction had a placebo event rate of 21% (Ballantyne et al., 2001; Pyorala et al., 1997). This event rate was reduced to 14% with simvastatin. In patients with the metabolic syndrome, the incidence of new infarctions

Options of Statin Therapy Does Not Reach its Goal

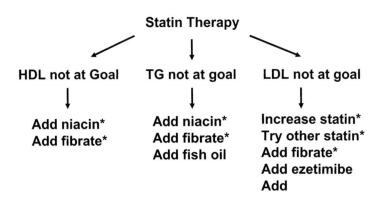

Fig. 4. Algorithm for selecting combination treatment.*Increased risk of myopathy. (Adapted from Grundy et al., 2004.)

was 36% and was even higher at 51% in people with diabetes. Treatment with simvastatin reduced the event rate by more than 50% in these groups. There are a number of different statin drugs on the market and the details of the differences are beyond the limits of this discussion. The reduction of cholesterol may not be adequate with the statin alone. Figure 4 provides an algorithm to select additional or alternative therapies.

FIBRATES

The fibrates gemfibrozil and fenofibrate act primarily to reduce triglycerides. They appear to activate PPAR-α in liver, which enhances the metabolism of triglycerides. Because elevation of triglycerides is a key feature of the metabolic syndrome, these agents may be important choices. Reductions of triglyceride by as much 25 to 30% are common and reductions of up to 50% have been seen. Gemfibrozil is lower in cost and there was a demonstration that cardiovascular events were reduced in two clinical studies (Manninen et al., 1988; Rubins et al., 1999).

NIACIN

Niacin or nicotinic acid produces significant improvements in almost all aspects of the lipid profile. It can lower LDL-cholesterol by 15%, triglycerides by 25 to 30%, and C-reactive protein by 15 to 25% as well as increase HDL-cholesterol by 25 to 30%. Why then is it not more widely used? One concern is that is may worsen glycemic control. However, recent clinical trials have shown this is not the case (Grundy et al., 2002). It also tends to be underutilized in some minds because it can produce flushing. This can be mitigated with aspirin and by increasing the niacin dose slowly.

EZETIMIBE

Ezetimibe reduces intestinal absorption of cholesterol by up to 50% and can reduce plasma LDL-cholesterol by 15 to 20%. It may also slightly raise the level of HDL-cholesterol and lower triglycerides and C-reactive protein (Ballantyne et al., 2003; Sager et al., 2003). It can also be used in combination with other lipid-lowering drugs.

Table 7
Blood Pressure Categories From Joint National Commission VII

Normal	<120/80
Prehypertension	120–139/80–89
Hypertension	>140/90
Stage 1	140–159/90–99
Stage 2	>160/100

TREATMENT OF HYPERTENSION

Diet and Exercise

Increased BP is a common component of the metabolic syndrome. Shown in Table 7 are the criteria for BP of the Joint National Commission VII. For the metabolic syndrome, a BP higher than 135/85 mmHg is used as the criteria. For people with diabetes, the goal is even lower at 130/80 mmHg. In the participants in the DPP, 53% had the metabolic syndrome (Table 2). In this group, hypertension was present in 45%.

Diet and exercise are effective in lowering BP. Even without weight loss, a diet rich in fruits and vegetables produced a significant reduction in BP. When this dietary pattern was modified by adding low-fat dairy products—the dietary approaches to stop hypertension (DASH) diet—the reduction in BP was even more substantial. The DASH diet also lowered BP at both normal and elevated levels of dietary sodium intake (Appel et al., 1997; Bray et al., 2004; Sacks et al., 2001). Because of these important effects on BP, the DASH diet has been included in the 2005 Dietary Guidelines (*see* Chapter 6).

In the Trials of Hypertension Prevention II, Stevens et al. (2001) reported a graded reduction in both systolic and diastolic BP with increasing weight loss. For a weight loss of more than −9.5 kg, the change in systolic and diastolic BP was −9.4/−8.4 mmHg. With a weight loss between −4.5 and −9.5 kg the BP declined −6.4/−6.4 mmHg, whereas a loss of −1.0 to 2.0 kg was associated with only a small change in BP of −4.4/−2.5 mmHg after 18 months of treatment with a behavioral weight-loss program. In a further follow-up, they reported that the participants in the weight-loss program who maintained their weight loss maintained a significantly lower BP as compared with individuals who regained their body weight. In the Swedish Obese Subjects study, Sjostrom et al. (1997) reported a nearly linear change in both systolic and diastolic BP with change in body weight.

Exercise is also effective in reducing BP (*see* Chapter 8), but the effect of diet is larger. In a study in hypertensive patients, Dengel et al. (1998) showed that aerobic exercise and diet improved BP in sedentary subjects who had hypertension but not diabetes.

Medications

Treatment of BP with medications is common. There are a number of drugs that are effective in reducing BP, including β-blocking drugs, thiazides, calcium channel blockers, α-blocking drugs, angiotensin-converting enzyme inhibitors (ACEIs), and angiotensin receptor antagonists. Monotherapy with any one of these drugs will produce a modest reduction in BP of −11/−5 to −6/−5 mmHg. This is comparable to the effect of the

DASH diet described earlier. Combinations of these antagonists and the DASH diet would appear to be an effective way to complement drug therapy with a demonstrably effective diet. Reviewing the effect of each of these individual anti-hypertensive agents is beyond the scope of this chapter.

ACEIS AND ANGIOTENSIN RECEPTOR BLOCKERS

ACEIs and angiotensin receptor blockers are probably the first choice for treating hypertension. In people with diabetes, they will reduce albuminuria. One of the ACEIs, ramipril, reduced risk of death from myocardial infarction, stroke, and cardiovascular death, as well as slowed the progression to type 2 diabetes in high-risk patients in the Heart Outcomes Prevention Evaluation (HOPE) study (Yusuf et al., 2000). Lisinopril, another ACEI, prevented diabetes more effectively than chlorthalidone or amlodipine, two other anti-hypertensive drugs, in the Anti-Hypertensive and Lipid Lowering Treatment to Prevent Heart Attack Trial, which was conducted in an older hypertensive population (ALLHAT, 2002). An angiotensin receptor blocker, losartan, slowed the onset of diabetes in the Losartan Intervention For Endpoint (LIFE) Reduction trial (Lindholm et al., 2002).

OTHER DRUGS

There are a number of other drugs, including β-blockers, thiazides, α-adrenergic antagonists and calcium channel blockers that can be used to control BP. Detailed discussion of these drugs is beyond the scope of this chapter.

REFERENCES

ALLHAT Officers and Coordinators for the ALLHAT Collaborative Research Group. The Antihypertensive and Lipid-Lowering Treatment to Prevent Heart Attack Trial. (2002). Major outcomes in high-risk hypertensive patients randomized to angiotensin-converting enzyme inhibitor or calcium channel blocker vs diuretic: The Antihypertensive and Lipid-Lowering Treatment to Prevent Heart Attack Trial (ALLHAT). JAMA 288(23):2981–2997.

Appel, L. J., et al. (1997). A clinical trial of the effects of dietary patterns on blood pressure. DASH Collaborative Research Group. N Engl J Med 336(16):1117–1124.

Ballantyne, C. M., et al. (2001). Influence of low high-density lipoprotein cholesterol and elevated triglyceride on coronary heart disease events and response to simvastatin therapy in 4S. Circulation 104(25):3046–3051.

Ballantyne, C. M., et al. (2003). Effect of ezetimibe coadministered with atorvastatin in 628 patients with primary hypercholesterolemia: a prospective, randomized, double-blind trial. Circulation 107(19): 2409–2415.

Bouchard, C., et al. (1994). The response to exercise with constant energy intake in identical twins. Obes Res 2(5):400–410.

Bray, G. A., et al. (2004). A further subgroup analysis of the effects of the DASH diet and three dietary sodium levels on blood pressure: results of the DASH-Sodium Trial. Am J Cardiol 94(2): 222–227.

Collins, R., et al. (2003). MRC/BHF Heart Protection Study of cholesterol-lowering with simvastatin in 5963 people with diabetes: a randomised placebo-controlled trial. Lancet 361(9374):2005–2016.

Dattilo, A. M. and Kris-Etherton, P. M. (1992). Effects of weight reduction on blood lipids and lipoproteins: a meta-analysis. Am J Clin Nutr 56(2):320–328.

Dengel, D. R., et al. (1998). Improvements in blood pressure, glucose metabolism, and lipoprotein lipids after aerobic exercise plus weight loss in obese, hypertensive middle-aged men. Metabolism 47(9):1075–1082.

Despres, J. P., et al. (2005). Effects of rimonabant on metabolic risk factors in overweight patients with dyslipidemia. N Engl J Med 353(20):2121–2134.

Ford, E. S. and Giles, W. H. (2003). A comparison of the prevalence of the metabolic syndrome using two proposed definitions. Diabetes Care 26(3):575–581.

Franco, C., et al. (2005). Growth hormone treatment reduces abdominal visceral fat in postmenopausal women with abdominal obesity: a 12-month placebo-controlled trial. J Clin Endocrinol Metab 90(3):1466–1474.

Fujimoto, W. Y. (2000). Background and recruitment data for the U.S. Diabetes Prevention Program. Diabetes Care 23 Suppl 2:B11–B13.

Grundy, S. M., et al. (2002). Efficacy, safety, and tolerability of once-daily niacin for the treatment of dyslipidemia associated with type 2 diabetes: results of the assessment of diabetes control and evaluation of the efficacy of niaspan trial. Arch Intern Med 162(14):1568–1576.

Grundy, S. M., et al. (2004) Implications of recent clinical trials for the National Cholesterol Education Program Adult Treatment Panel III guidelines. Circulation 110:227–239.

Hoffman, A. R., et al. (2004). Growth hormone (GH) replacement therapy in adult-onset gh deficiency: effects on body composition in men and women in a double-blind, randomized, placebo-controlled trial. J Clin Endocrinol Metab 89(5):2048–2056.

Kahn, R., et al. (2005). The metabolic syndrome: time for a critical appraisal: joint statement from the American Diabetes Association and the European Association for the Study of Diabetes. Diabetes Care 28(9):2289–3204.

Klein, S., et al. (2004). Absence of an effect of liposuction on insulin action and risk factors for coronary heart disease. N Engl J Med 350(25):2549–2557.

Knowler, W. C., et al. (2002). Reduction in the incidence of type 2 diabetes with lifestyle intervention or metformin. N Engl J Med 346(6):393–403.

Lindholm, L. H., et al. (2002). Cardiovascular morbidity and mortality in patients with diabetes in the Losartan Intervention For Endpoint reduction in hypertension study (LIFE):a randomised trial against atenolol. Lancet 359(9311):1004–1010.

Lonn, L., et al. (1994). Changes in body composition and adipose tissue distribution after treatment of women with Cushing's syndrome. Metabolism 43(12):1517–1522.

Lovejoy, J. C., et al. (1995). Oral anabolic steroid treatment, but not parenteral androgen treatment, decreases abdominal fat in obese, older men. Int J Obes Relat Metab Disord 19(9):614–624.

Manninen, V., et al. (1988). Lipid alterations and decline in the incidence of coronary heart disease in the Helsinki Heart Study. JAMA 260(5):641–651.

Marin, P., et al. (1993). Androgen treatment of abdominally obese men. Obes Res 1(4):245–251.

Masuzaki, H., et al. (2001). A transgenic model of visceral obesity and the metabolic syndrome. Science 294(5549):2166–2170.

Nam, S. Y., et al. (2001). Low-dose growth hormone treatment combined with diet restriction decreases insulin resistance by reducing visceral fat and increasing muscle mass in obese type 2 diabetic patients. Int J Obes Relat Metab Disord 25(8):1101–1107.

Orchard, T. J., et al. (2005). The effect of metformin and intensive lifestyle intervention on the metabolic syndrome: the Diabetes Prevention Program randomized trial. Ann Intern Med 142(8):611–619.

Pi-Sunyer, F. X., et al. (2006). Effect of rimonabant, a cannabinoid-1 receptor blocker, on weight and cardiometabolic risk factors in overweight or obese patients: RIO-North America: a randomized controlled trial. JAMA 295(7):761–775.

Pyorala, K., et al. (1997). Cholesterol lowering with simvastatin improves prognosis of diabetic patients with coronary heart disease. A subgroup analysis of the Scandinavian Simvastatin Survival Study (4S). Diabetes Care 20(4):614–620.

Rubins, H. B., et al. (1999). Gemfibrozil for the secondary prevention of coronary heart disease in men with low levels of high-density lipoprotein cholesterol. Veterans Affairs High-Density Lipoprotein Cholesterol Intervention Trial Study Group. N Engl J Med 341(6):410–418.

Sacks, F. M., et al. (2001). Effects on blood pressure of reduced dietary sodium and the Dietary Approaches to Stop Hypertension (DASH) diet. DASH-Sodium Collaborative Research Group. N Engl J Med 344(1):3–10.

Sager, P. T., et al. (2003). Effect of coadministration of ezetimibe and simvastatin on high-sensitivity C-reactive protein. Am J Cardiol 92(12):1414–1418.

Shimokata, H., et al. (1989). Studies in the distribution of body fat. III. Effects of cigarette smoking. JAMA 261(8):1169–1173.

Sjostrom, C. D., et al. (1997). Relationships between changes in body composition and changes in cardiovascular risk factors: the SOS Intervention Study. Swedish Obese Subjects. Obes Res 5(6):519–530.

Smith, S. R. and Zachwieja, J. J. (1999). Visceral adipose tissue: a critical review of intervention strategies. Int J Obes Relat Metab Disord 23(4):329–335.

Smith, S. R., et al. (2005). Effect of pioglitazone on body composition and energy expenditure: a randomized controlled trial. Metabolism 54(1):24–32.

Stamler, J., et al. (1986). Is relationship between serum cholesterol and risk of premature death from coronary heart disease continuous and graded? Findings in 356,222 primary screenees of the Multiple Risk Factor Intervention Trial (MRFIT). JAMA 256(20):2823–2828.

Stevens, V. J., et al. (2001). Long-term weight loss and changes in blood pressure: results of the Trials of Hypertension Prevention, phase II. Ann Intern Med 134(1):1–11.

Thorne, A., et al. (2002). A pilot study of long-term effects of a novel obesity treatment: omentectomy in connection with adjustable gastric banding. Int J Obes Relat Metab Disord 26(2):193–199.

Torgerson, J. S., et al. (2004). XENical in the prevention of diabetes in obese subjects (XENDOS) study: a randomized study of orlistat as an adjunct to lifestyle changes for the prevention of type 2 diabetes in obese patients. Diabetes Care 27(1):155–161.

Tuomilehto, J., et al. (2001). Prevention of type 2 diabetes mellitus by changes in lifestyle among subjects with impaired glucose tolerance. N Engl J Med 344(18):1343–1350.

Van Gaal, L. F., et al. (2005). Effects of the cannabinoid-1 receptor blocker rimonabant on weight reduction and cardiovascular risk factors in overweight patients: 1-year experience from the RIO-Europe study. Lancet 365(9468):1389–1397.

Villareal, D. T. and Holloszy, J. O. (2004). Effect of DHEA on abdominal fat and insulin action in elderly women and men: a randomized controlled trial. JAMA 292(18):2243–2248.

Wilson, P. W., et al. (1987). Coronary risk prediction in adults (the Framingham Heart Study). Am J Cardiol 59(14):91G–94G.

Wilson, P. W., et al. (2005). C-reactive protein and risk of cardiovascular disease in men and women from the Framingham Heart Study. Arch Intern Med 165(21):2473–2478.

Wing, R. R., et al. (2004). Achieving weight and activity goals among diabetes prevention program lifestyle participants. Obes Res 12(9):1426–1434.

Wood, P. D., et al. (1988). Changes in plasma lipids and lipoproteins in overweight men during weight loss through dieting as compared with exercise. N Engl J Med 319(18):1173–1179.

Yusuf, S., et al. (2000). Effects of an angiotensin-converting-enzyme inhibitor, ramipril, on cardiovascular events in high-risk patients. The Heart Outcomes Prevention Evaluation Study Investigators. N Engl J Med 342(3):145–153.

Yusuf, S., et al. (2005). Obesity and the risk of myocardial infarction in 27,000 participants from 52 countries: a case–control study. Lancet 366(9497):1640–1649.

11 Surgical Treatment for the Overweight Patient

KEY POINTS

- The number of surgical procedures done for extreme degrees of overweight has increased exponentially.
- Gastric bypass is the most commonly performed procedure in the United States and has proven success in long-term weight loss.
- It is associated with reduced food intake and altered gastrointestinal hormones.
- Laparoscopic techniques have largely replaced open surgical procedures.
- As with all surgical procedures there are short- and longer-term risks, including death, re-operation, infection, and metabolic derangements.
- Quality of life improves and use of health services, following the initial high costs, is reduced.
- Laparoscopic bariatric surgery has fewer postoperative problems and a more rapid post-operative recovery.
- There is less pain, fewer infections and hernia complications, as well as quicker postoperative recovery.

From: *The Metabolic Syndrome and Obesity*
By: G. A. Bray © Humana Press Inc., Totowa, NJ

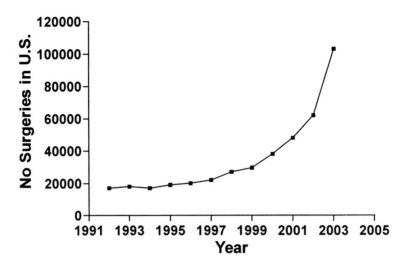

Fig. 1. Growth in number of bariatric operations.

INTRODUCTION

Although considered the "cornerstones" of treatment of overweight, the magnitude of the weight loss that can be achieved with behavioral, dietary, exercise, and pharmacological approaches is limited to about 10% of initial body weight. Moreover, when the treatment is "stopped" because the patient is dissatisfied with the failure to lose enough weight or the cost is more than they want to pay, weight is regained over several months to a level that is close to baseline—treatments only work when used. If your body mass index was 30 kg/m^2, a 10% weight loss would be to approximately 27 kg/m^2, which is still above the normal level of 25 kg/m^2. When overweight progresses to clinical overweight grade III, that is, a body mass index of higher than 40 kg/m^2, many patients seek surgical treatment in which much more weight loss is the usual rule. The use of surgical procedures to treat overweight patients is increasing at a rapid rate (Fig. 1). Using the Nationwide Inpatient Sample from 1998 to 2002 provided a quantitative estimate of bariatric surgical procedures. Between 1998 and 2002 the number of operations increased from 13,365 to 72,177, a more than fivefold increase. More than 80% of these were the so-called gastric bypass operations. Several other trends were noted in this paper: An increase from 81 to 84% women being operated on; privately insured patients rising from 75 to 83% of these patients; and patients aged 50 to 64 rising from 15 to 24% of these people. Length of hospitalization decreased from 4.5 to 3.3 days, and operative mortality ranged from 0.1 to 0.2%. Thus, consideration of this growing form of treatment is important both for the patient and for the physicians and other health professionals who will care for these patients.

Interest in bariatric surgery has grown considerably. On February 21, 2006, the Center for Medicare and Medicaid Services agreed to expand the coverage for bariatric surgery in the treatment of obesity. We can thus expect even more procedures to be done in the future. There are several sources of information that the reader can consult for additional details (Buchwald et al., 2004; Colquitt et al., 2005; Inge et al., 2004; Shekelle et al., 2004; Sjostrom, 2004).

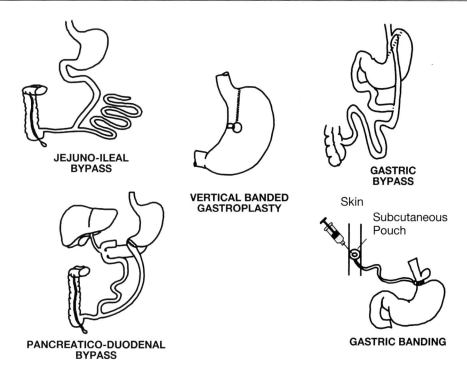

JEJUNO-ILEAL
BYPASS

VERTICAL BANDED
GASTROPLASTY

GASTRIC
BYPASS

Skin

Subcutaneous
Pouch

PANCREATICO-DUODENAL
BYPASS

GASTRIC BANDING

Fig. 2. Illustrations of operative procedures.

The operations used to treat obesity are generally referred to as "bariatric" procedures, a word derived from the Greek meaning "heavy." All of them involve some manipulation of the gastrointestinal (GI) track. Figure 2 shows some of the operations that are or have been used to treat the overweight patient.

DEVELOPMENT OF SURGICAL APPROACHES TO OBESITY

The earliest systematic use of surgery to treat obesity was published in 1963 by Payne et al. (1963). They separated the intestine at the mid-jejunum and connected the proximal end to the colon so that the content of the upper GI track was emptied into the colon. Weight loss with this procedure was rapid and subjects returned to nearly normal weight. However, there were serious problems with diarrhea and loss of potassium and other minerals. Believing that their patients had been "cured" of their obesity, the operations were reversed with rapid regain of the lost weight. The next approach was by the same group (DeWind and Payne, 1976) who pioneered a less drastic rearrangement of the GI track by coupling the jejunum to the distal segment of the ileum. These operations were very popular during the 1970s but fell into disuse as the number of complications continued to rise, and alternative gastric operations came into use.

Restrictive operations that reduce the volume of the stomach with various stapling procedures but leaving the flow of food from esophagus to duodenum appeared in 1979 (Pace et al., 1979) and 1980 (Gomez, 1979). They consisted of both transverse staple lines as well as vertical staple lines that in effect prolonged the esophagus in a procedure called the vertical-banded gastroplasty (VBG; Mason, 1982).

An alternative restrictive procedure consists of placing a plastic band around the stomach and, in some of the systems, providing a way to inflate it from a subcutaneous reservoir. The initial procedure was performed in 1976, but not published until 8 years later (Bo and Modalsli, 1983). This procedure is now widely used in Europe and has been approved by the Food and Drug Administration in the United States.

Three procedures have been developed that involve combinations of gastric and intestinal operations. The first of these is the gastric bypass originally developed by Mason and Ito (1967, 1969). In this procedure, a small gastric pouch is anastamosed to the distal limb of the jejunum, while the proximal limb is attached to the side of this loop a short way below the connection of the jejunum to the stomach. This is thus a restrictive and modest malabsorptive procedure. The next procedure is the biliopancreatic diversion, which was developed by Scopinaro and consists of two long intestinal segments, one draining contents from the stomach and the other the duodenal juices. They are connected near the ileo-cecal valve, thus reducing the length of intestine where food and intestinal juices are together and reducing absorption. The final procedure in this group is the distal gastric bypass, in which the jejunum replaces the duodenum in draining the lower stomach—the so-called biliopancreatic diversion with duodenal switch (Marceau et al., 1993).

All of these operations can now be done by laparoscopy, which has significantly reduced the operative morbidity and allowed more patients to have this procedures. These procedures were first undertaken by Fried and Peskova (1997) and Belachew et al. (1995). Gradually, these techniques spread.

INDICATIONS

The general outline for procedures for bariatric surgical procedures were outlined by a consensus conference at the National Institutes of Health Consensus Development Panel in 1991 and are summarized in Table 1 (N. A., 1991; N. A., 1992). Adult patients are eligible to be considered for these procedures if they have a BMI higher than 40 kg/m^2 or a higher than 35 kg/m^2 if they have serious co-morbidities such as sleep apnea, diabetes mellitus, or joint disease. For individuals less than 16 years of age, surgical and pediatric consultants should review each case separately (Inge et al., 2004), because operations that reduce caloric intake can slow weight gain when performed before an individual has achieved adult height. Similarly, bariatric surgery for individuals above 65 years of age should be considered on an individual basis, because the adaptation to the procedure may be more troublesome and difficult. Potential patients must have tried and failed nonsurgical weight-loss procedures. Patients and their significant others must understand the procedure and its complications and have acceptable surgical risks.

CONTRAINDICATIONS

Patients with major depression or psychosis should be carefully reviewed before being accepted. Binge-eating disorders, current drug and alcohol abuse, severe cardiac disease with prohibitive anesthetic risks, severe coagulopathy, or inability to comply with nutritional requirements, including life-long vitamin replacement. A large number of complications can occur in the postoperative period and it is thus desirable to have bariatric operations performed in a setting with comprehensive medical and nutritional

Table 1
Indications and Contraindications for Bariatric Surgery

Indications
BMI >40 kg/m^2 or BMI 35–39.9 kg/m^2 and life-threatening cardiopulmonary
 disease, severe diabetes, or lifestyle impairment.
Failure to achieve adequate weight loss with nonsurgical treatment.

Contraindications
History of noncompliance with medical care.
Certain psychiatric illnesses, such as personality disorder, uncontrolled depression,
 suicidal ideation, and substance abuse.
Unlikely to survive surgery.

support. To provide guidance in how to do this, The American Society of Bariatric
Surgeons developed guidelines for establishing Centers of Excellence for bariatric clinics
that are desirable to have in place (2003). In addition, a number of National Institutes
of Health-funded surgical centers have been established to advance the science and
care of patients needing bariatric surgery.

BARIATRIC SURGERY FOR PEDIATRIC PATIENTS

The rising prevalence of overweight among children and adolescence has seen an
increased interest in bariatric surgery for this age group (Inge et al., 2004). The principal
concern in this age group is the potential for reducing linear growth if a patient is operated
on before their adult height is reached. Criteria for adolescent patients are shown in
Table 2. The largest study in adolescents contained only 33 patients who underwent
several different procedures, thus providing little guidance (Sugerman et al., 2003).
The review of pediatrics suggests that the gastric bypass may be the most appropriate
procedure at the present time.

EFFECTIVENESS OF SURGICAL PROCEDURES

A number of studies compared bariatric procedures with each other and nonsurgical
techniques. Although no longer used, two randomized and two prospective non-
randomized trials have been published between 1977 and 1981 (Alden, 1977; Buckwalter,
1977; Griffen et al., 1977). The weight losses with the two procedures at 1 year were
similar, but the complications observed with the jejunoileal bypass over time were
more significant. In a comparison of the jejunoileal bypass against the horizontal gastroplasty, weight loss of 33% favored the jejunoileal bypass compared with the 16%
weight loss with the horizontal gastroplasty, but the side effects were less severe with
the gastroplasty (Deitel et al., 1982).

Jejunoileal bypass has also been compared with dietary treatment in the Danish Obesity
Project (N. A., 1979; Stokholm et al., 1982). There were 130 surgically treated patients
and 66 patients treated medically. After 2 years, the weight loss was 42.9 kg in the surgical
group and 5.9 kg in the diet group. The surgically operated patients had significant postoperative problems, but also had more improvement in blood pressure and quality of life.

The horizontal gastroplasty has been compared with the gastric bypass in several
studies (Sjostrom et al., 1999). In the largest of these studies, 204 patients weighing

Table 2
Criteria for Batriatric Surgery in Adolescents

Adolescents being considered for bariatric surgery should:
1. Have failed 6 months or more of organized attempts at weight management, as determined by their primary care provider.
2. Have attained or nearly attained physiological maturity.
3. Be very severely overweight (BMI ≥40 kg/m^2) with serious obesity-related comorbidities or have a BMI of higher than 50 kg/m^2 with less severe comorbidities.
4. Demonstrate commitment to comprehensive medical and psychological evaluations both before and after surgery.
5. Agree to avoid pregnancy for at least 1 year postoperatively.
6. Be capable of and willing to adhere to nutritional guidelines postoperatively.
7. Provide informed consent to surgical treatment.
8. Demonstrate decisional capacity.
9. Have a supportive family environmment.

112 kg were included and followed for 3 years. The weight loss at 3 years was 39 kg in the group treated by gastric bypass compared with 17 kg in the group receiving the gastroplasty (Hall et al., 1990). An additional problem with the horizontal gastroplasty operation is that more re-operations have been needed.

Horizontal gastroplasty has been compared with a very low-calorie diet (VLCD) in a 2-year study with follow-up for 5 years, but a dropout rate in excess of 50%. After 2 years, the weight loss was only 8.2 kg in the VLCD group compared with a robust 30.6-kg weight loss in the surgically treated group (Andersen et al., 1984; Andersen et al., 1988). At 5 years, success was expressed as losing more than 10% of initial weight. By this criterion, there was 16% success in the surgical group but only 3% in the VLCD group.

VBG has been compared with gastric bypass in a number of trials ranging up to 10 years in length (Howard et al., 1995; Sjostrom, 2004; Sjostrom et al., 2004). In the 10-year trial, individuals enrolled in the gastroplasty group lost about 16% of initial body weight compared with 24% for those in the gastric bypass group. Using different criteria, Howard et al. reported a loss of more than 75% of excess weight after 1 year in 18% of the patients with VBG compared with 60% for those with gastric bypass. Using a criterion of a weight loss to a BMI less than 35, MacLean et al. (1993) reported success for 83% of those with a gastric bypass and 43% for those with the VBG.

Two trials compared gastric bypass against nonsurgical treatment. In the first non-randomized trial, Martin et al. (1995) compared gastric bypass in 201 patients with VLCD and diet in 161 patients. After 6 years, the follow-up rate was 34.5% in the gastric bypass group and 19.7% in the VLCD-diet group. In the surgical group, BMI declined from 49.3 kg/m^2 at operation to a low of 31.8 kg/m^2 after 2 years and 33.7 kg/m^2 after 6 years. For the VLCD group, the corresponding data was a BMI of 41.2 kg/m^2 at baseline, 32.1 kg/m^2 after 2 years and 38.5 kg/m^2 after 6 years in those who returned for follow-up.

There is one trial comparing laparoscopic *roux-en-y* versus a mini-gastric bypass (Lee et al., 2005). In this trial, 40 subjects were randomized to each procedure and followed for a mean of 31.3 months. As expected, the operative time was shorter with the mini bypass procedure and the operative morbidity was higher in the *Roux-en-Y* procedure. Weight losses at 1 and 2 years were similar in the two groups. The authors conclude that the mini-gastric bypass is simpler and safer than the *Roux-en-Y* procedure.

The Swedish Obese Subjects (SOS) Trial is a second controlled, non-randomized trial directly comparing surgical and nonsurgical treatment for obesity, and is the largest trial comparing surgical versus medical treatment of morbid obesity (Karlsson et al., 1998; Sjostrom et al., 1992; Sjostrom et al., 2004; Torgerson and Sjostrom, 2001). A total of 6328 obese (BMI >34 kg/m^2 for men and >38 kg/m^2 for women) subjects were recruited, of whom 2010 underwent surgery for obesity (gastric banding, gastroplasty, or gastric bypass), whereas 2037 chose conventional treatment. Participants who underwent surgery were matched on a number of criteria to a group of 6322 overweight men and women in the SOS registry who were not operated on. The SOS study began slowly in 1987 and contributed significant new information about overweight individuals and the effects of surgical intervention. Before surgery, there was an average of 7.6 weight-loss attempts for the men and 18.2 for the women. The mean for the largest weight loss before surgery was 17.7 kg for the men and 18.2 kg for the women, but they were only able to maintain it for 7 to 10 months.

When the banding operation was compared with VBG and gastric bypass in the SOS study, Sjostrom et al. (2004) reported similar weight losses out to 10 years in the lap-band and VBG that was significantly less than that seen with the gastric bypass.

No randomized comparisons of the biliopancreatic diversion with other procedures have yet been published. However, there are two non-randomized comparisons. When 142 patients with the biliopancreatic diversion were compared with 93 patients undergoing a lap-band procedure, excess weight loss was 60% with the diversion operation against 48% for the lap-band (Bajardi et al., 2000). In a comparison of the diversion operation with a long-limb gastric bypass, BMI was reduced from 64 to 37 kg/m^2 in the diversion group compared with a decrease from 67 to 42 kg/m^2 (Murr et al., 1999). The biliopancreatic diversion appears to have more side effects than other procedures. Scopinaro, who originated the procedure, reported a low mortality of 0.5% with an excess body weight loss of 75%. Anemia occurring in spite of iron and folate replacement occurred in less than 5%, stomach ulcer during H$_2$-blocker therapy in 3.2%, and protein malnutrition in 3% (Scopinaro et al., 1996).

MECHANISMS FOR WEIGHT LOSS

There are at least two mechanisms that can account for the weight loss after bariatric surgery. The first of these is malabsorption. This was clearly an important component of the jejunoileal bypass (Bray, 1976), and is a prominent feature of the biliopancreatic diversion procedures. A second mechanism is altered hormonal secretion from the GI track. Glucagon-like peptide-1 (or enteroglucagon) is secreted from the lower intestinal track and has effects on GI function and on food intake (Kellum et al., 1990). More interest has been sparked by ghrelin, a small peptide released from the stomach that stimulates food intake. Cummings et al. (2002) reported that after bariatric surgery the level of this peptide was significantly reduced (Tritos et al., 2003), but there have been contradictory reports since. The final mechanism is a decrease in food intake. This was also present in the patients with jejunoileal bypass (Bray, 1976). In one report Lindroos et al. (1996) found no difference in energy intake between patients with gastric bypass

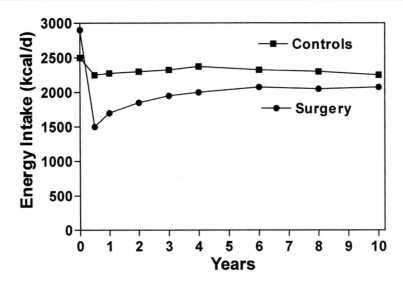

Fig. 3. Food intake following bariatric operations in the Swedish Obese Subjects study.

and those with gastroplasty, although those with gastroplasty lost less weight. In the SOS study food intake in the operated groups was less than in the control group at all time intervals (Fig. 3).

The lap-band procedure also reduces food intake and feelings of satiety. In one trial, Dixon et al. (2005) gave a test meal to individuals with a lap-band on two occasions, one with optimal restriction and one with reduced restriction. In the overweight control subjects with no bariatric procedure, the baseline levels of glucose, insulin, and leptin were higher, whereas ghrelin levels were lower. When they ate the test meal, the control subjects had a larger response of glucose and insulin, whereas the subjects with the lap-band had similar responses to both meals. Satiety, however, was less when the band was at the optimal restriction and there was less reduction in satiety when the band was not optimally inflated.

BENEFITS OF BARIATRIC SURGERY

Bariatric surgery produces more weight loss than conventional therapy for overweight, and the weight loss is more durable. After 2 years, weight reduction in the SOS study was 28 kg, which was significantly greater than the 0.5 kg in the matched registry patients (Torgerson and Sjostrom, 2001). After 10 years, control patients had gained an average of 1.4 kg compared with surgical patients who demonstrated persistent weight loss (Sjostrom et al., 2004; Fig. 4).

One randomized clinical trial compared intensive medical management versus laparoscopic insertion of an adjustable gastric band (lap-band system). Included in the trial were individuals who had a BMI between 30 and 35 kg/m², who also had co-morbid conditions such as hypertension, dyslipidemia, diabetes, obstructive sleep apnea, or gastroesophageal reflux disease, severe physical limitations, or clinically significant psychosocial problems. The intensive medical program consisted of a VLCD and behavior modification for 12 weeks followed by a transition phase over 4 weeks

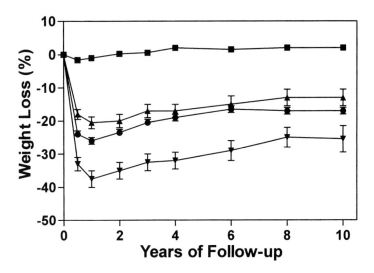

Fig. 4. Weight loss following bariatric operations in the Swedish Obese Subjects study.

combining some VLCD meals with 120 mg of orlistat and then orlistat 120 mg before all meals. Surgery was performed by two surgeons. Of the 40 patients in each group, 1 withdrew before surgery, leaving 39 at the end of 2 years, and 7 dropped out of the intensive intervention, leaving 33 patients who completed treatment. Both groups had an identical 13.8% weight loss at 6 months. The surgical group continued to lose weight and was 21.6% below baseline at 2 years. The nonsurgical group regained weight from 6 to 24 months, at which time they were on average only 5.5% below baseline weight. At 2 years, the surgically treated group had significantly greater improvements in diastolic blood pressure, fasting plasma glucose level, insulin sensitivity index, and HDL-cholesterol level. Quality of life improved more in the surgical group. Physical function, vitality, and mental health domains of the SF-36 were improved in the surgical group. Thus, laparoscopic insertion of an adjustable gastric band may be beneficial to some patients with weights below those usually recommended for this procedure (O'Brien et al., 2006).

Although there is a small death rate resulting from bariatric surgery, data are beginning to accumulate that the long-term benefits weigh in on the side of reduced mortality after bariatric surgery. Christou et al. (2004) compared 1035 patients who had undergone bariatric surgery with an age- and gender-matched severely obese case–control population. Patients who had bariatric surgery had a significantly lower rate of cardiovascular disease, cancer, endocrine disease, infectious, and psychiatric disorders than the case–control group. The overall mortality rate of 0.68% in the bariatric group was significantly lower than in the case–control group (6.17%, relative risk 0.11, 95% confidence interval 0.04–0.27). Mortality rates are influenced by the amount of surgical experience (Schauer et al., 2003; Wittgrove and Clark, 2000).

There are a number of reports showing improvement in the diseases associated with overweight. One of the most impressive has been sleep apnea. Even modest weight loss can benefit this disabling medical problem, and bariatric surgery has been particularly helpful (Dixon et al., 2001).

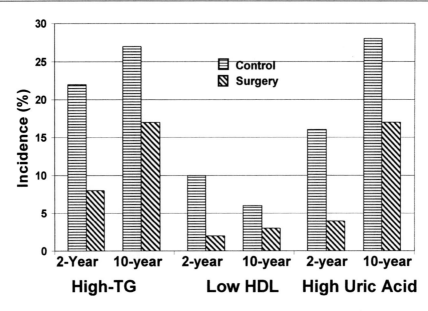

Fig. 5. Incidence of diabetes mellitus, low high-density lipoprotein-cholesterol and high uric acid at 2 and 10 years following bariatric surgery for obesity.

Next to the effects on sleep apnea is improvement in the prospects for patients with diabetes or those at high risk for developing it. Pories et al. (1992, 1995) were the first to note the marked effect on diabetes. Although there were design issues with these retrospective studies, they showed an annual incidence of 4.5% in the control group contrasted with only 1% in the surgically operated group. The SOS reported similarly impressive data. After 2 years of follow-up, the incidence of diabetes was 4.7% in the matched control group with no new cases in the surgical group. After 8 years, the incidence of diabetes in the control group was 18.5% compared with only 3.6% in the operated group. The incidence rate was related to the amount of weight lost. In the subgroup losing more than 12% of their initial body weight, there were no new cases, in contrast to 7% in those losing 2% and 9% in those gaining 4% (Fig. 5). This was reflected in the low odds ratio (OR) for diabetes (OR 0.10) and hyperinsulinemia (OR 0.1).

The incidence of other medical complications was also reduced. There was a linear reduction in the systolic and diastolic blood pressure with the degree of weight loss (Sjostrom et al., 1997) and the OR for incident hypertension was 0.38. Triglyceride and insulin levels also showed a linear decrease with weight loss (OR 0.28 for hypertriglyceridemia). The concentration of HDL-cholesterol increased linearly with weight loss (OR 0.28), but cholesterol did not decline significantly until weight loss had exceeded 25 kg (OR 1.24; Sjostrom et al., 1999).

Surgically treated patients required less medication for cardiovascular disease or diabetes than matched controls (Agren et al., 2002). Among those not already requiring such medications, surgery reduced the portion that required initiation of treatment, as well as the costs of medications (Narbro et al., 2002). Quality of life (Karlsson et al., 1998) was related primarily to the degree of weight loss. Psychiatric dysfunction also improved (Ryden et al., 2004).

Table 3
Complications from Laparoscopic Adjustable Gastric Band

- Revisional surgery up to 40%
- Acute stomal obstruction 2%
- Band erosion 0–3%
- Band slippage/prolapse up to 24%
- Port/tubing malfunction 0.4–7%
- Pouch/esophageal dilation up to 10%
- Infection at port site 0–9%

COMPLICATIONS FOLLOWING LAP-BAND BARIATRIC SURGERY

Despite its relative technical ease, laparoscopic adjustable gastric banding (LAGB) has been associated with several complications, which are summarized in Table 3. Laparoscopic procedures have significantly reduced rates of wound infections. One advantage of the lap-band is that it eliminates leakage at staple lines. There is no significant difference in leak rates between the open versus laparoscopic approach. An initial trial of LAGB in the United States showed disappointing weight-loss outcomes and high complication rates, associated with relatively high revisional surgery rate (40%; DeMaria et al., 2001). However, complications following LAGB were described far less frequently in Europe, Australia, and a more recent trial in the United States (Angrisani et al., 2003; O'Brien and Dixon, 2003). On average, approximately 13 to 15% of patients will require re-operation for various complications (Kothari et al., 2002). New standards for training and certification may ensure more standardized operative technique and optimal postoperative patient management, and this may lead to improved outcomes (Schneider et al., 2004). Occasionally, the stomach wall prolapses upward or downward through the band leading to gastric obstruction. In the registration trials submitted to the Food and Drug Administration (FDA Website), slippage occurred in 24% of patients but a lower incidence of 2 to 14% has been reported in subsequent studies (Ren et al., 2002; Rubenstein, 2002). If the tube becomes disconnected from the subcutaneous port, the compression of the band will be reduced. Port and tubing malfunction have occurred in 0.4 to 7.0% of patients (Dargent, 1999; Ren et al. 2002).

COMPLICATIONS FOLLOWING RESTRICTIVE BARIATRIC SURGERY

A list of some of the complications following restrictive gastric operations is shown in Table 4. Mortality rate varies from one center to another. As noted earlier, surgeons with more than 20–50 operations to their credit have significantly lower mortality. Wound infections were an important concern with the open procedures. Leaks around staple lines are a major life-threatening complication that can occur with VBG. Marginal (stomal) ulceration and stenosis with band erosion at the end of the esophageal extension, gastro-esophageal reflux disease, nausea and vomiting, and marginal ulcers are examples of problems with the lap-band and with laparoscopic or open gastroplasty. Regain of body weight is more common with gastroplasty than with gastric bypass or biliopancreatic diversion (Balsiger et al. 2000; Nightengale et al., 1991). Gastroesophageal reflux after VBG presents with classic symptoms such as burning pain, heartburn, aspiration, and

Table 4
Complications of Gastric Restriction Operations

- Disruption of staple line in vertical-banded gastric bypass 27–31%
- Stomal stenosis 20–33%
- Band erosion 1–7%
- Gastroesophageal reflux
- Recurrent vomiting 8–21%

Table 5
Complications of Gastric Bypass Operations

- Mortality 0–1%
- Deep vein thrombosis and pulmonary embolus 0–3.3%
- Leaks 0–5.1%
- Bleeding 0.6–4%
- Gastric remnant distension—rare
- Wound infection 10–15% with open and 3–4% with laparoscopic procedures
- Stomal stenosis 6–20%
- Marginal ulcers 0.6–3%
- Cholelithiasis up to 38%
- Ventral incisional hernia 0–1.8%
- Metabolic derangement (Fe; B_{12}; folate)

cough. It typically occurs as a late complication, as a result of stomal stenosis and pouch dilatation (Balsiger et al., 2000). Wound infection of 10 to 15% are significantly greater with gastric bypass procedures (Higa et al., 2000; Nguyen et al., 2001; Schauer et al., 2000) than the 3 to 4% seen with laparoscopic procedures. Peri-operative use of antibiotics (usually cefazolin) can reduce this problem (Pories et al., 1981).

COMPLICATIONS WITH MALABSORPTIVE OPERATIONS

Table 5 lists some of the complications associated with gastric bypass operations. Death following a *Roux-en-Y* gastric bypass ranges from 0 to 1% or somewhat more. (Pories et al., 1995; Schneider et al., 2003; Sugerman et al., 1989). In a recent assessment of deaths in the Medicare records, Flum et al. (2005) noted that among 16,155 patients undergoing these procedures between 1997 and 2002 the 30-day, 90-day, and 1-year mortality rates were 2.0, 2.8, and 4.6%, which are higher than the usual reported rates from surgical series. Men had higher early death rates than women. Death rates were also significantly higher among subjects over 65 years of age. After adjusting for sex and co-morbidity index, the odds of death within 90 days were fivefold higher in those over 75 years of age than in those 65 to 74 years.

Leaks around staple lines are a major life-threatening complication of gastric bypass and the biliopancreatic diversion. Leaks from the staple lines are the most serious complication and require immediate surgical intervention. They may be responsible for up to 50% of deaths (Regan et al., 2003). The quoted leak rate following gastric bypass is between 0 and 5.1%, with the average leak rate between 2 and 3% (Nguyen et al., 2001; Schauer et al., 2000; Westling and Gustavsson, 2001; Wittgrove and Clark, 2000).

Early symptoms of a suture line leak may be subtle, including a low-grade fever, respiratory distress, or an unexplained tachycardia (Hamilton et al., 2003). Exploratory surgery should be performed without delay.

Hospitalization following *Roux-en-Y* gastric bypass is significantly increased. Between 1995 and 2004 there were 60,077 gastric bypass operations performed in California with 11,659 performed in 2004 alone (Zingmond et al., 2005). The hospitalization rate was 7.9% in the year preceding the *Roux-en-Y* gastric bypass and 19.3% in the year following. Among the 24,678 patients for whom 3-year data are available, 8.4% were admitted in the year before surgery, 20.2% in the first year after bariatric surgery, 18.4% in the second year, and 14.9% in the third year. The authors conclude that hospitalization in the years following gastric bypass is related to the surgery.

Another early postoperative risk common to all procedures is pulmonary embolus (Melinek et al., 2002). The incidence of deep vein thrombosis and pulmonary embolism varies between 0 to 3.3% with laparoscopic bypasses (Nguyen et al., 2001; Schauer et al., 2000; Westling and Gustavsson, 2001; Wittgrove and Clark, 2000) and 0.3 to 1.9% with open bypasses (Fobi et al., 1998; Griffen, 1979; Hall et al., 1990). In an autopsy series (Melinek et al., 2002), pulmonary embolism was the cause of death in 30% of patients. In addition 80% had silent pulmonary emboli despite prophylactic treatment with anti-coagulants. Risk factors associated with fatal PE include severe venous stasis disease, BMI higher than 60 kg/m^2, truncal adiposity, and obesity-hypoventilation syndrome (Sapala et al., 2003). Use of heparin prophylactically would appear to be a desirable postoperative procedure in obese patients having this operation. Prophylactic use of heparin may be desirable in high-risk patients.

Ventral hernias occur in up to 24% of patients who have open operations but its occurence is reduced to an incidence of 0 to 1.8% with laparoscopic surgery (Higa et al., 2000; Nguyen et al., 2000; Nguyen et al., 2001; Pories et al. 1995; Wittgrove and Clark, 2000). The *Roux-en-Y* procedure also carries a risk of internal hernias, because the anatomical changes provide new holes through which bowel can be squeezed (Champion and Williams, 2003). These internal hernias have been described in 0 to 5% of patients undergoing laparoscopic bariatric surgery (Higa et al., 2000; Nguyen et al., 2001). Surgery is required.

Development of gall stones is a common problem with rapid weight loss and thus cholelithiasis is to be expected following surgical procedures for overweight. Gall stone disease has been reported to develop in as many as 38% of patients within 6 months of surgery (Shiffman et al., 1991). The risk of gall stones can be reduced to as low as 2% by using bile salt (ursodeoxycholic acid) for 6 months following surgery (Sugerman et al., 1995).

The metabolic and nutritional derangements can pose significant problems following malabsorptive procedures. Life-long use of vitamins and minerals are important. Malabsorption of iron, vitamin B12, and folate are the most likely problems. Malabsorption of fat soluble vitamins, protein, and thiamine may also occur and can manifest itself clinically.

INTRAGASTRIC BALLOON

The intragastric balloon (Bioenterics® Intragastric Balloon, Inamed) is a temporary alternative for weight loss in moderately obese individuals. It consists of a soft, saline-filled balloon placed endoscopically that promotes a feeling of satiety and restriction. It is currently not available for use in the United States, but is undergoing extensive testing in Europe and Brazil. Mean excess weight loss is reported to be 38% and 48% for 500- and 600-mL balloons, respectively (Roman et al., 2004). However, the results of a Brazilian multicenter study indicate weight loss is transient, with only 26% of patients maintaining more than 90% of the excess weight loss out over 1 year (Sallet et al., 2004). Side effects include nausea, vomiting, abdominal pain, ulceration, and balloon migration.

GASTRIC STIMULATION OR GASTRIC PACING

Gastric pacing as a technique for weight loss was pioneered in pigs, in which repeated stimulation produced significant weight loss (Cigaina et al., 1996). The first clinical trial included 24 overweight human beings with a BMI higher than 40 kg/m^2. Over the 9 months of the trial, BMI was reduced 4.7 kg/m^2 with no significant side effects (Cigaina et al., 1996). In a follow-up study of 11 patients with an initial BMI of 46.0 kg/m^2 who lost 3.6 kg in the 2 months after implantation of the pacemaker but before it was turned on, there was a further 6.8 kg weight loss after 6 months of electrical stimulation. Following a test meal, there was a smaller rise in cholecystokinin, and lower levels of somatostatin, glucagon-like peptide-1, and leptin, although it is unclear whether this was secondary to the stimulation or weight loss. In a summary of experience on more than 200 patients who had gastric implantation, Shikora (2004) noted that some patients responded well, whereas others did not. An algorithm was developed based on baseline age, gender, body weight, BMI, and response to pre-operative questionnaires. With this algorithm, the selection rate for the procedure was 18 to 33%. When this algorithm is applied, excess weight loss is up to 40% in 12 months, compared with a 4% excess weight gain in the control group. More data are needed.

LIPOSUCTION AND OMENTECTOMY

Liposuction, also known as lipoplasty or suction-assisted lipectomy, is the most common aesthetic procedure performed in the United States with more than 400,000 cases performed annually (Klein et al., 2004). Although not generally considered to be a bariatric procedure, removal of fat by aspiration after injection of physiological saline has been used to remove and contour subcutaneous fat. Because the techniques have improved, it is now possible to remove significant amounts of subcutaneous adipose tissue without affecting the amount of visceral fat. In a study to examine the effects of this procedure, Klein et al. (2004) studied seven overweight women with diabetes and eight overweight women with normal glucose tolerance before and after liposuction. One week after assessing insulin sensitivity, the subjects underwent large-volume tumescent liposuction, which consists of removing more than 4 L of aspirate injected into the fat beneath the skin. There was a significant loss of subcutaneous fat, as expected, but no change in the visceral fat. Subjects were reassessed 10 to 12 weeks after the surgery when the women without diabetes had lost –6.3 kg of body weight and –9.1 kg of body fat, which reduced body fat by –6.3%. The women with diabetes had a similar response with a weight loss of –7.9 kg, a reduction in body fat of –10.5 kg, and reduction in percent fat of –6.7%. Waist circumference was also significantly reduced.

In spite of these significant reductions in body fat, there were no changes in blood pressure, lipids, cytokines (tumor necrosis factor-α, interleukin-6), or C-reactive protein. There was also no improvement in insulin sensitivity, suggesting that removal of subcutaneous adipose tissue without visceral fat reduction has little influence on the risk factors related to being overweight.

Omentectomy is the direct removal of the intra-abdominal fat by surgical means. One randomized controlled trial in 50 overweight subjects compared the effect of an adjustable lap-band alone with a lap-band plus removal of the omentum (Thorne et al., 2002). Of the original 50 patients, 37 were re-evaluated 2 years after the surgery. The reduction in body weight was 27 kg in the lap-band group and 36 kg in the lap-band plus omentectomy group ($p = 0.07$). Both glucose and insulin improved more in the subjects with omentectomy than in those without it. This study complements the one by Klein et al. described above by showing that removal of extra visceral fat can have a small but significant effect, whereas decreasing subcutaneous fat alone has little impact.

REFERENCES

Agren, G., et al. (2002). Long-term effects of weight loss on pharmaceutical costs in obese subjects. A report from the SOS intervention study. Int J Obes Relat Metab Disord 26(2):184–192.

Alden, J. F. (1977). Gastric and jejunoileal bypass. A comparison in the treatment of morbid obesity. Arch Surg 112(7):799–806.

American Society of Bariatric Surgery. (2003). Bariatric Centers of Excellence. ASBS Newsletter. Spring: 4.

Andersen, T., et al. (1984). Randomized trial of diet and gastroplasty compared with diet alone in morbid obesity. N Engl J Med 310(6):352–356.

Andersen, T., et al. (1988). Long-term (5-year) results after either horizontal gastroplasty or very-low-calorie diet for morbid obesity. Int J Obes 12(4):277–284.

Angrisani, L., et al. (2003). Lap Band adjustable gastric banding system: the Italian experience with 1863 patients operated on 6 years. Surg Endosc 17(3):409–412.

Bajardi, G., et al. (2000). Surgical treatment of morbid obesity with biliopancreatic diversion and gastric banding: report on an 8-year experience involving 235 cases. Ann Chir 125(2):155–162.

Balsiger, B. M., et al. (2000). Gastroesophageal reflux after intact vertical banded gastroplasty: correction by conversion to Roux-en-Y gastric bypass. J Gastrointest Surg 4(3):276–281.

Balsiger, B. M., et al. (2000). Bariatric surgery. Surgery for weight control in patients with morbid obesity. Med Clin North Am 84(2):477–489.

Belachew, M., et al. (1995). Laparoscopic placement of adjustable silicone gastric band in the treatment of morbid obesity: how to do it. Obes Surg 5(1):66–70.

Bo, O. and Modalsli, O. (1983). Gastric banding, a surgical method of treating morbid obesity: preliminary report. Int J Obes 7(5):493–499.

Bray, G. A. (1976). The Obese Patient: Major Problems in Internal Medicine. Philadelphia: WB Saunders.

Buchwald, H., et al. (2004). Bariatric surgery: a systematic review and meta-analysis. JAMA 292(14): 1724–1737.

Buckwalter, J. A. (1977). A prospective comparison of the jejunoileal and gastric bypass operations for morbid obesity. World J Surg 1(6):757–768.

Champion, J. K. and Williams, M. (2003). Small bowel obstruction and internal hernias after laparoscopic Roux-en-Y gastric bypass. Obes Surg 13(4):596–600.

Christou, N. V., et al. (2004). Surgery decreases long-term mortality, morbidity, and health care use in morbidly obese patients. Ann Surg 240(3):416–423; discussion 423–424.

Cigaina, V. V., et al. (1996). Long-term effects of gastric pacing to reduce feed intake in swine. Obes Surg 6(3):250–253.

Colquitt, J., et al. (2005). Surgery for morbid obesity. Cochrane Database Syst Rev (4):CD003641.

Cummings, D. E., et al. (2002). Plasma ghrelin levels after diet-induced weight loss or gastric bypass surgery. N Engl J Med 346(21):1623–1630.

Dargent, J. (1999). Laparoscopic adjustable gastric banding: lessons from the first 500 patients in a single institution. Obes Surg 9(5):446–452.

Deitel, M., et al. (1982). Intestinal bypass and gastric partitioning for morbid obesity: a comparison. Can J Surg 25(3):283–289.

DeMaria, E. J., et al. (2001). High failure rate after laparoscopic adjustable silicone gastric banding for treatment of morbid obesity. Ann Surg 233(6):809–818.

DeWind, L. T. and Payne, J. H. (1976). Intestinal bypass surgery for morbid obesity. Long-term results. JAMA 236(20):2298–2301.

Dixon, A. F., et al. (2005). Laparoscopic adjustable gastric banding induces prolonged satiety: a randomized blind crossover study. J Clin Endocrinol Metab 90(2):813–819.

Dixon, J. B., et al. (2001). Sleep disturbance and obesity: changes following surgically induced weight loss. Arch Intern Med 161(1):102–106.

Flum, D. R., et al. (2005). Early mortality among Medicare beneficiaries undergoing bariatric surgical procedures. JAMA 294(15):1903–1908.

Fobi, M. A., et al. (1998). Gastric bypass operation for obesity. World J Surg 22(9):925–935.

Food and Drug Administration Website. FDA trial summary of safety and effectiveness data: the lap-band adjustable gastric banding system. Retrieved 2 March, 2006. Available from: www.fda.gov/cdrh/pdf/P000008b.doc.

Fried, M. and Peskova, M. (1997). Gastric banding in the treatment of morbid obesity. Hepatogastro-enterology 44(14):582–587.

Gomez, C. A. (1979). Gastroplasty in morbid obesity. Surg Clin North Am 59(6):1113–1120.

Griffen, W. O., Jr. (1979). Gastric bypass for morbid obesity. Surg Clin North Am 59(6):1103–1112.

Griffen, W. O., Jr., et al. (1977). A prospective comparison of gastric and jejunoileal bypass procedures for morbid obesity. Ann Surg 186(4):500–509.

Hall, J. C., et al. (1990). Gastric surgery for morbid obesity. The Adelaide Study. Ann Surg 211(4):419–427.

Hamilton, E. C., et al. (2003). Clinical predictors of leak after laparoscopic Roux-en-Y gastric bypass for morbid obesity. Surg Endosc 17(5):679–684.

Higa, K. D., et al. (2000). Complications of the laparoscopic Roux-en-Y gastric bypass: 1,040 patients—what have we learned? Obes Surg 10(6):509–513.

Howard, L., et al. (1995). Gastric bypass and vertical banded gastroplasty: a prospective randomized comparison and 5-year follow-up. Obes Surg 5(1):55–60.

Inge, T. H., et al. (2004). Bariatric surgery for severely overweight adolescents: concerns and recommendations. Pediatrics 114(1):217–223.

Karlsson, J., et al. (1998). Swedish obese subjects (SOS)—an intervention study of obesity. Two-year follow-up of health-related quality of life (HRQL) and eating behavior after gastric surgery for severe obesity. Int J Obes Relat Metab Disord 22(2):113–126.

Kellum, J. M., et al. (1990). Gastrointestinal hormone responses to meals before and after gastric bypass and vertical banded gastroplasty. Ann Surg 211(6):763–770; discussion 770–771.

Klein, S., et al. (2004). Absence of an effect of liposuction on insulin action and risk factors for coronary heart disease. N Engl J Med 350(25):2549–2557.

Kothari, S. N., et al. (2002). Lap-band failures: conversion to gastric bypass and their preliminary outcomes. Surgery 131(6):625–629.

Lee, W. J., et al. (2005). Laparoscopic Roux-en-Y versus mini-gastric bypass for the treatment of morbid obesity: a prospective randomized controlled clinical trial. Ann Surg 242(1):20–28.

Lindroos, A. K., et al. (1996). Weight change in relation to intake of sugar and sweet foods before and after weight reducing gastric surgery. Int J Obes Relat Metab Disord 20(7):634–643.

MacLean, L. D., et al. (1993). Results of the surgical treatment of obesity. Am J Surg 165(1):155–60; discussion 160–162.

Marceau, P., et al. (1993). Biliopancreatic diversion with a new type of gastrectomy. Obes Surg 3(1):29–35.

Martin, L. F., et al. (1995). Comparison of the costs associated with medical and surgical treatment of obesity. Surgery 118(4):599–606; discussion 606–607.

Mason, E. E. (1982). Vertical banded gastroplasty for obesity. Arch Surg 117(5):701–706.

Mason, E. E. and Ito, C. (1967). Gastric bypass in obesity. Surg Clin North Am 47(6):1345–1351.

Mason, E. E. and Ito, C. (1969). Gastric bypass. Ann Surg 170(3):329–339.

Melinek, J., et al. (2002). Autopsy findings following gastric bypass surgery for morbid obesity. Arch Pathol Lab Med 126(9):1091–1095.

Murr, M. M., et al. (1999). Malabsorptive procedures for severe obesity: comparison of pancreaticobiliary bypass and very very long limb Roux-en-Y gastric bypass. J Gastrointest Surg 3(6):607–612.

N. A. (1979). Randomised trial of jejunoileal bypass versus medical treatment in morbid obesity. The Danish Obesity Project. Lancet 2(8155):1255–1258.

N. A. (1991). NIH conference. Gastrointestinal surgery for severe obesity. Consensus Development Conference Panel. Ann Intern Med 115(12):956–961.

N. A. (1992). Gastrointestinal surgery for severe obesity: National Institutes of Health Consensus Development Conference Statement. Am J Clin Nutr 55(2 Suppl):615S–619S.

Narbro, K., et al. (2002). Pharmaceutical costs in obese individuals: comparison with a randomly selected population sample and long-term changes after conventional and surgical treatment: the SOS intervention study. Arch Intern Med 162(18):2061–2069.

Nguyen, N. T., et al. (2000). A comparison study of laparoscopic versus open gastric bypass for morbid obesity. J Am Coll Surg 191(2):149–155; discussion 155–157.

Nguyen, N. T., et al. (2001). Laparoscopic versus open gastric bypass: a randomized study of outcomes, quality of life, and costs. Ann Surg 234(3):279–289; discussion 289–291.

Nightengale, M. L., et al. (1991). Prospective evaluation of vertical banded gastroplasty as the primary operation for morbid obesity. Mayo Clin Proc 66(8):773–782.

O'Brien, P. E. and Dixon, J. B. (2003). Lap-band: outcomes and results. J Laparoendosc Adv Surg Tech A 13(4):265–270.

O'Brien, P. E., et al. (2006). Treatment of mild to moderate obesity with laparoscopic adjustable gastric banding or an intensive medical program: a randomized trial. Ann Intern Med 144(9):625–633.

Pace, W. G., et al. (1979). Gastric partitioning for morbid obesity. Ann Surg 190(3):392–400.

Payne, J. H., et al. (1963). Metabolic observations in patients with jejunocolic shunts. Am J Surg 106: 273–289.

Pories, W. J., et al. (1992). Is type II diabetes mellitus (NIDDM) a surgical disease? Ann Surg 215(6): 633–642; discussion 643.

Pories, W. J., et al. (1995). Who would have thought it? An operation proves to be the most effective therapy for adult-onset diabetes mellitus. Ann Surg 222(3):339–350; discussion 350–352.

Pories, W. J., et al. (1981). Prophylactic cefazolin in gastric bypass surgery. Surgery 90(2):426–432.

Regan, J. P., et al. (2003). Early experience with two-stage laparoscopic Roux-en-Y gastric bypass as an alternative in the super-super obese patient. Obes Surg 13(6):861–864.

Ren, C. J., et al. (2002). US experience with the LAP-BAND system. Am J Surg 184(6B):46S–50S.

Roman, S., et al. (2004). Intragastric balloon for "non-morbid" obesity: a retrospective evaluation of tolerance and efficacy. Obes Surg 14(4):539–544.

Rubenstein, R. B. (2002). Laparoscopic adjustable gastric banding at a U.S. center with up to 3-year follow-up. Obes Surg 12(3):380–384.

Ryden, A., et al. (2004). A comparative controlled study of personality in severe obesity: a 2-y follow-up after intervention. Int J Obes Relat Metab Disord 28(11):1485–1493.

Sallet, J. A., et al. (2004). Brazilian multicenter study of the intragastric balloon. Obes Surg 14(7):991–998.

Sapala, J. A., et al. (2003). Fatal pulmonary embolism after bariatric operations for morbid obesity: a 24-year retrospective analysis. Obes Surg 13(6):819–825.

Schauer, P., et al. (2003). The learning curve for laparoscopic Roux-en-Y gastric bypass is 100 cases. Surg Endosc 17(2):212–215.

Schauer, P. R., et al. (2000). Outcomes after laparoscopic Roux-en-Y gastric bypass for morbid obesity. Ann Surg 232(4):515–529.

Schneider, B. E., et al. (2003). Laparoscopic gastric bypass surgery: outcomes. J Laparoendosc Adv Surg Tech A 13(4):247–255.

Schneider, B. E., et al. (2004). How to implant the laparoscopic adjustable gastric band for morbid obesity. Contemporary Surgery 60(6):256–264.

Scopinaro, N., et al. (1996). Biliopancreatic diversion for obesity at eighteen years. Surgery 119(3): 261–268.

Shekelle, P. G., et al. (2004). Pharmacological and surgical treatment of obesity. Evid Rep Technol Assess (Summ)(103):1–6.

Shiffman, M. L., et al. (1991). Gallstone formation after rapid weight loss: a prospective study in patients undergoing gastric bypass surgery for treatment of morbid obesity. Am J Gastroenterol 86(8): 1000–1005.

Shikora, S. A. (2004). Implantable gastric stimulation for the treatment of severe obesity. Obes Surg 14(4):545–548.

Sjostrom, C. D., et al. (1997). Relationships between changes in body composition and changes in cardiovascular risk factors: the SOS Intervention Study. Swedish Obese Subjects. Obes Res 5(6):519–530.

Sjostrom, C. D., et al. (1999). Reduction in incidence of diabetes, hypertension and lipid disturbances after intentional weight loss induced by bariatric surgery: the SOS Intervention Study. Obes Res 7(5): 477–484.

Sjostrom, L. (2004). Surgical treatment of obesity: An overview and results from the SOS Study. In: Handbook of Obesity: Clinical Applications, edited by Bray, G. and Bouchard C. New York: Marcel Dekker; pp. 359–389.

Sjostrom, L., et al. (1992). Swedish obese subjects (SOS). Recruitment for an intervention study and a selected description of the obese state. Int J Obes Relat Metab Disord 16(6):465–479.

Sjostrom, L., et al. (2004). Lifestyle, diabetes, and cardiovascular risk factors 10 years after bariatric surgery. N Engl J Med 351(26):2683–2693.

Stokholm, K. H., et al. (1982). Correlation between initial blood pressure and blood pressure decrease after weight loss: A study in patients with jejunoileal bypass versus medical treatment for morbid obesity. Int J Obes 6(3):307–312.

Sugerman, H. J., et al. (1989). Weight loss with vertical banded gastroplasty and Roux-Y gastric bypass for morbid obesity with selective versus random assignment. Am J Surg 157(1):93–102.

Sugerman, H. J., et al. (1995). A multicenter, placebo-controlled, randomized, double-blind, prospective trial of prophylactic ursodiol for the prevention of gallstone formation following gastric-bypass-induced rapid weight loss. Am J Surg 169(1):91–96; discussion 96–97.

Sugerman, H. J., Sugerman, E. L., et al. (2003). Bariatric surgery for severely obese adolescents. J Gastrointest Surg 7(1):102–107; discussion 107–108.

Thorne, A., et al. (2002). A pilot study of long-term effects of a novel obesity treatment: omentectomy in connection with adjustable gastric banding. Int J Obes Relat Metab Disord 26(2):193–199.

Torgerson, J. S. and Sjostrom, L. (2001). The Swedish Obese Subjects (SOS) study—rationale and results. Int J Obes Relat Metab Disord 25(Suppl 1):S2–S4.

Tritos, N. A., et al. (2003). Serum ghrelin levels in response to glucose load in obese subjects post-gastric bypass surgery. Obes Res 11(8):919–924.

Westling, A. and Gustavsson, S. (2001). Laparoscopic vs open Roux-en-Y gastric bypass: a prospective, randomized trial. Obes Surg 11(3):284–292.

Wittgrove, A. C. and Clark, G. W. (2000). Laparoscopic gastric bypass, Roux-en-Y- 500 patients: technique and results, with 3-60 month follow-up. Obes Surg 10(3):233–239.

Zingmond, D. S., et al. (2005). Hospitalization before and after gastric bypass surgery. JAMA 294(15): 1918–1924.

Index

Printed in the United States of America